# Simulation in Surgical Training and Practice

*Editors*

KIMBERLY M. BROWN
JOHN T. PAIGE

SURGICAL CLINICS OF NORTH AMERICA

www.surgical.theclinics.com

*Consulting Editor*
RONALD F. MARTIN

August 2015 • Volume 95 • Number 4

**ELSEVIER**

1600 John F. Kennedy Boulevard • Suite 1800 • Philadelphia, Pennsylvania, 19103-2899

http://www.surgical.theclinics.com

**SURGICAL CLINICS OF NORTH AMERICA Volume 95, Number 4**
**August 2015 ISSN 0039–6109, ISBN-13: 978-0-323-39356-0**

Editor: John Vassallo, j.vassallo@elsevier.com
Developmental Editor: Colleen Viola



*Surgical Clinics of North America* (ISSN 0039–6109) is published bimonthly by Elsevier Inc., 360 Park Avenue South, New York, NY 10010-1710. Months of publication are February, April, June, August, October, and December. Business and Editorial Offices: 1600 John F. Kennedy Blvd., Suite 1800, Philadelphia, PA 19103-2899. Periodicals postage paid at New York, NY and additional mailing offices. Subscription prices are $370.00 per year for US individuals, $627.00 per year for US institutions, $180.00 per year for US students and residents, $455.00 per year for Canadian individuals, $793.00 per year for Canadian institutions, $510.00 for international individuals, $793.00 per year for international institutions and $250.00 per year for Canadian and foreign students/residents. To receive student/resident rate, orders must be accompanied by name of affiliated institution, date of term, and the *signature* of program/residency coordinator on institution letterhead. Orders will be billed at individual rate until proof of status is received. Foreign air speed delivery is included in all *Clinics* subscription prices. All prices are subject to change without notice. POSTMASTER: Send address changes to *Surgical Clinics*, Elsevier Health Sciences Division, Subscription Customer Service, 3251 Riverport Lane, Maryland Heights, MO 63043. **Customer Service (orders, claims, online, change of address): Telephone: 1-800-654-2452 (U.S. and Canada); 314-447-8871 (outside U.S. and Canada). Fax: 314-447-8029. E-mail: journalscustomerservice-usa@elsevier.com (for print support); journalsonline support-usa@elsevier.com (for online support)**.

*Reprints*. For copies of 100 or more, of articles in this publication, please contact the Commercial Reprints Department, Elsevier Inc., 360 Park Avenue South, New York, New York 10010-1710. Tel. 212-633-3874, Fax: 212-633-3820, E-mail: reprints@elsevier.com.

*The Surgical Clinics of North America* is also published in Spanish by McGraw-Hill Interamericana Editores S.A., P.O. Box 5-237 06500 Mexico D.F. Mexico; and in Portuguese by Interlivros Edicoes Ltda., Rua Comandante Coelho 1085, CEP 21250, Rio de Janeiro, Brazil; and in Greek by Paschalidis Medical Publications, Athens Greece.

*The Surgical Clinics of North America* is covered in *MEDLINE/PubMed (Index Medicus), EMBASE/Excerpta Medica, Current Contents/Clinical Medicine, Current Contents/Life Sciences, Science Citation Index*, and *ISI/BIOMED*.

# Contributors

## CONSULTING EDITOR

**RONALD F. MARTIN, MD**
Staff Surgeon, Department of Surgery, Marshfield Clinic, Marshfield, Wisconsin; Clinical Associate Professor, University of Wisconsin School of Medicine and Public Health, Madison, Wisconsin; Colonel (ret.), Medical Corps, United States Army Reserve

## EDITORS

**KIMBERLY M. BROWN, MD, FACS**
Director, Laboratory for Surgical Training, Assessment and Research; Section Chief, Hepatobiliary-Pancreatic Surgery; Associate Professor, Department of Surgery, University of Texas Medical Branch, Galveston, Texas

**JOHN T. PAIGE, MD, FACS**
Associate Professor of Clinical Surgery; Director of Wound Care, Department of Surgery, LSU Health Sciences Center, School of Medicine, LSU Health New Orleans School of Medicine, New Orleans, Louisiana

## AUTHORS

**ROBERT D. ACTON, MD**
Associate Professor of Surgery and Pediatrics, Division of Pediatric Surgery, Department of Surgery, University of Minnesota, Minneapolis, Minnesota

**JEAN BISMUTH, MD**
Department of Surgery, Houston Methodist, Houston, Texas

**KIMBERLY M. BROWN, MD, FACS**
Director, Laboratory for Surgical Training, Assessment and Research; Section Chief, Hepatobiliary-Pancreatic Surgery; Associate Professor, Department of Surgery, University of Texas Medical Branch, Galveston, Texas

**JUSTIN A. CHARLES, BS**
Department of Surgery, Walter Reed National Military Medical Center, Uniformed Services University, Bethesda, Maryland

**SHEILA W. CHAUVIN, PhD, MEd**
Professor, Department of Medicine and School of Public Health; Director, Office of Medical Education Research and Development, School of Medicine; Director, Academy for the Advancement of Educational Scholarship, LSU Health New Orleans School of Medicine, New Orleans, Louisiana

**TIFFANY COX, MD**
Minimally Invasive Surgery Fellow, Department of Surgery, Carolinas Medical Center, Charlotte, North Carolina

**ANNE-LISE D. D'ANGELO, MD**
Department of Surgery, University of Wisconsin School of Medicine and Public Health, Madison, Wisconsin

**BRIAN J. DUNKIN, MD, FACS**
Professor of Surgery; Medical Director, Houston Methodist Institute for Technology, Innovation, and Education (MITIE), Houston, Texas

**CASSIDY DURAN, MD**
Department of Surgery, Houston Methodist, Houston, Texas

**DEBORAH D. GARBEE, PhD, APRN, ACNS-BC**
Acting Associate Dean of Professional Practice, Community Service and Advanced Nursing Practice, Department of Graduate Nursing Education, LSU Health New Orleans School of Nursing, New Orleans, Louisiana

**AIMEE K. GARDNER, PhD**
Assistant Professor of Surgery, Associate Director of Education, Department of Surgery, UT Southwestern Medical Center, Dallas, Texas

**LOUISE HULL, PhD**
Department of Surgery and Cancer, Patient Safety Translational Research Center, St Mary's Hospital, Imperial College London, London, United Kingdom

**SOLVEIG IMSDAHL, BA**
Department of Surgery, Walter Reed National Military Medical Center, Uniformed Services University, Bethesda, Maryland

**DANIEL JONES, MD**
Professor of Surgery, Beth Israel Deaconess Medical Center, Harvard Medical School, Boston, Massachusetts

**JAMES R. KORNDORFFER Jr, MD, MHPE**
Department of General Surgery, Tulane University School of Medicine, New Orleans, Louisiana

**KATHERINE E. LAW, MS**
Department of Industrial and Systems Engineering, University of Wisconsin-Madison, Madison, Wisconsin

**PETER W. LUNDBERG, MD**
Department of General Surgery, Tulane University School of Medicine, New Orleans, Louisiana

**SOPHIA K. McKINLEY, MD, EdM**
Department of Surgery, Massachusetts General Hospital, Harvard Medical School, Boston, Massachusetts

**JULIA METZNER, MD**
Associate Professor, Department of Anesthesiology and Pain Medicine, University of Washington, Seattle, Washington

**ADNAN MOHSIN, BS**
Surgical Skills and Simulation Laboratory Coordinator, Department of Surgery, University of Nevada School of Medicine, Las Vegas, Nevada

**JOHN T. PAIGE, MD, FACS**
Associate Professor of Clinical Surgery; Director of Wound Care, Department of Surgery, LSU Health Sciences Center, LSU Health New Orleans School of Medicine, New Orleans, Louisiana

**DAWN TAYLOR PETERSON, PhD**
Department of Pediatrics, Office of Interprofessional Simulation, University of Alabama School of Medicine, Birmingham, Alabama

**ROY PHITAYAKORN, MD, MHPE (MEd), FACS**
Department of Surgery, Massachusetts General Hospital, Harvard Medical School, Boston, Massachusetts

**BRENT A. PONCE, MD**
Division of Orthopaedic Surgery, Department of Surgery, University of Alabama School of Medicine, Birmingham, Alabama

**JOHN R. PORTERFIELD Jr, MD, MSPH**
Division of Gastrointestinal Surgery, Department of Surgery, University of Alabama School of Medicine, Birmingham, Alabama

**CARLA M. PUGH, MD, PhD**
Department of Surgery, University of Wisconsin School of Medicine and Public Health; Department of Industrial and Systems Engineering, University of Wisconsin-Madison, Madison, Wisconsin

**DAVID A. ROGERS, MD, MHPE**
Division of Pediatric Surgery, Department of Surgery, University of Alabama School of Medicine, Birmingham, Alabama

**JOSE D. ROJAS, RT, PhD**
Associate Professor and Chair, Department of Respiratory Care, University of Texas Medical Branch, School of Health Professions, Galveston, Texas

**BRIAN K. ROSS, PhD, MD**
Professor, Department of Anesthesiology and Pain Medicine, University of Washington, Seattle, Washington

**DREW N. RUTHERFORD, MS**
Department of Surgery, University of Wisconsin School of Medicine and Public Health, Madison, Wisconsin

**DANIEL J. SCOTT, MD**
Professor and Vice Chair of Education, Department of Surgery, UT Southwestern Medical Center, Dallas, Texas

**NICK SEVDALIS, PhD**
Health Service and Population Research Department, Center for Implementation Science, King's College London, London, United Kingdom

**NEAL SEYMOUR, MD**
Chief, Division of General Surgery, Vice Chair, Department of Surgery, Surgery Residency Program Director, Professor, Tufts University School of Medicine, Boston, Massachusetts; Director, Baystate Simulation Center—Goldberg Surgical Skills Lab, Springfield, Massachusetts

**MALACHI G. SHEAHAN, MD**
Division of Vascular and Endovascular Surgery, The Claude C. Craighead Jr. Professor and Chair, Department of Surgery, LSU Health Sciences Center, New Orleans, Louisiana

**ELLIOTT SILVERMAN, PA-C, MSHS**
Assistant Professor of Surgery; Director, Surgical Skills and Training; Associate Program Director, Surgical Education Simulation Fellowship, Department of Surgery, Walter Reed National Military Medical Center, Uniformed Services University, Bethesda, Maryland; The Choral Arts Society of Washington, Washington, DC

**DIMITRIOS STEFANIDIS, MD, PhD, FACS, FASMBS**
Department of Surgery, Research and Surgical Director, Carolinas Simulation Center, Carolinas Medical Center, Associate Professor of Surgery, Carolinas Healthcare System, Charlotte, North Carolina

**MALLORY A. STELLATO, BS**
Department of Surgery, Walter Reed National Military Medical Center, Uniformed Services University, Bethesda, Maryland

**SHAWN TSUDA, MD**
Associate Professor, Department of Surgery, University of Nevada School of Medicine, Las Vegas, Nevada

**SCOTT A. TUCKER, MA**
The Choral Arts Society of Washington, Washington, DC

**KENT R. VAN SICKLE, MD, FACS**
Chief, Division of General and Minimally Invasive Surgery, Department of Surgery, University of Texas Health Science Center at San Antonio, San Antonio, Texas

**MERCY D. WAGNER, MD**
Department of Surgery, Walter Reed National Military Medical Center, Uniformed Services University, Bethesda, Maryland

**MARJORIE LEE WHITE, MD, MPPM, MA**
Division of Emergency Medicine, Department of Pediatrics, University of Alabama School of Medicine, Birmingham, Alabama

**ROSS E. WILLIS, PhD**
Director of Surgical Education, Department of Surgery, University of Texas Health Science Center at San Antonio, San Antonio, Texas

# Contents

**Foreword** xiii

Ronald F. Martin

**Preface** xvii

Kimberly M. Brown and John T. Paige

## Training & Practice

**Applying Educational Theory to Simulation-Based Training and Assessment in Surgery** 695

Sheila W. Chauvin

Considerable progress has been made regarding the range of simulator technologies and simulation formats. Similarly, results from research in human learning and behavior have facilitated the development of best practices in simulation-based training (SBT) and surgical education. Today, SBT is a common curriculum component in surgical education that can significantly complement clinical learning, performance, and patient care experiences. Beginning with important considerations for selecting appropriate forms of simulation, several relevant educational theories of learning are described.

**Concepts for Developing Expert Surgical Teams Using Simulation** 717

Aimee K. Gardner and Daniel J. Scott

This article investigates how simulation-based training can enhance the effectiveness of surgical teams. First, a description of team training within surgical settings is provided. Then, empirical work from a variety of fields is introduced to describe common characteristics of expert teams, with a specific focus on training surgical teams in simulated settings. Finally, methods and suggestions for evaluation of simulation-based team training are discussed.

**Simulation and Faculty Development** 729

David A. Rogers, Dawn Taylor Peterson, Brent A. Ponce, Marjorie Lee White, and John R. Porterfield Jr

As members of the faculty, surgeons take on a variety of roles related to the use of simulation. Surgeons will continue to interact with simulation as learners given the emerging role of simulation in continuing medical education. Surgeons who regularly teach others will also be using simulation because of its unique properties as an instructional method. Leading a simulation effort requires vision, creativity in resource management, and team leadership skills. Surgeons can use simulation to innovate in surgical patient care and in surgical education.

**Simulation for Maintenance of Certification** **893**

Brian K. Ross and Julia Metzner

Maintenance of certification (MOC) is a process through which practitioners are able to show continuing competence in their areas of expertise. Simulation plays an increasingly important role in the assessment of students and residents, as well as in the initial practice certification for health care professionals. The use of simulation as an assessment tool in MOC has been sluggish to be universally accepted. This article discusses the role of simulation in health care education, how simulation might be effectively applied in the MOC process, and the future role of simulation in the MOC process.

**Index** **907**

# SURGICAL CLINICS OF NORTH AMERICA

## FORTHCOMING ISSUES

*October 2015*
**Cancer Screening and Genetics**
Christopher L. Wolfgang, *Editor*

*December 2015*
**Inflammatory Bowel Disease**
Kerry L. Hammond, *Editor*

*February 2016*
**Development of a Surgeon: Medical School through Retirement**
Ronald F. Martin and Paul J. Schenarts, *Editors*

## RECENT ISSUES

*June 2015*
**Surgical Approaches to Esophageal Disease**
Dmitry Oleynikov, *Editor*

*April 2015*
**Perioperative Management**
Paul J. Schenarts, *Editor*

*February 2015*
**Caring for the Geriatric Surgical Patient**
Fred A. Luchette, *Editor*

*December 2014*
**Surgical Infections**
Robert G. Sawyer and Traci L. Hedrick, *Editors*

## ISSUE OF RELATED INTEREST

*Neurosurgery Clinics of North America*
April 2015 (Vol. 26, Issue 2)
**Quality Improvement in Neurosurgery**
John D. Rolston, Seunggu J. Han, and Andrew T. Parsa, *Editors*
Available at: www.neurosurgery.theclinics.com

**THE CLINICS ARE AVAILABLE ONLINE!**
Access your subscription at:
www.theclinics.com

# Foreword

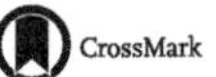

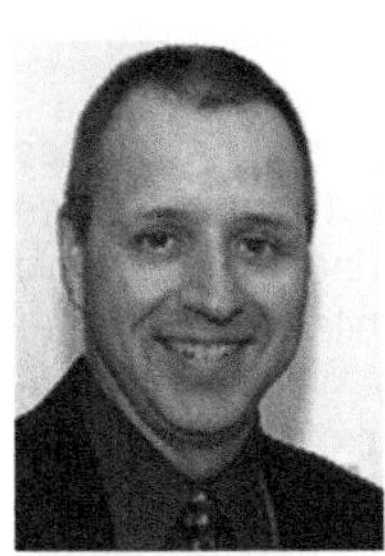

Ronald F. Martin, MD
*Consulting Editor*

I would like to think that I am not that old. My residents would like to disagree. When I speak with colleagues of my vintage at various meetings, it appears that I am not alone in facing this difference in perspective. From a chronologic standpoint, I am not that old, certainly not compared with the patient population I care for. Viewed through the prism of a surgical career, however, I am getting a bit old—not ancient, but definitively older. While I suspect this has always been the case for anyone going through his or her career in surgery, it may be possible that we have a slightly greater divide at present than previously. In addition to the usual breakdown of one's career by thirds—first third, building capability and credibility; second third, doing the heavy lifting and fostering change; and last third, transition to role of mentor and senior statesperson prior to retirement—at this particular time, we also have one other divide—those who did some or all of their training prior to the widespread use of videoscopic devices. And I might add that, as an offshoot of the videoscopic era, we also have those who trained before and after *simulation*.

By way of full disclosure, I did in fact do much, though not all, of my training prior to the widespread use of videoscopic tools. Also, other than using a few mannequins for the various lifesaver/life-support courses, I preceded simulation as a requirement for training—in my civilian job anyway. I am also an avid supporter of using simulated environments and situations to improve training opportunity and efficiency. I do, however, feel that we do not always consider simulation in the right light, and as such we may be losing our path a bit on the big scale.

A few years ago, I was at a national meeting when a very well-known professor was giving a presentation about the use of simulation in the training of surgeons. He made the argument that surgeons could not be trained without simulation. I was astonished enough that I questioned this proposition at the microphone. My only rebuttal was that he and I were both trained as surgeons before simulation was used for training as was pretty much everybody who trained us—and that we seemed to do all right clinically. I don't think my logic convinced him. This left me to consider something about this topic—we are not necessarily using logic at all; we are using belief. It is possible that we are simply framing the problem improperly, and we are asking the wrong questions. The question isn't can we or can't we train surgeons without

Surg Clin N Am 95 (2015) xiii–xv
http://dx.doi.org/10.1016/j.suc.2015.06.001
0039-6109/15/$ – see front matter 

simulation; of course we can! We have been doing it for most of history. The question should be: can we train surgeons better by using simulation? Could we make patients safer by using simulation? Could we even make training less expensive or more efficient by using simulation?

One concept that might help us address the issues above is to separate the process of *simulation* from *skills practice*. The best distinction I have heard to discern between the two is that one can practice skills (central line placement, suturing, laparoscopic skills, and so on) by oneself with some gadgets or spare parts, while simulation requires others to participate either as observers or as team members. While I am confident not all would agree with those distinctions, they serve a useful division as skills can represent limited part(s) of some technical adventure and simulation focuses on interaction(s) between a person or persons and responsive elements. There are clearly some instances in which the line blurs, but overall it may be a helpful clarification.

If one lends any credence to the above concept, the next logical extension is what one uses the tools for. A trainee is having trouble with a technical aspect of an operation, say laparoscopic knot tying; so then off to the skills lab. Tie a million knots if he likes, maybe he will get better. If a team is having trouble with trauma resuscitations, then off to the simulation center and respond to a trauma code while being remotely observed and learn through effective debriefing. Both concepts can benefit from coaching as well. In short, the best use for simulated environments or tasks is to help solve a problem that is otherwise difficult, unsafe, or expensive to solve by other means. The problem was never that we were globally deficient in simulation (human patients are incredibly high-fidelity "simulators" for other human patients) but rather how we could incorporate what non-real-patient simulation exists into our global training paradigm—which parenthetically does not end with residency or fellowship.

As I stated earlier, I believe in simulation. As some of you who have followed our series may know, I spent a fair bit of time in military service. Compared with the civilian sector, the military is far more advanced and dependent on simulation for training. Military simulation takes on a whole new meaning in terms of scope and fidelity as well. In my military career, I was involved in training environments that ranged from as big as the laptop I was working on to bicoastal exercises that involved thousands of personnel and many millions of dollars worth of equipment for sustained periods of time. Those types of exercises are very useful for training people and for reducing lack of familiarity with equipment and procedures. However, as anyone who has actually been to a real shooting war will tell you, no battle plan survives contact with the enemy. Similarly, whatever gear you used in training and whatever systems you got used to will have to be modified when placed in a hostile or austere environment. Thus, it has always been. We need to be reality-based in our understanding of the limits and benefits of simulation as they translate to actual patient care.

Organized surgery continues to expand its requirement for documented simulation proficiency in order to be admissible to high-stakes exams for surgeons. We currently require candidates to have taken and passed exams in Advanced Cardiac Life Support, Advanced Trauma Life Support, and Fundamentals of Laparoscopic Surgery for eligibility to take the Qualifying Exam for the American Board of Surgery (ABS). Shortly, we will be adding the exam for Fundamentals of Endoscopic Surgery (FES) to that list. The growing list is adding great cost and burden to training programs, and it is unclear, at least to me, that the costs warrant the incremental benefit we are getting in terms of making patients safer. Perhaps time will prove me wrong on this, but for now, there is a growing concern that we are adding in layer upon layer of testing without necessarily having the data to support its mandatory inclusion. Perhaps the most controversial of the above is the FES provision. Present ABS data shared with the Association of Program Directors in Surgery in Seattle this spring suggested that only 20% of people who finish Categorical General Surgery Residency Programs actually go on to perform any endoscopy as part of their clinical practice, yet all will be required to take the FES exam in order to seek ABS certification. I will let you, dear reader, consider that requirement for yourself.

As I stated earlier, I am a supporter of simulations and skills training. They can both be useful tools to help individuals or teams become proficient at many things while reducing unnecessary risks to actual patients. Simulation in all its forms is not a panacea for all ills. It will not correct the shift in delayed skill acquisition for trainees—that is, a systemic problem that incorporates medical schools, liability issues, financial constraints, and public demands and expectations. Simulation will not replace the need to interact with actual humans both in and out of the operating room to become proficient as a surgeon. Simulation will not eliminate the anxiety (or joy) of the attending surgeon when teaching trainees. Simulation and skills training, however, are highly likely to be useful in solving or helping to solve subsets of problems that we all encounter when training or when incorporating new technology or procedures into our environments.

If we are going to use simulation wisely and *surgically* (to borrow a profoundly overused adjective used in the manner of the media) to address our training and development issues, then we must understand how to frame the questions and to critically and honestly evaluate how these programs are helping or not. We must have ways of showing where the investment of time and treasure translates into patient and community benefit. To that end, Drs Brown and Paige have assembled an impressive collection of articles to help you do just that. Whether you run a training program, are in a training program, or work nowhere even close to a training program, there is something in here for you. Simulation is here to stay. If I read the tea leaves right, I would also submit that its use for initial ABS Board of Certification wouldn't be where its requirement ends. I would not be surprised at all to see documentation of simulation training be required for individual maintenance of certification or institutional certification—all the more reason to understand its uses and limitations.

I am indebted once again to Dr Brown for her willingness to contribute to this series and I welcome and thank very much Dr Paige for his efforts. It is their and their colleagues' hard work that makes this series what it is.

Ronald F. Martin, MD
Department of Surgery
Marshfield Clinic
1000 North Oak Avenue
Marshfield, WI 54449, USA

E-mail address:
martin.ronald@marshfieldclinic.org

# Preface

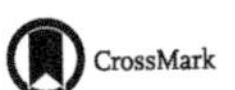

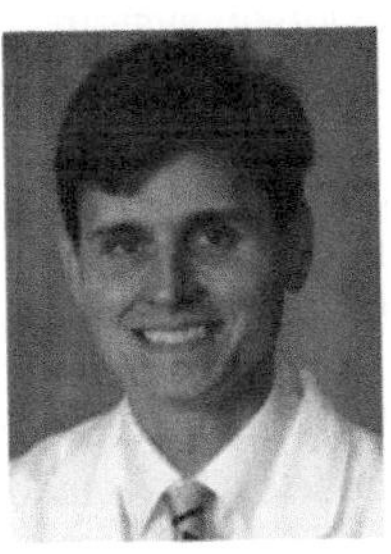

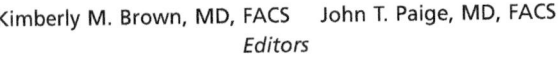

Kimberly M. Brown, MD, FACS    John T. Paige, MD, FACS
*Editors*

"See one. Do one. Teach one." During our years of training, this mantra encompassed the essence of the Halstedian apprenticeship model of surgical residency and education. Combined with two years of bench work in the pursuit of basic science knowledge, it formed the cornerstone of access to a competitive fellowship and a successful career as an academic surgeon—regardless whether the surgeon ever set foot in a lab once finished with residency.

In the last two decades, the field of surgery has recognized and begun to value new avenues of education and training as well as new ways to learn the critical thinking skills required for scientific investigation. Training programs are now more than ever employing objectives-based, proficiency-driven curricula with deliberate practice to accelerate the learning curve before the "Do one" of old, ushering an era of "See one; practice many; do one." Furthermore, the notion of surgical education as a scholarly endeavor has gradually taken hold, and with the energy and drive of bright surgical minds, trainees now benefit from our improved understanding of how people acquire the knowledge, skills, and attitudes required to be excellent surgeons. In addition, residents and faculty are now pursuing the study of educational methods, assessment tools, and other aspects of education as the substance of academic work. Fellowships and graduate degree programs now exist to teach the science of health care education, and many universities offer education-based tracks in their promotion and tenure processes.

The recognition of simulation as a highly effective tool to teach a variety of technical and nontechnical skills to students, residents, and practicing surgeons has been critical in this transformation. The value of simulation is now widely accepted and integrated into health care training, from undergraduate medical education through continuing medical education, across and among professions, and within health systems. We have moved beyond validating simulators and now understand that the process of gathering validity evidence for an educational activity is an ongoing process grounded in similar scientific principles to the evidence a clinician would consider when choosing a treatment for a patient. Academics are now applying more rigorous criteria to the study of simulation and its impact on the knowledge, skills, and attitudes, as well as the health care outcomes at the patient and population level.

Surg Clin N Am 95 (2015) xvii–xviii
http://dx.doi.org/10.1016/j.suc.2015.06.002
0039-6109/15/$ – see front matter 

In addition, we have a broader perspective of the applications of simulation throughout health care. Simulation-based training has helped uncover the importance of human factors engineering in designing systems that facilitate desired behaviors or outcomes and that actively discourage unsafe or inappropriate actions. We are learning more about the impact of teaching methods and developing the skills of those educators who teach using simulation.

As a result of more rigorous scientific study of how technical skills are acquired, and the accumulation of validity evidence around specific assessment tools, simulation is used in several high-stakes examinations in undergraduate medical education and for professional certifications. This is truly an educational achievement, to test a person's skills through the performance of those skills, instead of just their ability to answer multiple choice questions.

It has been a pleasure to work with our talented authors in bringing together this issue of *Surgical Clinics of North America* dedicated to the applications of Simulation in Surgical Training and Practice. From nuts and bolts to educational theory, from traditional uses of simulation to innovative applications, this issue provides the reader with perspective on the breadth of simulation's influence in surgical education and practice today, and insights into where simulation is heading tomorrow.

Kimberly M. Brown, MD, FACS
Laboratory for Surgical Training
Assessment, and Research
Hepatobiliary-Pancreatic Surgery
Department of Surgery
University of Texas Medical Branch
301 University Boulevard
Galveston, TX 77555-0737, USA

John T. Paige, MD, FACS
School of Medicine
Department of Surgery
LSU Heath Sciences Center
LSU Health New Orleans School of Medicine
1542 Tulane Avenue, Room 734
New Orleans, LA 70112, USA

E-mail addresses:
kim.brown@utmb.edu (K.M. Brown)
jpaige@lsuhsc.edu (J.T. Paige)

# Applying Educational Theory to Simulation-Based Training and Assessment in Surgery

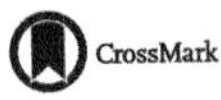

Sheila W. Chauvin, PhD, MEd

**KEYWORDS**

- Simulation-based training • Instructional design • Assessment
- Educational learning theory

**KEY POINTS**

- To optimize effective, cost-efficient use of simulation, good alignment among learning objectives, teacher and learner features, fidelity and replicability of simulators and simulation environment, and assessment processes is necessary.
- Consider the level of the learners, prior knowledge and experiences, and targeted learning outcomes and be judicious in determining the appropriate level of fidelity and complexity for simulation.
- To achieve mastery, learners must first learn fundamental knowledge and skills, then practice integrating them until fluent and automatic, and finally, learn when and how to apply what they learned appropriately in various contexts.
- Establishing evidence of validity and reliability is never finished and requires diligence in examining how assessment measures and processes interact with assessment situations across time, individuals, settings, and purposes to produce data.
- The selection and preparation of assessors are critical to the validity and reliability of data, because an assessment is only as good as the person doing it.

## INTRODUCTION

Considerable progress has been made regarding the range of simulator technologies and simulation formats. Similarly, results from research in human learning and behavior have facilitated the development of best practices in simulation-based training (SBT) and surgical education.[1–4] Today, SBT routinely complements actual clinical learning and patient care experiences in surgical education.

---

Disclosure: The author has nothing to disclose.
Office of Medical Education Research and Development, Louisiana State University Health Sciences Center – New Orleans, School of Medicine, 2020 Gravier Street, Suite 657, New Orleans, LA 70112, USA
*E-mail address:* schauv@lsuhsc.edu

Surg Clin N Am 95 (2015) 695–715
http://dx.doi.org/10.1016/j.suc.2015.04.006 surgical.theclinics.com
0039-6109/15/$ – see front matter 

Beginning with important considerations for selecting appropriate forms of simulation, several relevant educational theories of learning are described, followed by a practical overview of the ADDIE model that offers a systematic approach to curriculum and instructional design.[5–7] Definitions of key terms and important principles provide guidance for designing and using assessments. Additional key resources are identified and referenced for further reading and application in designing effective SBT and assessment in surgical education.

## SIMULATORS AND SIMULATION

McGaghie[8(p9)] offers a useful definition for simulation:

> In broad, simple terms, a simulation is a person, device, or set of conditions that attempts to present (education and) evaluation problems authentically. Students or trainees are required to respond to the problems as they would under natural circumstances. Frequently, a trainee receives performance feedback as if in a real situation.

McGaghie also notes commonalities between simulation-based teaching and assessment methods (**Box 1**).

*Simulation* refers to the design and process of teacher and learner interaction. *Simulator* refers to the actual device, object, or person used to mimic the relevant real-life elements in a simulation-based instructional or assessment activity. A simulator could be a paper case, a role-play exercise, or a teacher's use of "what if" questions in the discussion of a real patient case. A more complex simulation might involve the single or combined use of other types of simulators (eg, live simulated patient/actor, anatomic trainer, cadaver, and/or computerized or mannequin-based human patient simulator).

To optimize effective and cost-efficient use of simulation, good alignment among the learning objectives, teacher and learner features, simulator(s), and overall purpose of the activity or process is necessary. Underestimating the level of fidelity (realism) can result in not achieving intended learning outcomes and wasting time and expertise. Overestimating fidelity might result in achieving learning outcomes but wasting

**Box 1**
**Common features between simulation-based training and assessment methods**

- Learners can be situated in complex scenarios.
- Learners experience cues and consequences that accurately reflect real-life experience.
- Learners respond to simulated situations similarly to how they would in real-life.
- Simulation does not completely replicate real life (ie, fidelity) due to its limitations (eg, cost, technological capacity, time, assessment requirements, ethics, and safety).
- A wide variety of simulation formats facilitate individual or group learning and performance.
- Simulations can involve a variety of simulator technology in single or combined use (eg, a simple inanimate, anatomic model, programmable module, and/or high-fidelity, physiologically responsive, mannequin-based human patient simulator).
- Use of simulation can reflect decisions and consequences that can range from low- to high-stakes impact on the learner.

*Adapted from* McGaghie WC. Simulation in professional competence assessment: basic considerations. In: Tekian A, McGuire CH and McGaghie WC, editors. Innovative simulations for assessing professional competence. Chicago: Department of Medical Education, University of Illinois at Chicago; 1999.

resources when lower fidelity would have been equally effective. Also, overestimating simulation fidelity may not achieve intended learning outcomes due to cognitive and sensory overload. Learners can be overloaded by unnecessary stimuli and have insufficient cognitive processing capacity to use prior knowledge and experience to make sense of new learning.[9–12] Therefore, consider the level of the learners, prior knowledge and experiences, and targeted learning outcomes and be judicious in determining the level of fidelity and complexity for simulation.

## EDUCATIONAL THEORIES AND MODELS OF LEARNING

Theoretic models provide generalizable explanations of natural phenomenon confirmed through observations, experimentation, and logical reasoning across various settings. These explanations produce generalized statements or principles that can guide action and activities (eg, teaching and learning). Custers and Boshuizen[13] differentiate psychological and educational theories of learning. Psychological theories reflect processes that occur within a learner's mind, whereas, educational theories of learning extend beyond a learner's mind to also include teacher and learner characteristics, actions, interactions, teaching methods, and physical and psychosocial elements of the learning environment. Several educational taxonomies and theoretic models are described that provide guiding principles for designing and implementing SBT.

## TAXONOMIES OF LEARNING AND THINKING

Taxonomies are useful in deciding the level at which to initiate and advance learning to higher levels of thinking and expertise. Two frequently used taxonomies are discussed.

### *Bloom's Taxonomy*

Bloom and colleagues[14] published a taxonomy comprising 3 domains for developing learner assessments. Over the decades, Bloom's taxonomy has been been used as much if not more for developing specific educational goals, learning objectives/outcomes, and corresponding educational activities and materials. As shown in **Table 1**, all 3 domains are applicable to surgical education for designing teaching, learning, and assessment using simulation-based methods.

Anderson and Krathwohl[15] updated the cognitive domain of Bloom's taxonomy. As shown in **Table 2**, they reversed the 2 highest levels and redefined synthesis to

**Table 1**
**Bloom's taxonomy in the cognitive, affective, and psychomotor domains**

| Level | Cognitive (Knowledge) | Affective (Attitude) | Psychomotor (Skills) |
|---|---|---|---|
| 1 | Recall (information) | Receive (awareness) | Imitate |
| 2 | Understand (comprehend) | Respond (react) | Manipulate (follow directions) |
| 3 | Apply (use) | Value (understand and act) | Develop precision |
| 4 | Analyze | Organize (in terms of personal value system) | Articulate (combine, integrate skills) |
| 5 | Synthesize | Internalize value system (characterize, adopt behaviors associated with value[s]) | Naturalize (automate, become expert) |
| 6 | Evaluate (judge) | — | — |

*Adapted from* Bloom B, Engelhart MD, Furst EJ, et al. Taxonomy of educational objectives: handbook 1, the cognitive domain. New York: Longman; 1956.

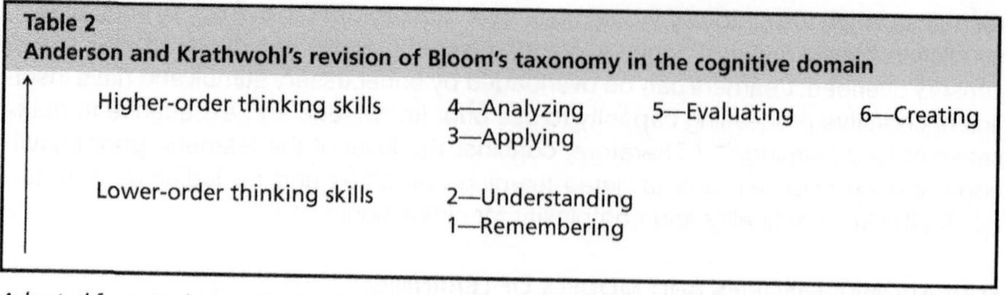

**Table 2**
**Anderson and Krathwohl's revision of Bloom's taxonomy in the cognitive domain**

| | | | |
|---|---|---|---|
| Higher-order thinking skills | 4—Analyzing<br>3—Applying | 5—Evaluating | 6—Creating |
| Lower-order thinking skills | 2—Understanding<br>1—Remembering | | |

*Adapted from* Anderson LW, Krathwohl DR, editors. A taxonomy for learning, teaching, and assessing: a revision of Bloom's taxonomy of educational objectives. New York: Longman; 2001.

explicitly *reflect* the aspect of creating as a higher level ability than *evaluation*. They also posited that levels 4 to 6 occur more as simultaneous than hierarchical functions. Finally, the labels were revised to reflect verb forms to emphasize levels as active processes. Regardless of the version used, a first step is to decide whether training or assessment reflects lower- or higher-order thinking, because this can inform the selection of appropriate simulator and simulation formats. Next, the levels within a domain can be used to further refine selection and development processes.

### *Miller's Pyramid*

Miller's[16] assessment framework, shown in **Fig. 1**, was conceptualized for clinical competence, particularly in medical education. Beginning at the bottom of the pyramid, *Knows* reflects the initial acquisition of factual knowledge. *Knows how* reflects the ability to explain or describe. *Shows how* reflects the ability to apply knowledge and skills to a real-life situation. *Does* reflects the ability to routinely perform targeted ability(ies). Performance at this highest level reflects integrating knowledge, skills, and attitudes in everyday practice that includes approaching and solving ill-structured and evolving patient problems.

## THEORIES AND MODELS OF LEARNING

Many educational theories and models relevant to SBT are available but beyond the scope of this article. Some models focus on individual learning, whereas others target

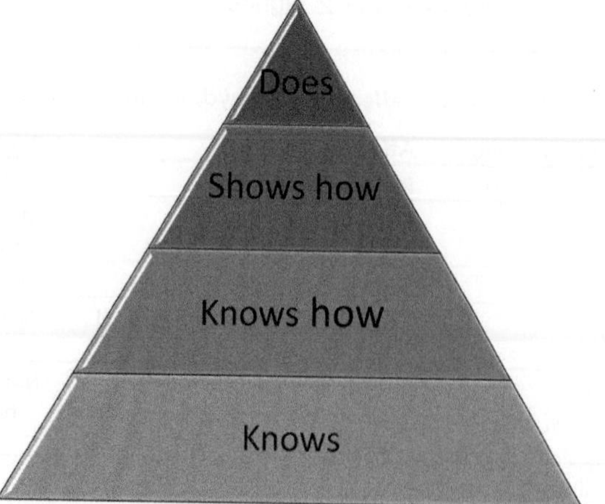


**Fig. 1.** Miller's pyramid for assessing clinical competence. (*Adapted from* Miller GR. The assessment of clinical skills/competence/performance. Acad Med 1990:65;S63–6.)

social and group aspects of learning processes. Several are described that are particularly relevant to SBT.

### *Adult Learning Theory*

Knowles and colleagues[17] introduced *andragogy* to differentiate adult learning from that in children (ie, pedagogy). Their theory conceptualized adult learners as intrinsically motivated and driven by independent, self-directed application of new learning to relevant, real-life situations. Candy[18] identified more than 100 characteristics associated with self-directed learning. Of these, the following were deemed most important:

- Confident and competent learning behavior
- Curious, open, creative, self-motivated
- Disciplined and methodical
- Analytical, logical, and reflective
- Collaborative and interdependent with others
- Responsible and persistent, and self-aware.

**Box 2** summarizes 7 best practices that are representative of active, adult learning. To maximize learning benefits in SBT, learners need to safely and comfortably identify gaps in their knowledge and skills. Learners can begin by identifying relevant information they know already, then identify what else they need to learn and why. Teachers' effective use of questions helps learners clarify, expand, and enhance learning and resolve misunderstandings and mistakes. Learners should be encouraged to reflect on their own and each other's learning to provide feedback, assess learning progress, and gain insights regarding how they can build on learning achievements. SBT is well-suited to provide such thinking and learning processes during realistic and hands-on learning. Teachers must communicate specific expectations for both learners and teachers.

### *Experiential Learning Theory*

Shown in **Fig. 2**, Kolb and Fry[19,20] conceptualized learning as a 4-stage process, grounded in individual or group real-life experiences that can begin at any stage. Kolb's experiential learning cycle includes the following stages:

**Box 2**
**Education principles for designing and implementing effective teaching and learning**

1. Provide learners with a safe and respectful learning environment in which learners are comfortable experimenting with new learning, expressing themselves, learning from mistakes, and learning with and from each other.
2. Engage learners directly in planning content, curriculum, and methods for learning and assessment.
3. Motivate and facilitate intrinsic motivation by engaging learners in identifying their own learning needs.
4. Allow learners to have some control over their learning processes (eg, formulating, selecting, or prioritizing their own learning objectives).
5. Engage learners in identifying preferred learning strategies and resources.
6. Support learners in taking responsibility for implementing their personal learning plans.
7. Facilitate learners' development of critical reflection and responsibility for self-directed learning and improvement.

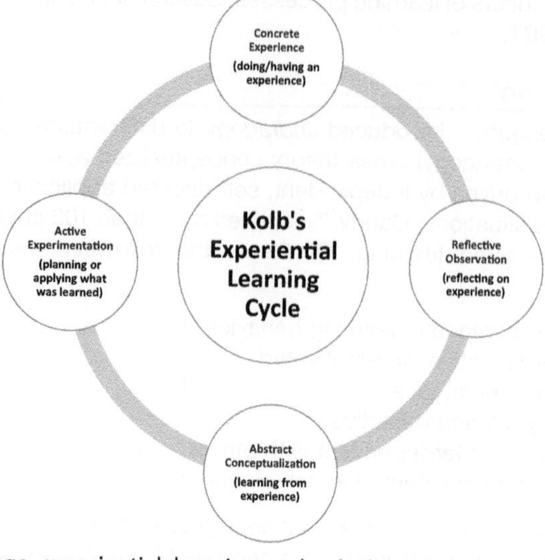


**Fig. 2.** Kolb's 4-stage experiential learning cycle. (*Adapted from* Kolb DA. Experiential learning. Englewood Cliffs (NJ): Prentice Hall; 1984.)

1. Concrete experience
2. Observation during and reflection on experience to form concepts
3. Formulation of concepts, generalizations, principles, and rules
4. Testing or experimentation with these concepts, generalizations, principles, and rules in new situations

Houle[21(p221)] noted that this type of learning results from "education that occurs as a direct participation in the events of life." Such events can be formal academic learning or real-life experience. In surgical education, learning is influenced by the types of patient problems encountered in real life and through simulation experiences that provide greater focus and control over what actually happens. Both real-life and simulated scenarios support learners' use of Kolb's 4-stage process and facilitate active engagement in testing and reflecting on experiences to enhance learning. To maximize learning, careful attention to the use of effective questioning and coaching behaviors facilitate active learning (see **Box 2**).[22]

### *Constructivist, Zone of Proximal Development, and Self-Efficacy Theories*

Constructivist theory conceptualizes learners as active, self-directed learners and emphasizes learners' use of prior learning and experiences to construct and reconstruct new meanings, knowledge, skills, and perspectives. Learners decide when and how they modify their knowledge and abilities based on their experiences and engagement with others. The following 4 principles are critical to effective teaching and learning within a constructivist perspective[10,23,24]:

- Teachers are guides who facilitate learning, not transmitters of information.
- Teachers must structure learning experiences so learners have opportunities to identify inconsistencies between their current understandings and new experiences, so new meaning and knowledge can be constructed.
- Learning activities must engage learners actively in using relevant problems and situations.

- Sufficient time for in-depth exploration and resolution of inconsistencies is critical for construction and reflection on new knowledge and understandings.

Within constructivist theory, cognitive and social perspectives are important. How individuals understand things and make sense reflects their developmental level, thinking processes, and preferences for learning. From a social perspective, emphasis is on how social interactions with others (eg, real-life or SBT) influence a learner's construction of new meanings, knowledge, skills, and perspectives.[23,24]

Vygotsky[25] introduced the theoretic perspective of a zone of proximal development (ZPD), where learning progress can be optimized. This ZPD is the sweet spot just beyond a learner's current abilities that is challenging yet achievable with help. Vygotsky emphasized the critical role of social interaction in learning. Engaging learners with others who are just beyond their stage of development (ie, near-peer) can facilitate using the ZPD for advancing learning while minimizing failure.

Through systematic use of modeling and coaching, near-peers and teachers can serve as models from whom less-experienced learners can observe and plan initial performance. Near-peers also benefit through offering explanations and engaging in peer coaching to refine performance. Teachers use effective coaching and feedback strategies to assist individual learners. As knowledge and skills are achieved and integrated, the teacher can *fade*, or gradually reduce, direct support/instruction and coaching/feedback to facilitate independent practice. The purposeful use of the ZPD, with modeling, coaching, feedback, and fading, is often referred to as *scaffolding*.[2,23,26,27]

Bandura[28] recognized how individuals' self-judgments influenced their actions. These judgments, called self-efficacy, represented learners' self-perceptions and beliefs about their abilities to respond to different situations effectively. Such self-perceptions may or may not be accurate, but they are real to individuals and can either limit or facilitate the extent to which they seek, act on, and succeed in tasks.

Bandura[28] identified 4 sources of information that form perceptions of self-efficacy: actual achieved performance, observation of others, verbal persuasion, and physiologic state. That is, personal experiences of success increase self-efficacy for similar types of tasks. Observations of others performing tasks successfully can positively influence self-efficacy for being able to perform an unfamiliar task. Receiving encouraging feedback, preperformance guidance, and effective mentoring and coaching (ie, verbal persuasion) can enhance self-efficacy for attempting new tasks or experiences. Feeling safe and supported in a learning environment (ie, physiologic state in real-life or simulation) can positively influence individuals' self-efficacy and the likelihood for participation and successful performance. The integration of adult and active learning principles and experiential and constructive theories can optimize the ZPD to promote learning. Positive self-efficacy facilitates safe learning environments and promotes motivation and persistence, even when learning is challenging.

### *Mastery Teaching and Learning, Reflection, and Deliberate Practice*

Mastery models are grounded in the recognition that everyone can learn. Some people learn faster or slower than others. With careful monitoring and effective instruction and feedback, mastery can be achieved. The mastery learning model developed first by Bloom[29] and later expanded by Block and Burns[30] includes 6 consistently aligned features. Hunter created a mastery Teaching model of lesson design[31,32] that included similar steps. See **Box 3** for a summary of these models.

Such models emphasize focused and systematic instruction, practice, monitoring, immediate feedback, and gradual fading strategies to achieve independent practice. Progression to the next level of learning occurs only after meeting mastery criteria.

**Box 3**
**Mastery learning and mastery teaching models**

| Mastery Learning (Bloom and Block and Burns) | Mastery Teaching (Hunter) |
| --- | --- |
| • Baseline, diagnostic assessment<br>• Clear and sequenced learning objectives reflecting increasing difficulty<br>• Involvement in specific objectives-based learning activities<br>• Established minimum mastery criteria for each instructional unit that must be achieved before advancing to the next unit<br>• Formative assessment at the end of each unit<br>• Corrective feedback and continued practice and learning in an instructional unit until the mastery criteria are met. | • Anticipatory set—establish motivation, assess readiness for learning, and introduce learning<br>• Learning objectives—communicate learning targets and learner expectations<br>• Instruction—objectives-based instruction and modeling of expected outcome(s)<br>• Check for understanding—monitor and adjust teaching to facilitate learning<br>• Guided practice—provide support, assistance, coaching, and scaffolding of task, as needed<br>• Independent practice—provide learners' opportunity perform independently, observe carefully, and provide specific feedback |

*Data from* Refs.[29–32]

McGaghie and colleagues[33] have provided a critical review of such SBT mastery learning that is a good resource for further reading.

Reflective practice is associated with developing expertise and is an essential element of ongoing learning and improvement. Flavell[34] and Bransford, and colleagues[2] noted the importance of learners' development of metacognitive abilities (eg, predicting, monitoring, and reflecting on thinking, actions, and perspectives) as important strategies for the development of expertise and transfer of learning to everyday practice and new situations.

In Schon's[35,36] model of reflective practice, *reflection-in-action* occurs during experiences and *reflection-on-action* occurs after experiences. In SBT, reflection-in-action can occur during *think-aloud* communications about what and why one is thinking or doing during procedures training or team-based patient scenarios. Reflection-on-action typically occurs during after-action debriefing discussions. Reflection can also be used effectively in preparatory briefings or discussions to bring to consciousness relevant knowledge and prior experiences before engaging in the SBT experience.

In more recent times, focused practice with focused feedback has been further studied, with particular attention to the development of expertise. Ericcson and colleagues[37,38] conceptualized *deliberate practice* as the engagement of highly motivated learners in intense, concentrated practice that is guided by explicit performance outcomes. Advancement to another task or learning objective occurs when mastery criteria are met, much like the mastery teaching/learning models, only more focused and explicit to performance tasks. Once a learner is able to perform a task in a real-life setting (ie, Miller's *does* competency level [see **Fig. 1**]), then deliberate practice techniques can be used to refine abilities. That is, using focused repetitive practice, close monitoring and assessment, and explicit frequent feedback facilitates accuracy, fluency, and advancement to expert performance. The specific use of simulation in deliberate practice to achieve mastery has been demonstrated.[33,39]

To summarize the various educational theories, **Box 4** provides 7 evidence-based principles of effective teaching,[1] that, when used in combination with effective learning principles (see **Box 2**), provides an evidence-based framework for achieving effective SBT.

Issenberg, and colleagues[40] identified 10 key findings from their systematic review targeting features and uses of high-fidelity medical simulations that lead to most effective learning. These findings also serve as a set of guiding principles for optimizing the effective design and use of SBT in surgical education (**Table 3**). A systematic approach to curriculum and instructional design is described.

**Box 4**
**Seven evidence-based principles of effective teaching**

1. Learners' need to access sufficient and appropriate prior knowledge enhances their learning.
2. How learners organize knowledge influences how they learn and apply what they know (eg, strive to weave tapestry instead of cheesecloth-type neural associations among concepts, principles, and generalizations).
3. Learners' motivation generates, directs, and sustains what they do to learn (ie, goals play a key role; both value and expectancies are critical features of motivation). Value relates to learners' interest and perceived importance and expectancy relates to the learners' perception of the extent to which the goal is attainable (ie, reasonable expectation).
4. To develop mastery, learners must first learn fundamental skills within a targeted domain, then practice integrating them to the point of fluency and reasonable automaticity, and finally, learn when to apply what they have learned appropriately in various contexts (ie, 3 elements of mastery). The novice to expert trajectory is based on 2 dimensions: competence and consciousness. The 2-D model yields 4 levels of expertise: unconscious incompetence (ie, unaware of errors and what one needs to know), conscious incompetence (ie, aware of knowledge and skill deficiencies), conscious competence (ie, aware of and attentive to necessary knowledge and skills), and unconscious competence (ie, knowledge and skills are integrated and automatic, do not require explicit attention to perform).
5. Deliberate practice (ie, goal-directed, focused practice with specific feedback) is critical to learning. Goals direct practice, help evaluate the observed performance, and give appropriate and specific feedback that in turn guides additional practice and achievement of goal-related performance (ie, mastery).
6. Learners' current level of development interacts with the learning environment (eg, social, emotional, and intellectual climate) and these features influence learning (teacher-learner and learner-learner interactions, safe climate, and focused on learning with and from each other—cooperation and collaboration vs competition), clear communication of expectations, and performance standards and reduce anonymity (ie, recognition of learners and enhancing accountability, professional learning environment, reveal inconsistencies, and embrace conflict as opportunity for growth and learning).
7. To become self-directed learners, individuals must learn to assess the demands of a given task, accurately self-assess their knowledge and skills, plan how to proceed with the task, self-monitor progress, and adjust strategies as needed (role of metacognition, as a process of thinking and reflecting on and directing one's own thinking.

*Adapted from* Ambrose SA, Bridges MW, DiPietro M, et al. How learning works: seven research-based principles for smart teaching. San Francisco: Jossey-Bass; 2010; and Bransford JD, Brown AL, Cocking RR. How people learn: brain, mind, experience, and school. Washington, DC: National Academy Press; 2000.

**Table 3**
**Education principles for designing and implementing simulation-based teaching and learning experiences using high-fidelity simulations**

| Education Principle | Annotation |
|---|---|
| 1. Define specific, observable learner outcomes and benchmarks. | Learners are more likely to master expected outcomes that are clear and appropriate for their level of learning. |
| 2. Establish the simulator is a valid teaching/learning tool. | Using simulators and a simulation learning environment that authentically reflect real life promotes suspended disbelief and facilitates transfer of learning from training to real-life practice. |
| 3. Integrate simulation-based experiences into the overall curriculum/program. | Learners and faculty are more likely to take simulation experiences more seriously if they are well integrated into the curriculum, performance assessment, and everyday educational activities. Simulation should be used for deliberate practice opportunities and transfer to actual patient care. |
| 4. Simulation experiences should complement multiple learning methods. | Integrate simulation opportunities with the range of methods used in the curriculum (eg, small group tutorials, independent learning stations, and faculty-facilitated scenarios for individuals and teams). |
| 5. Learning using simulation should occur in controlled learning environments. | Simulation exercises should be safe for learners and learning-focused experiences that can take advantage of teachable moments and opportunities to correct mistakes and refine abilities through deliberate practice. |
| 6. Ensure that simulators can support a wide range of patient problems and situations. | Using simulators and simulation experiences to sample broadly from the array of patient problems and situations can strengthen the overall curriculum and educational program. This is particularly important for rare or limited access to important patient situations in the real-life setting. |
| 7. Design and use simulations to provide standardized, reproducible experiences that can accommodate learners' individualized needs. | Even when training groups or teams of learners, provide individualized learning in SBT sessions. |
| 8. Maximize use of simulation for opportunities to engage in deliberate practice. | The deliberate and repetitive cycles of focused practice with focused and frequent feedback is a necessary component to developing expertise. |
| 9. As learners achieve one level of learning, they should be progressively challenged to perform at higher levels of difficulty. | Scaffolding the level of challenge motivates and sustains learner engagement and persistence when the press for achievement is reasonable and attainable. |
| 10. Provide learners with purposeful and effective feedback during simulation-based training. | Feedback is the single most important element in SBT to promote effective learning. Feedback should be specific to the learner and to the task/performance, timely, and provided in a way that encourages continued effort. Feedback should also be given in a way that maintains learner dignity and helps the learner monitor and self-assess progress toward mastery. |

*Adapted from* Issenberg SB, McGaghie WC, Petrusa ER, et al. BEME guide no. 4: features and uses of high-fidelity medical simulations that lead to effective learning. Dundee (United Kingdom): AMEE; 2004.

## ADDIE: A SYSTEMATIC APPROACH TO CURRICULUM AND INSTRUCTIONAL DESIGN

Organized as an ongoing cycle and shown in **Fig. 3**, the ADDIE model is comprised of 5 components: assess, design, develop, implement, and evaluate.[5,41,42]

The ADDIE model is effective for developing and refining SBT programs, regardless of the selected simulator technology or the extent to which SBT is used with more traditional instruction methods (eg, lecture or small group discussion). The ADDIE model also supports educational design as a collaborative process among faculty, learners, content experts, and educational and assessment consultants. Collaboration is critical to effective SBT and long-term sustainability, especially given the associated high costs (eg, people, time, technology, and money). **Box 5** provides additional details for each ADDIE component.

The quality of assessment tools and processes has a direct impact on the extent to which results are usable for making sound and defensible decisions about learner progress and program/curriculum effectiveness. Relevant assessment principles and strategies are highlighted.

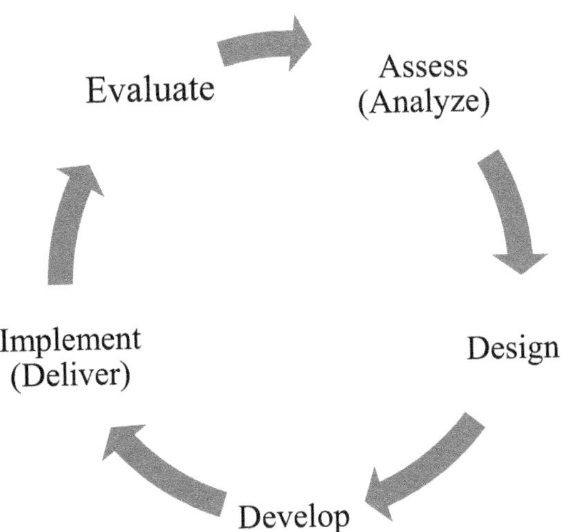


**Fig. 3.** The ADDIE model of curriculum and instructional design.

**Box 5**
**Components of the ADDIE model for curriculum and instructional design**

*Assess/Analyze*

- Needs assessment: Using appropriate methods, gather relevant information about specific needs, including those of learners, course/program, accreditation, and school. Needs assessment processes also target issues of resource availability, feasibility, receptivity to innovation and change, and organizational support.

*Design*

- Context: Define the educational context in which the curriculum or course will be implemented, including the learner group(s) and the context or target to which the learning to transfer (eg, specific knowledge, competency, or behaviors) is expected.
- Goals: Identify and clearly state the major goals to be addressed by the curriculum or course.
- Learning objectives: Develop specific, learner-centered and observable objectives (or expected learning outcomes) that will lead to achievement of each major curriculum

goals. The process of developing goals and objectives will help to identify the learning context that will be best for achieving the intended education and training outcomes.

- Assessment: Early in the instructional design process, envision how learning goals and intended objectives/outcomes can be assessed. Develop the assessment framework and define assessment methods for both processes and outcomes. Knowledge assessments might include multiple-choice item tests. Technical and procedural skills would likely require direct observation by trained assessors and the use of standards-based checklists.
- Facilitators: identify individual and organizational features that can facilitate or support the curriculum or course.
- Obstacles: Identify potential challenges and obstacles at the individual and organizational levels and realistic coping strategies to address and overcome them.
- Content: Define the core content and the scope and sequence in which they will be presented that is appropriate to the learner group and the goals, objectives, and educational setting. Specify any knowledge and skill prerequisites and assure that learners can achieve these prior to the planned simulation-based experience.

*Develop*

- Methods: Identify and develop methods and associated activities for the teaching and learning process and for conducting formative (informal) and summative (formal, graded) assessments, including the sequence and timing of these activities.
- Resources and materials: Develop teaching, learning and assessment materials. Acquire necessary resources for implementation (eg, equipment, supplies, space, personnel, images, laboratory reports, props, and so forth) and to achieve sufficient fidelity (realism).

*Implement*

- Pilot study: Conduct a pilot or field test of the simulation-based curriculum or module, including assessment procedures (typically small-scale implementation).
- Refine and finalize: Use results of the pilot study to make necessary adjustments or refinements to the curriculum, scenarios, context features, questions and debriefing prompts, facilitator guide, and supporting materials (eg, cases, scenarios, curriculum materials, and assessment instruments).
- Implement: Implement the full-scale curriculum, course, or training session or series.

*Evaluate*

- Although the evaluate component is listed last, it is actually the component that occurs throughout each cycle. The evaluate component includes, but is not limited to, the following types of activities:
- Conduct assessments of learner performance and program effectiveness.
- Examine formative and summative results in terms of intended processes and outcomes of the educational program (ie, program evaluation).
- Provide feedback to faculty, learners, and other stakeholders.
- Use results and feedback process to identify areas in need of redesign, refinement, and/or expansion. Include relevant stakeholders in using results for both formative (improvement) and summative (decision-making) purposes.
- Begin the ADDIE cycle again to achieve desired enhancement and/or expansion.

## ASSESSMENT PRINCIPLES

A full discussion of assessment and evaluation is beyond the scope of this article. This section provides key terms and principles for thinking about and engaging with others to design and use assessment effectively.

**Box 6**
**Features of formative versus summative processes**

| Feature | Formative | Summative |
| --- | --- | --- |
| Purpose | To facilitate improvement | To decide success/achievement |
| Format | Informal, nongraded | Formal, graded, or scored |
| Context | Embedded within teaching and learning activities | Separate or outside of teaching and learning activities |
| Data/evidence | Specific, discrete performance (eg, low-inference judgments) | Combined/integrated behaviors or performance over a time period (eg, high-inference judgments) |
| Consequence | Low, limited impact on learner's or program's future | High, potential for significant impact on learner's or program's future |

### *Common Terms Important in Assessment and Evaluation*

Although distinct, the terms, *assessment* and *evaluation*, are often used synonymously. Differentiating these terms can be helpful in considering which data are gathered already and which data are needed to make decisions about learners. At the most basic level, assessment involves the specific measurements, tools, and procedures used to systematically gather information about a person's behavior, performance, or achievement of targeted learning outcomes.[43–46] When things are examined about a curriculum or program, this is typically referred to as evaluation. Thus, assessment focuses on individuals and evaluation focuses on programs.[47,48] One model used frequently in evaluating training programs is Kirkpatrick's[49] 4 levels (reaction, learning, behavior change, and impact). An extensive array of program evaluation models and theories is available in the literature and via the American Evaluation Association (http://www.eval.org).[50,51]

### *Formative Versus Summative*

The terms, *formative* and *summative*, reflect distinct purposes for using detailed input regarding evidence of process, performance, or characteristics. Formative purposes include specific observations, evidence, and feedback regarding how learning and performance are *progressing* toward expected levels of achievement and/or outcomes. Formative assessments support descriptive and corrective feedback for facilitating improvement. Summative purposes for assessment, evaluation, and feedback target data-based decision-making (eg, whether a learner has met required criteria to advance to the next education level or whether a program has met required accreditation standards) (**Box 6**).

When using criteria-based assessments and evaluations for summative decisions, it is important to use an appropriate method for setting decision standards. Although such a discussion is beyond the limits of this article, an excellent introduction is available by Yudkowsky and colleagues.[52]

## VALIDITY AND RELIABILITY

Establishing evidence of validity and reliability is a necessary element for achieving quality assessments and appropriate use of results. Validity is the extent to which data are accurate and representative for a particular purpose/decision. Instead of asking the question, Is this a valid instrument? the question should be asked, Are these data/results valid for the intended propose/decision? For example, data gathered using a direct observation checklist may be valid for assessing residents' abilities in a specific simulation-based exercise and providing feedback but not valid for assessing third-year medical students' abilities in the clinical setting during a general surgery clerkship as a component of summative assessment (ie, grade).[53]

Reliability refers to the consistency or dependability of data. Reliability estimates reflect the extent to which assessment would produce the same data if repeated with the same individuals. Assessment data may be reliable (ie, consistent and replicable) but not valid (ie, inaccurate and not representative). Assessment data cannot be valid if they are not reliable. For example, assessing an individual's visual acuity with a standard eye examination may be highly reliable but not valid as an assessment for reading an MRI correctly.

Establishing evidence of validity and reliability is an ongoing process that is never done. Educators must be diligent in examining how assessment methods and measures interact with assessment situations across time, individuals, settings, and purposes to produce data. When selecting established assessment instruments and procedures, it is important to review the primary evidence reported for validity and reliability. Consider and evaluate the extent to which the prior uses of the assessment(s) are similar to intended assessment activities (eg, purpose, learners, content and skills, task demand, setting, and consequences).

Additional research may be necessary to strengthen validity evidence for use of an instrument for a selected purpose, particularly if use of an assessment instrument or procedure differs in important ways (eg, learner or setting characteristics) from its prior application(s). Even when similar, sufficient evidence of validity and reliability of the data is necessary to assure quality, rigor, and appropriate use of assessments. When it is necessary to adapt or develop new instruments, **Table 4** provides a step-by-step overview of the process. The higher the consequences of assessment (eg, for learners, the educational program, and society), the stronger the evidence of validity and reliability should be.[53]

### *Establishing Validity*

Kane[54] explained validity as systematic, multifaceted investigative processes through which data are gathered and evidence provided to define constructs of assessment. Such evidence is also used to argue for or against a particular interpretation of assessment results. Early approaches to establishing validity evidence used various activities to establish the following types of validity: face, content, criterion (predictive and concurrent), and discriminant. Messick[53] argued that all forms of validity represent a collective, unified framework of construct validity. Today, a unified validity framework is more commonly used that consists of 6 aspects of validity: content, substantive, structural, generalizability, external, and consequential (**Table 5**). Sweet and colleagues[55] have reported stakeholder support for use of this framework in surgical technical skills training.

When designing and using assessments involving simulation, each aspect of validity becomes important.[56,57] Elements of the structure and fidelity of simulation formats are as important to effective assessment as they are to teaching/learning processes. Published standards of best practice in assessment provide additional guidance.[43] Downing and Yudkowsky,[58] Hawkins and Holmboe,[59] and Johnson and colleagues[60] are other useful resources for designing and using assessment.

**Table 4**
**Guidelines for developing and using performance-based assessments**

| Stage | Activities |
| --- | --- |
| Predevelopment | Analyze and establish purposes and goals.<br>Design an assessment plan or blueprint:<br>• Fit assessment types to objectives (eg, formats, low vs high inference).<br>• Describe assessment types and implementation/administration procedures.<br>• Identify resources needed up front and to maintain.<br>• Finalize assessment plan with stakeholders. |
| Development | Develop assessment:<br>• Best practices, literature review, expert panel are common sources for gathering validity evidence.<br>• How should assessment questions or instructions be presented to learners/assessees (eg, announced or unannounced assessments)?<br>• Which stimuli are needed to prompt learners?<br>• What will be the learner's response mode?<br>• What are the criteria for judging responses/performances?<br>• Which scale structure is appropriate for assessing performances (eg, rating scale, anchors, or number of levels/scale points)?<br>• What are examples of performances for each level of response?<br>• Refine assessment instrument and administration as indicated.<br>Develop assessment administration directions:<br>• Standardize an assessment situation that can be replicated.<br>• Complete and accurate (pilots and field testing are essential)<br>• Modify and finalize directions based on field test results.<br>• Collect example behaviors.<br>• Use example behaviors to score responses according to criteria.<br>• Develop preliminary scoring guide.<br>• Develop an appeals guide.<br>Pilot assessment and use results to refine instrument.<br>Retest and submit to expert panel for final review.<br>Finalize instrument. |
| Preassessment administration | Identify or select assessors, administration support staff.<br>Train and certify assessors and staff:<br>• Retrain/recalibrate assessors who do not meet assessor certification standards.<br>Pilot assessment administration and use results to refine assessment administration (including assessors).<br>Inform learners of assessment expectations and orient them to the assessment process. |
| Assessment administration | Implement assessment:<br>• Finalize assessment schedule and logistics planning (who, when, where, and so forth).<br>• Use an objective coordinator (not an assessor) to examine implementation processes.<br>• Monitor and recalibrate, as needed, to ensure validity and reliability. |
| Postassessment administration | Implement scoring protocol.<br>Establish and maintain secure storage of confidential assessment data.<br>Establish and maintain a management system of results (eg, database)<br>Summarize and prepare score reports (eg, individual, cohort, and assessor).<br>Use assessment results to inform future programming and teaching/learning methods.<br>Evaluate effectiveness of assessment implementation:<br>• Debrief regarding processes and value of assessment activities.<br>• Examine measurement qualities of assessment (eg, validity and reliability issues).<br>• Revisit and revise assessment components as indicated. |

**Table 5**
**Six aspects of a unified framework of validity as conceptualized**

| Validity | Example Evidence | Example Methods |
|---|---|---|
| Content | • Assessment items, instrumentation, simulation tasks, and scenarios reflect relevant and representative content; technical quality. | • Best practice(s) in targeted domain<br>• Literature review<br>• Content expert review |
| Substantive | • Assessment includes sufficient representation of relevant knowledge, skills, and abilities in the domain(s) of interest.<br>• Simulated scenario includes sufficient prompts/triggers to illicit representative relevant responses, maneuvers, and behaviors. | • Best practice(s) in targeted domain<br>• Use of established standards or algorithms (eg, breast imaging protocol)<br>• Task analysis<br>• Content expert review<br>• Direct observation of real-life practice and/or experts |
| Structural | • Assessment process and scoring criteria fit the cognitive, psychomotor, and effective domains and underlying constructs of the domain(s) of interest. | • Assessment structure representative of real-life abilities<br>• Instrument development and refinement (eg, content, structure, wording, order, response scales, labels, scoring protocols)<br>• Implementation issues (eg, assessor training and calibration, administration procedures, timing, setting, preparation of learners/assessees) |
| Generalizability | • Assessment scores represent targeted abilities across settings, tasks, and groups, not limited to the particular assessment task or context in which it is administered. | • Statistical analysis (eg, factor analysis, generalizability analysis) |
| External | • Relationships between assessment scores and other measures of the targeted domain reflect expected values. | • Criterion-related validity studies (predictive and concurrent)<br>• Discriminant validity studies (eg, assessment discriminates between novice and expert performances) |
| Consequential | • Intended and unintended effects of assessment scores are accurate and appropriate.<br>• Assessment addresses issues of bias, fairness, justice, and aspects of correct and incorrect decisions (ie, false-positive and false-negative decisions).<br>• Assessment is reasonable and provides sufficient sampling, opportunity for assessee to perform. | • Compliance with the Standards for Educational and Psychological Testing (AERA, APA, NCME, 1999)<br>• Standard setting methods (eg, Angoff) (Yudkowsky and colleagues, 2009) |

*From* Kane M. Validation. In: Brennan RL, editor. Educational measurement. 4th edition. New York: American Council on Education and Greenwood; 2006. p. 17–64.

### *Establishing Reliability*

In measurement, *true score* represents a person's actual ability, whereas, *observed score* is the result obtained using the selected assessment tool that includes both true score and error. All assessments contain some degree of measurement error resulting from variation across assessors, assessees, occasions, settings, and/or use of assessment items/measurement. The goal of establishing reliability is to maximize true score and minimize error, so results can be dependable and trusted for making decisions.

The reliability of assessments can be strengthened through good practices for instrument development and sufficient evidence of validity.[43,45,46,60] The reliability of assessments involving simulation is also influenced by the features and replicability of the simulator functioning and the simulation format across repeated implementations.[60,61] Attending carefully to the details of the simulation context (eg, setting, preparation, fidelity of simulators, and simulation format) can enhance the replicability of experiences and assessment strategies. Finally, pilot and field testing is essential to achieving quality assessments.

Producing high-quality instruments and clear, complete assessor guidelines is an important training component. Clear behavior descriptions, performance criteria, and scoring options on observation checklists, rating scales, and scoring rubrics enhance accuracy and consistency within and across assessors. Again, **Table 4** and Johnson and colleagues[60] provide guidance and examples. Gable and Wolf[62] and Colton and Covert[63] are specific resources for instrument development in nontechnical, affective, and social constructs (eg, professional behavior, teamwork, beliefs, and values). Whereas Stufflebeam[64] and Bichelmeyer[65] provide excellent guidance to developing checklists in program evaluation, both of these are also applicable to learner assessment.

The reliability and validity of assessment can also be enhanced during instrument development by determining whether low-inference or high-inference assessment items are appropriate for the target and purpose of assessment. Low-inference items reflect clear descriptions of discrete behaviors or processes (eg, made first incision correctly and without hesitation) or specific outcomes (eg, recognized a specific change in status of a patient simulator) that can be easily and directly observed and assessed. Low-inference items may be more effective in certain situations because there is less opportunity for variation in interpretation. Alternatively, high-inference items reflect global assessments in which the assessor must identify and interpret multiple behaviors to make an overall inference about the extent that an item was observed and achieved.

### *Assessors and Assessments*

The selection and preparation of assessors are critical to the validity and reliability of data, because assessment is only as good as the person doing it. Rigorous training, calibration, and recalibration of assessors contribute directly to minimizing variation within and among assessors. Consider that for each item or rating in an observation-based assessment, assessors execute a minimum of the following steps that at each step has potential for error:

- Observe a behavior/response.
- Interpret the behavior.
- Compare the interpreted behavior to the item (also involves interpreting the item wording).
- Record a rating or assessment decision (eg, numeric rating or dichotomous decision).

Design and format of an assessment tool can also contribute to errors. Ensuring the layout or visual design of instruments is clear and easy to use can prevent errors.

Scoring procedures and clear rules for optimal assessor position and performance in the assessment environment can minimize or alleviate sources of assessor error. Johnson and colleagues[60] provide specific suggestions for achieving effective assessor training for observation-based assessments and for assessing products of performance-based assessments (eg, using scoring rubrics for portfolios, patient write-ups, and written/constructed responses).

*Assessor drift* is a particular threat to validity and reliability. Without appropriate training and routine calibration, assessors are more likely over time to drift or deviate from the intended implementation and interpretation of observed behaviors and criteria. For example, assessor drift can result when an assessor gradually shifts from adhering to assessment criteria to that of personal preference for doing a procedure that alters how behaviors are observed, interpreted, and scored.

Assessors are also subject to *halo* and *pitchfork* (or *dove* and *hawk*) effects. That is, by not adhering closely to the standard assessment protocol and criteria, assessors could tend toward being harder or easier in their assessments or drift in one or the other direction as they complete multiple assessments (eg, due to fatigue or the influence of performances of previous assessees). Personal qualities of an individual being assessed, recent observations or encounters with assessees (positive or negative), or physical features of a product (eg, attractiveness of portfolio layout not related to content) can also cause assessors to be more or less harsh and drift from the established criteria.

## SUMMARY

In summary, increased options in simulators and simulation formats have contributed to enhanced and greater use of simulation in surgery education. The careful selection and alignment of simulation choices with specific learning objectives for targeted learners and a systematic and collaborative approach to instructional design (eg, ADDIE model) can contribute to well-integrated SBT in the overall surgical education curriculum. Additionally, grounding SBT in educational best practices guided by evidence-based principles (eg, active, experiential, and learner-driving engagement in relevant situations and problems) facilitates effective learning progress and transfer from training to real-life practice. Integrating SBT within the larger surgical education program enhances the complementarity between real-life clinical and simulated learning experiences.

Two additional resources are recommended that complement and provide additional details and suggestions to the overviews provided in this article. First, grounded in the key findings of Issenberg and colleagues,[40] Cannon-Bowers and colleauges[4] provide several relevant sets of findings from the empirical evidence in learning and human performance research. Second, a best-evidence guide on simulation in health care by Motola and colleagues[66] provides another excellent resource that expands on the content of this article.

In this article, key principles of assessment best practice are summarized along with important strategies for optimizing the development and use of assessment involving simulation. There are many more important details that were beyond the scope of this article, so interested readers are encouraged to access the suggested references and, when necessary, seek consultation of colleagues having appropriate assessment and measurement expertise. Assessment is serious and tedious work, so engaging individuals with experience can be incredibly helpful.

## REFERENCES

1. Ambrose SA, Bridges MW, DiPietro M, et al. How learning works: seven research-based principles for smart teaching. San Francisco (CA): Jossey-Bass; 2010.

2. Bransford JD, Brown AL, Cocking RR. How people learn: brain, mind, experience, and school. Washington, DC: National Academy Press; 2000.
3. Haskell RE. Transfer of learning: cognition, instruction, and reasoning. San Diego (CA): Academic Press; 2001.
4. Cannon-Bowers JA, Bowers C, Procci K. Optimizing learning in surgical simulations: guidelines from the science of learning and human performance. Surg Clin North Am 2010;90:583–603.
5. Goldstein LL. Training in organizations. 3rd edition. Pacific Grove (CA): Brooks/Cole; 1993.
6. Kraiger K. Creating, implementing, and managing effective training and development: state-of-the-art lessons for practice. San Francisco (CA): Jossey-Bass; 2002.
7. Rothwell WJ, Butler MN, Hunt DL, et al. The handbook of training technologies: an introductory guide to facilitating learning with technology – from planning to evaluation, Instructional Technology and Training Series. San Francisco: John Wiley; 2006.
8. McGaghie WC. Simulation in professional competence assessment: basic considerations. In: Tekian A, McGuire CH, McGaghie WC, editors. Innovative simulations for assessing professional competence. Chicago: Department of Medical Education, University of Illinois at Chicago; 1999. p. 7–22.
9. Miller GA. The magical number seven, plus or minus two: Some limits on our capacity for processing information. Psychol Rev 1956;63:81–97.
10. Mayer RE. Applying the science of learning to medical education. Med Educ 2010;44:543–9.
11. Grunwald T, Corsbie-Massay C. Guidelines for cognitively efficient multimedia learning tools: educational strategies, cognitive load, and interface design. Acad Med 2006;81:213–23.
12. Van Merriënboer JJ, Sweller J. Cognitive load theory in health professions education: design principles and strategies. Med Educ 2010;44:85–93.
13. Custers EJ, Boshuizen HP. The psychology of learning. Ch. 5. In: Norman GR, van der Vleuten CP, Newble DI, editors. International handbook of research in medical education. Dordrecht (The Netherlands): Kluwer Academic Publishers; 2002. p. 163–203.
14. Bloom B, Engelhart MD, Furst EJ, et al. Taxonomy of educational objectives: handbook 1, the cognitive domain. New York: Longman; 1956.
15. Anderson LW, Krathwohl DR. A taxonomy for learning, teaching, and assessing: a revision of bloom's taxonomy of educational objectives. New York: Longman; 2001.
16. Miller GR. The assessment of clinical skills/competence/performance. Acad Med 1990;65:S63–7.
17. Knowles M. Andragogy in action: applying modern principles of adult learning. San Francisco (CA): Jossey-Bass; 1984.
18. Candy PC. Self-direction for lifelong learning: a comprehensive guide to theory and practice. San Francisco (CA): Jossey-Bass; 1991.
19. Kolb DA, Fry R. Toward an applied theory of experiential learning. In: Cooper C, editor. Theories of group processes. London: John Wiley; 1975. p. 33–58.
20. Kolb DA. Experiential learning. Englewood Cliffs (NJ): Prentice Hall; 1984.
21. Houle C. Continuing learning in the professions. San Francisco (CA): Jossey-Bass; 1980.
22. Kaufmann DM, Mann KV, Jennett P. Teaching and learning in medical education: how theory can inform practice. In: Understanding medical education series. London: Association for the Study of Medical Education; 2000.

23. Jonassen D. Designing constructivist learning environments. Ch. 10. In: Reigeluth CM, editor. Instructional-design theories and principles, vol. II. Mahwah (NJ): Lawrence Erlbaum Associates; 1999. p. 215–39.
24. Kaufmann DM. Applying educational theory in practice. Ch. 1. In: Cantillon P, Hutchinson L, Wood D, editors. ABC of learning and teaching in medicine. 2nd edition. London: BMJ Books; 2010. p. 1–4.
25. Vygotsky LS. Mind in society: the development of higher psychological processes. Cambridge (MA); New York: The Harvard University Press; Oxford University Press; 1978. Originally published 1930.
26. Wood DJ, Middleton R. A study of assisted problem-solving. Br J Psychol 1975; 66(2):181–91.
27. Wood DJ. How children think and learn. 2nd edition. Oxford (United Kingdom): Blackwell Publishers; 1998.
28. Bandura A. Social foundations of thought and action: a social cognitive theory. Englewood Cliffs (NJ): Prentice Hall; 1986.
29. Bloom B. Mastery learning. In: Block JH, editor. Mastery learning: theory and practice. New York: Holt, Rinehart & Winston; 1971. p. 47–63.
30. Block JH, Burns RH. Mastery learning. In: Shulman LS, editor. Review of research in education, vol. 4. Itasca (IL): Peacock; 1971. p. 3–49.
31. Hunter MC. Teaching is decision-making. Educ Leader 1979;37(1):62–7.
32. Hunter MC. Mastery teaching. El Segundo (CA): TIP Press; 1982.
33. McGaghie WC, Issenberg SB, Barsuk JH, et al. A critical review of simulation-based mastery learning with translational outcomes. Med Educ 2014;48(4):375–85.
34. Flavell JH. Metacognitive aspects of problem-solving. In: Resnick L, editor. The nature of intelligence. Hillsdale (NJ): Erlbaum; 1976. p. 231–6.
35. Schon DA. The reflective practitioner: how professionals think. New York: Basic Books; 1983.
36. Schon DA. Educating the reflective practitioner: toward a new design for teaching and learning in the professions. San Francisco (CA): Jossey-Bass; 1987.
37. Ericcson KA, Krampe RT, Tesch-Römer C. The role of deliberate practice in the acquisition of expert performance. Psychol Rev 1993;100:363–406.
38. Ericcson KA. Deliberate practice and the acquisition and maintenance of expert performance in medicine and related domains. Acad Med 2004;79:S70–81.
39. Ericcson KA. An expert-performance perspective of research on medical expertise: the study of clinical performance. Med Educ 2007;41:1124–30.
40. Issenberg SB, McGaghie WC, Petrusa ER, et al. BEME Guide no. 4: Features and Uses of High-Fidelity Medical Simulations that Lead to Effective Learning. Dundee (UK): AMEE; 2004.
41. Diamond RM. Designing and improving courses and curricula in higher education. San Francisco (CA): Jossey-Bass; 1989.
42. Rothwell WJ, Kazanas HC. Mastering the instructional design process: a systematic approach. 2nd edition. San Francisco (CA): Jossey-Bass; 1998.
43. American Educational Research Association, American Psychological Association, National Council on Measurement in Education. Standards for educational and psychological testing. Washington, DC: American Educational Research Association; 2014.
44. Freeman R, Lewis R. Planning and implementing assessment. London: Routledge-Falmer; 1998.
45. Downing SM, Yudkowsky R. Introduction to assessment in the health professions. In: Downing SM, Yudkowsky R, editors. Assessment in health professions education. New York: Routledge; 2009. p. 1–20.

46. Hawkins RE, Holmboe ES. Constructing an evaluation system for an educational program. In: Holmboe ES, Hawkins RE, editors. Practical guide to the evaluation of clinical competence. Philadelphia: Mosby; 2008. p. 216–37.
47. Goldie J. AMEE education guide no. 29: evaluating educational programs. Med Teach 2006;28:210–24.
48. Mehrens WA. Measurement and evaluation in education and psychology. 4th edition. New York: Holt, Rinehart & Winston; 1991.
49. Kirkpatrick DL. Evaluating training effectiveness: the four levels. San Francisco (CA): Bennett-Koehler; 1994.
50. Stufflebeam DL, Shinkfield AJ. Evaluation theory, models, and applications. San Francisco (CA): Jossey-Bass; 2007.
51. Worthen BR, Sanders JR, Fitzpatrick JL. Program evaluation: alternative approaches and practical guidelines. 2nd edition. White Plains (NY): Longman; 1997.
52. Yudkowsky R, Downing SM, Tekian A. Standard setting. In: Downing SM, Yudkowsky R, editors. Assessment in health professions education. New York: Routledge; 2009. p. 119–48.
53. Messick S. Validity. In: Linn RL, editor. Educational measurement. 3rd edition. New York: American Council on Education and Macmillan; 1989. p. 13–104.
54. Kane M. Validation. In: Brennan RL, editor. Educational measurement. 4th edition. New York: American Council on Education and Greenwood; 2006. p. 17–64.
55. Sweet RM, Hananel D, Lawrenz F. A unified approach to validation, reliability and educational study design for surgical technical skills training. Arch Surg 2010; 145(2):197–201.
56. Norcini JJ, McKinley DW. Assessment methods in medical education. Teach Teach Educ 2007;23:239–50.
57. Scalese RJ, Issenberg SB. Simulation-based assessment. In: Holmboe ES, Hawkins RE, editors. Practical guide to the evaluation of clinical competence. Philadelphia: Mosby-Elsevier; 2006. p. 179–200.
58. Downing SM, Yudkowsky R, editors. Assessment in health professions education. New York: Routledge; 2009.
59. Holmboe ES, Hawkins RE, editors. Practical guide to the evaluation of clinical competence. Philadelphia: Mosby; 2008.
60. Johnson RL, Penny JA, Gordon B. Assessing performance: designing, scoring, and validating performance tasks. New York: Guildford Press; 2009.
61. McGaghie WC, Issenberg SB. Simulations in assessment. In: Downing SM, Yudkowsky R, editors. Assessment in health professions education. New York: Routledge; 2009. p. 245–68.
62. Gable RK, Wolf MB. Instrument development in the affective domain: measuring attitudes and values in corporate and school settings. 2nd edition. Boston: Kluwer Academic Publishers; 1993.
63. Colton D, Covert RW. Designing and constructing instruments for social research and evaluation. San Francisco (CA): Jossey-Bass; 2007.
64. Stufflebeam DL. Guidelines for developing evaluation checklists: the checklists development checklist (CDC). 2000. Available at: http://www.wmich.edu/evalctr/archive_checklists/guidelines_cdc.pdf. Accessed November 20, 2014.
65. Bichelmeyer B. Checklist for formatting checklists. 2003. Available at: http://www.wmich.edu/evalctr/archive_checklists/cfc.pdf. Accessed November 20, 2014.
66. Motola I, Devine LA, Chung HS, et al. Simulation in healthcare education: a best evidence practical guide. AMEE education guide no. 82. Med Teach 2013;35:e1511–30. Available at: http://informahealthcare.com/doi/pdf/10.3109/0142159X.2013.818632. Accessed November 20, 2014.

# Concepts for Developing Expert Surgical Teams Using Simulation

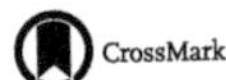

Aimee K. Gardner, PhD*, Daniel J. Scott, MD

**KEYWORDS**

• Team training • Teamwork • Simulation • Surgical teams

**KEY POINTS**

- Surgical education research has shown the value of incorporating simulation into training programs.
- Simulation-based team training programs need to have a firm foundation in the science of team performance and effectiveness.
- Characteristics of expert teams have been identified by researchers in other domains and can be applied to simulation-based training programs for surgical teams.

Historically, simulation-based training among surgical trainees has focused on technical skills,[1] perpetuating a model in which team members practice their tasks separately rather than as an interdependent unit.[2] However, it is not sufficient that team members be solely technical experts; they must also be experts in social interactions that lead to adaptive and coordinated action. Indeed, more than 2 decades of research in numerous domains has demonstrated that it takes more than a set of experts to make an expert team.[3–5] Recently, research in surgical education has pointed to the critical nature of team dynamics, suggesting that adverse events in surgery may often derive from an aspect of team system design.[6–8] These and other reports have prompted educators to explore and develop simulation-based team training strategies that will sculpt trainees into well-rounded and competent surgeons.

This article investigates how simulation-based training can enhance the effectiveness of surgical teams. First, a description of team training in surgical settings is provided. Then, empirical work from a variety of fields is introduced to describe common characteristics of expert teams, with a specific focus on application to training surgical teams within simulated settings. Finally, methods and suggestions for evaluation of simulation-based team training are discussed.

---

The authors have no relevant disclosures.
Department of Surgery, UT Southwestern Medical Center, 5323 Harry Hines Boulevard, Dallas, TX 75390, USA
* Corresponding author.
*E-mail address:* aimee.gardner@utsouthwestern.edu

Surg Clin N Am 95 (2015) 717–728
http://dx.doi.org/10.1016/j.suc.2015.03.001
surgical.theclinics.com
0039-6109/15/$ – see front matter 

## WHAT IS TEAM TRAINING?

Although team training has been recognized and embraced as a critical component for the preparation of effective health care teams,[9,10] ambiguity regarding what is meant by team training still exists. Even terms such as teams, teamwork, and team effectiveness mean different things to different specialties.[1] Not only are there subtle distinctions across different care environments for each of these but variation also exists within specialties. Within surgical settings, for example, trauma resuscitation teams differ from procedure-based surgical teams, which differ from transplant teams. Similarly, the competencies required for effective teamwork and performance vary based on the settings and goals. Thus, a short clarification of the terms is warranted so that a better understanding of team training can be achieved.

Traditionally, teams are defined as identifiable groups of 2 or more individuals working independently toward a shared goal that requires coordination of effort and resources to achieve mutually desired outcomes.[11] An important characteristic of teams is that they consider themselves and are seen by others as distinct social entities working within a larger organization and are, therefore, differentiated from groups.[12] In surgical settings, for example, interprofessional trauma teams would comprise a team, whereas the trauma nurses would be a group.

Teamwork, on the other hand, describes the actual cognitions, behaviors, and attitudes that make interdependent performance possible.[13] For example, teams must appropriately and successfully exhibit essential knowledge (cognitions), skills (behaviors), and feelings (attitudes) in a dynamic environment. These are the processes that are synergistically combined to yield successful team performance.

Finally, team effectiveness refers to the evaluative judgments regarding the results of performance relevant to set criteria. These can be subjective (eg, self-report assessments, observer opinion) or objective (eg, time to intubation, adverse events). The criteria and tools to assess effectiveness must be valid and appropriate for the team level of measurement (see later discussion).

In sum, a team provides the input, teamwork is the process, and team effectiveness is the outcome. Simulation-based training, therefore, is the mechanism by which appropriate teamwork processes can be identified and instigated, and by which team effectiveness can be measured and improved. Fortunately for surgical educators, empirical work has shown commonalities in how expert teams think, feel, and act (ie, the process), even when working on seemingly dissimilar tasks within diverse contexts. See later discussion for a summary of these commonalities within the context of surgical teams, followed by the development of an overarching model capturing the key components and mechanisms that can inform simulation-based training endeavors for surgical trainees. Simulation designers can capitalize on these findings to better understand how to create surgical team training scenarios, what processes to assess and when, and what outcomes to measure.

## TEAM-BASED THEORIES AND PRINCIPLES AND/OR CHARACTERISTICS OF EXPERT TEAMS

Research on team effectiveness from domains outside of surgery can inform the understanding and ability to purposefully design simulation-based team training programs. Expert teams have distinct patterns in how they think, act, and feel. See later discussion for an overview of each of these characteristics of expert teams and recommendations for the design and evaluation of simulation-based training programs in surgical settings.

## How Expert Teams Think

### Team mental models

Team mental models (TMMs) represent team members' shared, organized understanding and mental representation of knowledge about key elements of the team's relevant environment.[14] TMMs represent the extent to which team members are "on the same page." These shared knowledge structures are beneficial for teams because teams are able to execute behaviors that would be difficult or impossible to perform without shared knowledge. A common illustration of this concept is the "no-look pass" in basketball in which a player passes the ball to a teammate without looking at the recipient, which would signal the defense where the pass is going. Both team members need to share expectations for the pass to be successful. They must agree that such a maneuver is possible, that it will be beneficial for the team, and have shared knowledge of where each of them is on the court. Similarly, teams in surgical settings need to have a shared understanding of goals of the procedure, believe that it can be performed successfully, be able to anticipate each other's needs, and engage in purposeful and coordinated action without superfluous communication.

Research in other domains has demonstrated that greater sharing of mental models among teams leads to better team performance[15,16]; however, there is a paucity of empirical work on this construct in the surgical simulation literature. Engaging in team-based training in a simulated environment likely catalyzes the process by which surgical teams are able to develop these shared knowledge structures because they learn to develop shared goals, anticipate each other's needs, coordinate efficient action, and improve their perceptions of group effectiveness. Purposeful design and evaluation of team-based scenarios to elicit these processes are needed. Additionally, TMMs may be used as a diagnostic measure to delineate expert from novice teams in surgical settings. For example, patterns of expert TMMs can be used as a baseline from which to compare novice teams, with the ultimate goal of training novice teams until they hold TMMs similar to those of experts. Being able to document team-based understanding and behaviors in a standardized setting might be a fruitful avenue in moving toward competency-based assessment in surgery.

### Transactive memory

Transactive memory is a similar team-level concept that describes the differentiated set of knowledge structures distributed across team members, coupled with the understanding of who possesses particular sets of knowledge.[17–19] Team transactive memory represents team members' understanding of who has which expertise so that members can focus resources on their own respective tasks and engage in more efficient coordination and communication (ie, they know who knows what and use that knowledge to decide who will do what). In the operating room (OR), this collective team awareness is crucial. Surgeons, nurses, and anesthesiologists need to agree on who holds what expertise, trust that one another will perform the assigned task efficiently, and tacitly coordinate their individual efforts in a way that these practices will enhance team effectiveness. Unfortunately, team cognition about members' roles and expertise can vary greatly among teams because each individual enters the scene with different knowledge, experience, skill set, and ability level. However, placing surgical teams in simulated scenarios can speed up the emergence of this process because these cognitions are believed to become more accurate with multiple performance episodes among teams.[18] Preliminary work within trauma teams supports these suggestions. One study found that interprofessional groups had significant increases in team transactive memory before and after participating in 4 simulated trauma scenarios. Additionally, improvements in transactive memory were positively related to observer-rated performance using a trauma performance checklist consisting of 22 graded and 6 timed items.[20] These findings support the use of simulation within surgical team settings to enhance transactive memory structures among teams.

Finally, expert teams differ from novice teams in situation awareness (SA).[21] SA refers to the team's perception of environmental elements, comprehension of their significance, and ability to project future activities.[22] In surgical settings in which large amounts of information exist in a complex and dynamic environment, developing and maintaining SA can be an extremely difficult task. As noted in several domains, novice teams have substantial problems in building SA.[21,23,24] Compared with expert teams, novices are unable to take in key information, manage distractions and high workload, monitor effectively, and project future events.[23] Simulation-based training researchers have investigated this process in military,[25,26] aviation,[23] anesthesiology,[27] and trauma[24] domains.

Although these studies have shown differences between expert and novice teams, it remains unclear how best to design simulation scenarios to enhance SA in traditional surgical team settings. It has been noted that SA can build up and change with time as trainees gain more exposure to situations and their outcomes,[28] warranting the integration of simulation-based training. Thus, development of curricula and scenarios in which surgical teams are trained to discriminate between relevant and irrelevant information, manage distractions, work under high stress, monitor progress, and anticipate future events would be valuable. Changes in SA among team members could be assessed during simulations with temporary freezes using the SA global assessment technique[29] and these metrics could be investigated periodically and related to other performance outcomes. Ultimately, SA could be assessed with eye-tracking equipment and give insight into expert and novice team differences in visual attention to future-oriented information (eg, vitals, patient anatomy), proactive allocation of resources, and vulnerability to distracting stimuli. Team SA could be measured by the amount of congruence of visual attention across members (ie, team members dedicating resources to the same environmental features for the same amount of time). To optimize the ability of simulation-based training to assess, predict, train, and improve surgical teams, it is imperative to understand and measure team cognitive constructs.

## *How Expert Teams Feel*

Attitudes refer to those internal states that affect individual choices and/or decisions to act in a certain way.[30] Among teams, these are the mental states that are associated with the team. Mutual trust and collective efficacy are the original team attitude competencies that have received extensive empirical support for contributing to team effectiveness and performance. A summary of each, within the context of surgical-team training settings, follows.

### *Mutual trust*

Mutual trust describes the "shared perception that individuals in the team will perform particular actions important to its members and will recognize and protect the rights and interests of all the team members engaged in their joint endeavor."[31] Trust is essential to team-based behaviors such as communication and backup behavior. Without mutual trust, team resources (eg, attention, communication) may be superfluously consumed by checking up on team members to ensure they are adequately performing. Additionally, this attitude plays a fundamental role in coordination because team members need to believe that they are safe to focus on their own assigned tasks, and that they are safe to ask for and provide assistance when needed. Previous studies have demonstrated that trust in interdependent working relationships develops with time, based on ongoing interaction and the experience of working together.[32,33] This process likely occurs because the interactions and experiences allow team members to learn and assess one another. Simulation, then, can serve as a proxy for this process because simulation training allows team members to establish these judgments. Thus, team training scenarios should be designed to allow each member of the surgical team to have the opportunity to demonstrate their competence and expertise so that other team members are able to develop appropriate perceptions of trust. Monitoring the development and maintenance of trust among surgical teams is also warranted because breaches or decays in trust may foreshadow declining performance.

#### *Collective efficacy*

Collective efficacy is the shared belief among team members that they are capable of successfully meeting their task demands. It reflects a sense of confidence among team members. Teams with high collective efficacy are believed to choose more challenging goals, expend greater effort, and persist longer in the face of adversity than teams with lower collective efficacy.[34] Collective efficacy certainly emerges through repeated successes with a stable team. That is, observing fellow teammates perform behaviors that are perceived as helpful with respect to team performance should instill a sense of confidence about the team's capability. Thus, placing surgical teams in simulated scenarios in which they have the opportunity to master tasks and experience success in overcoming obstacles will allow this shared perception to emerge. Verbal self-guidance (VSG) training is a specific technique that has been shown to increase efficacy at the team level and subsequently enhance team performance.[35,36] VSG training for surgical teams would consist of teams watching another team successfully perform the task, then performing the task themselves with each team member thinking aloud during tasks and/or decisions and overtly repeating the instructions needed to complete the task, and finally performing the task as they would in a real setting. This intervention is effective because it enhances team member perceptions of one another, enhances development of team shared mental models, and contributes to overall team self-regulation.[36] Additional ways to create training situations that will elicit collective efficacy have also been identified, such as implementing shared team goals and providing feedback at the group level.[37] These attitudes contribute to the process of team performance. As such, they are necessary, but not sufficient, conditions for team effectiveness. These constitute some of the processes by which individual and team competencies are interwoven to produce expert team performance.

### *How Expert Teams Act*

Extensive lists of generalizable teamwork behaviors (or skills) have been created that include task organization, mutual performance monitoring, flexibility, compensatory behavior, and information exchange, among others.[13,30] In fact, across numerous domains, much more team-based theoretic and empirical work has been devoted to behaviors compared with attitudes and cognitions.[30] This trend is likely due to the simple reason that team behaviors are more easily measured. To avoid an exhaustive discussion on all of these behaviors, a brief snapshot of behaviors that are particularly relevant for simulation-based training is provided.

#### *Team leadership*

Team leadership is essential for team effectiveness. Leaders influence team effectiveness by facilitating team actions and making sure that teams have all of the required resources for optimal performance. In this way, leaders help members achieve a synergy in which collective effort far outweighs the sum of individual abilities or efforts. Team leaders accomplish this synergy by planning team duties, coordinating team actions, delegating roles, resolving conflicts, providing coaching and feedback, and ensuring that monitoring and information sharing takes place.[38] Within the context of interprofessional surgical teams, this role arguably most frequently belongs to the surgeon. Thus, identifying ways in which simulation can be used to identify and enhance the leadership skills of surgeons is essential.

Using simulations and behavioral assessment techniques for the selection and development of potential leaders is a common strategy in the business world.[39] Additionally, the military has been using simulation for these purposes for decades and many of their techniques can be adopted for surgery. For example, military organizations place officer candidates in turbulent environments and assess the decision effectiveness of potential leaders with different personality traits and decision styles under varying degrees of information, uncertainty, and complexity.[40] Their ability to communicate and direct team processes is evaluated and can be used as a selection and/or diagnostic tool. Similarly, surgical trainees can be placed in several scenarios that are strategically designed to trigger the desired leadership behaviors. Based on their performance, a more focused simulation-based training program can be developed and/or instituted to address any gaps. Thus, surgeons can be assessed and their leadership and crisis management capabilities can be developed in a simulation rather than discovering competency deficits in the clinical environment. Proactively using simulation for team leadership will also help avoid the Darwinian approach to leadership, which is that the fittest will somehow emerge as leaders.

### *Coordination*

Coordination refers to a team's ability to integrate their collective set of interdependent tasks. Coordination is believed to enhance team effectiveness because it creates accountability, predictability, and a common understanding among team members.[41] Teams that have efficient coordination behaviors sequence their tasks so that downtime is minimized (ie, team members do not have to wait for someone else's input to do their task), pass information to one another in a timely and efficient manner, and synchronize actions without overt and/or unnecessary communication. In health care settings, timeouts, checklists, mnemonics, and protocols are frequently implemented to help facilitate these processes. However, in situations in which standard procedures are insufficient to coordinate the work of saving patients, teams must rely on their own abilities to organize patient care activities.

Simulation-based training can help surgical teams improve coordination competencies because it provides a venue for interdependent teams to come together and interact. As noted by Okhuysen and Bechky,[41] 5 mechanisms need to be in place to develop coordination among teams: proximity, roles, routines, objects and representations, and plans and rules. Thus, for simulation-based training to successfully enhance coordination among teams, the design of training must bring together the relevant team members (proximity); allow for the identification of the roles and tasks expected of each team member (roles); permit patterns of behavior to be repeated (routines); provide teams with appropriate technologies or objects that can provide the necessary instrumental or symbolic patient information to teams (objects and representations); and provide teams with the ability to make plans, define responsibilities, and allocate resources (plans and rules). Training designers need to ensure that these criteria are met to achieve optimal results from team-training programs.

***Communication***

Communication is likely the one team behavior that has received the most attention among simulation-training programs in surgery. This trend is not unwarranted. Forty-three percent of surgical failures have been attributed to communication failures.[11] Further research of teamwork in the operating theater has shown that communications were often too late, incomplete, or not received by those concerned and were left unresolved.[12] This work has prompted several strategies to foster the development and refinement of communication strategies among surgical teams. For example, researchers have found that design of enhanced displays[42] and preoperative checklists and team briefings[43] can enhance communication within the OR. Indeed, communication has been identified as an essential area in need of improvement for surgeons.[44] Simulation serves as a fruitful modality for training this crucial team competency because it places team members in contexts that require adequate communication, can highlight the outcomes of inadequate communication, and can be easily recorded for analysis and assessment.

## HOW TO MEASURE TEAM EFFECTIVENESS

Measuring team performance is an essential step to developing simulation-based training programs. A well-designed assessment process helps validate curricula, highlights systematic differences between ineffective and effective teams, provides valuable diagnostic data at the individual and team level, and can serve as a needs assessment for future training endeavors. Simulation-based team training without team performance measurement results in unguided practice for teams, which limits the effectiveness of the team and the resources spent on training.[45]

The complexity of surgical teams makes meaningful measurement difficult. A traditional assumption within training settings is that improving team-member performance will improve team performance. With that mindset, many training designers choose to train surgeons individually within simulated settings with confederate actors serving as nurses, anesthesiologists, and other personnel. The expectation is that this setting allows generic teamwork processes and attitudes to emerge, which can then be generalized to team members in actual patient care settings. However, when measuring team effectiveness among surgical teams, focusing on individual contributions without an acknowledgment of the collective product might be short-sighted. For example, how each team member completes his or her work within the team may be largely affected by the speed, accuracy, and motivation of other team members. Although team outcomes are easily decomposed into individual contributions, there still exists a group level effect that should be considered in assessments of performance in the simulation setting. Likewise, only measuring the team as a whole assumes that each member contributed equally to collective performance, which negates individual contributions. Thus, in many situations, skills and behaviors must be measured at multiple levels to adequately understand and improve team performance. Future research should investigate the utility of each training and assessment approach on team outcomes in actual clinical settings.

Unfortunately, there is no one-size-fits-all solution to team performance measurement and evaluation. The idiosyncrasies of surgical teams most often require that the collection and analysis of data be unique to the context of the simulation-training program. However, best practices in team performance measurement for simulation-based training for health care have been identified, as shown in **Box 1**.[45] These recommendations provide scientifically-grounded guidance for developing team performance measures that can be applied to several training needs.

**Box 1**

**Summary of best practices in team performance measurement for simulation-based training in health care**

Ground measures in theory

- Use theory to answer questions about what to measure
- Capture aspects of Input → Process → Output models of team performance

Design measures to meet specific learning outcomes

- Clearly articulate the purpose (ie, specific learning outcomes) of measurement at the beginning of the development process
- Design the measurement system to capture information necessary for making decisions about the learning outcomes (eg, have they been met?)

Capture competencies

- Explicitly link performance measures to the individual and team competencies targeted for training

Measure multiple levels of performance

- Performance measures must be sensitive to the differences in individual and team performance

Link measures to scenario events

- Link performance measures to opportunities to perform (ie, events) in the simulation
- Event-based measurement affords greater structure and standardization for observers

Focus on observable behaviors

- Focusing on behaviors decreases the "drift" of observer's periodic ratings (observers are less likely to develop idiosyncratic scoring)
- Measuring observable behavior provides a fine level of granularity that is necessary for providing corrective feedback

Incorporate multiple measures from different sources

- Different measurement sources provide unique information
- Generate a plan for rapidly integrating multiple sources of measurement

Capture performance processes in addition to outcomes

- Team performance measurement should provide information not only about the end result of performance but about how the team reached that performance outcome
- Team performance measurement should provide information on how to correct team processes

Create diagnostic power

- Team performance measurement should provide information about the causes of effective and ineffective performance

Train observers and structure observation protocols

- Establish and implement a program of training and evaluation to ensure observers are accurately and reliably rating performance
- Provide structured protocols to ease the information burden of observation

Facilitate debriefs and training remediation after training

- Team performance measurement should be quickly translate into feedback and decisions about required future training.

*From* Rosen MA, Salas E, Wilson KA, et al. Measuring team performance in simulation-based training: adopting best practices for healthcare. Sim Healthcare 2008;3:33–41; with permission.

## EXISTING WORK IN THESE AREAS

Although many opportunities still exist to further explore simulation-based training within the context of surgical teams, a few groups have published studies that embody some of the concepts previously covered. For example, numerous projects have demonstrated the value of simulation-based team training on communication skills of participants, whether those trainees be intact interprofessional OR teams,[10,46–48] endoscopic teams,[49] surgeons working with one another among confederate nurses and anesthesiologists,[50] or undergraduate students working together.[51,52] In fact, a study from Forse and colleagues[53] documented excellent retention of communication skills 9 months following interprofessional simulation-based team training for all OR staff. Thus, the value of using simulation for training communication skills among teams has been demonstrated.

Simulation-based team training to enrich other highlighted teamwork processes has been explored to a lesser extent within the surgical education literature. Preliminary work, however, has shown that simulation can enhance cognitive processes among teams, such as shared mental models,[47,51] situational awareness,[52] and transactive memory.[20] Simulation has also been shown to increase coordination behaviors[48] and efficacy among teams.[54] Additional studies in these and other areas are needed to validate these concepts within surgical education.

## SUMMARY

Work within surgical education and research has shown the value of incorporating team training into simulation programs. Importantly, simulation-based team training within surgery needs to have a firm foundation in the science of team performance and effectiveness. Simulation programs need to be developed in a systematic fashion that allow educators to elucidate and investigate processes that contribute to surgical team effectiveness.

## REFERENCES


1. Weaver SJ, Feitosa J, Salas E, et al. The theoretical drivers and models of team performance and effectiveness for patient safety. In: Salas E, Frush K, editors. Improving patient safety through teamwork and team training. New York: Oxford University Press; 2013.
2. Bleakley A, Boyden J, Hobbs A, et al. Improving teamwork climate in operating theatres: the shift from multiprofessionalism to interprofessionalism. J Interprof Care 2006;20(5):461–70.
3. Hackman JR. Groups that work (and those that don't). San Francisco (CA): Jossey-Bass; 1990.
4. Cannon-Bowers JA, Salas E, editors. Making decisions under stress: implications for individual and team training. Washington, DC: APA; 1998.
5. Salas E, Stagl KC, Burke CS. 25 year of team effectiveness in organizations: research themes and emerging needs. In: Cooper CL, Robertson IT, editors. International review of industrial and organizational psychology. New York: Wiley; 2004.
6. Kohn LT, Corrigan JM, Donaldson MS. To err is human: building a safer health system. Washington, DC: National Academy Press; 1999.
7. Brennan TA, Leape LL, Laird NM, et al. Incidence of adverse events and negligence in hospitalized patients. Results of the Harvard Medical Practice Study I. N Engl J Med 1991;324:370–6.

8. Vincent C, Taylor-Adams S, Stanhope N. Framework for analyzing risk and safety in clinical medicine. BMJ 1998;316:1154–7.
9. Greiner AC, Knebel E, Institute of Medicine, editors. Health professions education: a bridge to quality. Washington, DC: National Academies Press; 2003.
10. Paige JT, Kozmenko V, Yang T, et al. High-fidelity, simulation-based, interdisciplinary operating room team training at the point of care. Surg 2009;145:138–46.
11. Salas E, Dickinson TL, Converse SA, et al. Toward an understanding of team performance and training. In: Swezy RW, Salas E, editors. Teams: their training and performance. Norwood (NJ): Ablex; 1992.
12. Cohen SG, Bailey DR. What makes teams work: group effectiveness research from the shop floor to the executive suite. J Manag 1997;23:238–90.
13. Salas E, Rosen MA, Burke CS, et al. The wisdom of collectives in organizations: an update of the teamwork competencies. In: Salas E, Goodwin GF, Burke CS, editors. Team effectiveness in complex organizations. New York: Taylor & Francis; 2009.
14. Klimoski R, Mohammed S. Team mental model: construct or metaphor? J Manage 1994;20:403–37.
15. Marks MA, Sabella MJ, Burke CS, et al. The impact of cross-training on team effectiveness. J Appl Psychol 2002;87:3–13.
16. Smith-Jentsch KA, Mathieu JE, Kraiger K. Investigating linear and interactive effects of shared mental models on safety and efficiency in a field setting. J Appl Psychol 2005;90:523–35.
17. Wegner DM. Transactive memory: a contemporary analysis of the group mind. In: Mullen B, Goethals GR, editors. Theories of group behavior. New York: Springer-Verlag; 1986.
18. Liang DW, Moreland R, Argote L. Group versus individual training and group performance. The mediating factor of transactive memory. Pers Soc Psychol Bull 1995;85:331–48.
19. Moreland RL, Argote L, Krishnan R. Socially shared cognition at work: transactive memory and group performance. In: Nye JL, Brower AM, editors. What's social about social cognition? Research on socially shared cognition in small groups. Thousand Oaks (CA): Sage; 1996.
20. Gardner AK, Ahmed RA. Transforming trauma teams through transactive memory: can simulation enhance performance? Simulat Gaming 2014;4:356–70.
21. Endsley MR. Expertise and situation awareness. In: Ericsson KA, Charness P, Feltovich P, et al, editors. The Cambridge handbook of expertise and expert performance. New York: Cambridge University Press; 2006.
22. Endsley MR. Toward a theory of situation awareness in dynamic systems. Hum Fact 1995;37:32–64.
23. Endsley MR, Garland DJ, Shook RW, et al. Situation awareness problems in general aviation. Marietta (GA): SA Technologies; 2000.
24. Hogan MP, Pace DE, Hapgood J, et al. Use of human patient simulation and the situation awareness global assessment technique in practical trauma skills assessment. J Trauma 2006;61:1047–52.
25. Patrick J, James N, Ahmed A, et al. Observational assessment of situation awareness, team differences and training implications. Ergonomics 2006;15: 393–417.
26. Saner LD, Bolstad CA, Gonzalez C, et al. Measuring and predicting shared situation awareness in teams. J Cogn Eng Decis Mak 2009;3:280–308.
27. Zhang Y, Drews FA, Westenskow DR, et al. Effects of integrated graphical displays on situation awareness in anaesthesiology. Cogn Tech Work 2002;4:82–90.

28. Mohammed S, Hamilton K, Lim A. The incorporation of time in team research: past, current, and future. In: Salas E, Goodwin GF, Burke CS, editors. Team effectiveness in complex organizations: cross-disciplinary perspective and approaches. New York: Taylor & Francis/Routledge; 2009.
29. Endsley MR. SAGAT: a methodology for the measurement of situation awareness. Hawthorne (CA): Northrop Corporation; 1987.
30. Cannon-Bowers JA, Tannenbaum SI, Salas E, et al. Defining competencies and establishing team training requirements. In: Guzzo R, Salas E, editors. Team effectiveness and decision-making in organizations. San Francisco (CA): Jossey-Bass; 1995. p. 333–80.
31. Webber SS. Leadership and trust facilitating cross-functional team success. J Manag Dev 2002;21:201–14.
32. Rotter JB. Interpersonal trust, trustworthiness, and gullibility. Am Psychol 1980; 35:1–7.
33. Rempel JK, Holmes JG, Zanna MP. Trust in close relationships. J Pers Soc Psychol 1985;49:95–112.
34. Bandura A. Social foundations of thought and action. Englewood Cliffs (NJ): Prentice Hall; 1986.
35. Meichenbaum DH. Cognitive behavior modification: an integrative approach. New York: Plenum Press; 1977.
36. Brown TC. The effect of verbal self-guidance training on collective efficacy and team performance. Person Psychol 2003;56:935–64.
37. Tasa K, Taggar S, Seijts GH. The development of collective efficacy in teams: a multilevel and longitudinal perspective. J Appl Psyc 2007;92:17–27.
38. Alonso A, Dunleavy DM. Building teamwork skills in healthcare: the case for communication and coordination competencies. In: Salas E, Frush K, editors. Improving patient safety through teamwork and team training. New York: Oxford University Press; 2013.
39. Salas E, Wildman JL, Piccolo RF. Using simulation-based training to enhance management education. Acad Manag Learn Educ 2009;8:559–73.
40. Hunsaker PL. Using social simulations to assess and train potential leaders to make effective decisions in turbulent environments. Career Dev Int 2007;12:341–60.
41. Okhuysen GA, Bechky BA. Coordination in organizations: an integrative perspective. Acad Manag Ann 2009;3:463–502.
42. Parush A, Kramer C, Foster-Hunt T, et al. Communication and team situation awareness in the OR: implications for augmentative information display. J Biomed Inform 2011;44:477–85.
43. Lingard L, Regehr G, Orser B, et al. Evaluation of a preoperative checklist and team briefing among surgeons, nurses, and anesthesiologists to reduce failures in communication. Arch Surg 2008;143:12–7.
44. Kim S, Dunkin BJ, Paige JT, et al. What is the future of training in surgery? Needs assessment of national stakeholders. Surg 2014;156:707–17.
45. Rosen MA, Salas E, Wilson KA, et al. Measuring team performance in simulation-based training: adopting best practices for healthcare. Sim Healthcare 2008;3: 33–41.
46. Awad SS, Fagan SP, Bellows C, et al. Bridging the communication gap in the operating room with medical team training. Am J Surg 2005;190:770–4.
47. Paige JT, Aaron DL, Yang T, et al. Improved operating room teamwork via SAFETY prep: a rural community hospital's experience. World J Surg 2009;33:1181–7.
48. Paige JT, Kozmenko V, Morgan B, et al. From the flight deck to the operating room: an initial pilot study of the feasibility and potential impact of true

interdisciplinary team training using high-fidelity simulation. J Surg Educ 2007;64:369–77.

49. Zheng B, Denk PM, Martinec DV, et al. Building an efficient surgical team using a bench model simulation: construct validity of the Legacy Inanimate System for Endoscopic Team Training (LISETT). Surg Endosc 2008;22:930–7.
50. Powers KA, Rehrig ST, Irias N, et al. Simulated laparoscopic operating room crisis: an approach to enhance surgical team performance. Surg Endosc 2008;22:885–900.
51. Garbee DD, Paige JT, Barrier K, et al. Interprofessional teamwork among students in simulated codes: a quasi-experimental study. Nurs Educ Perspect 2013;34:339–44.
52. Garbee DD, Paige JT, Bonanno LS, et al. Effectiveness of teamwork and communication education using an interprofessional high-fidelity human patient simulation critical care code. J Nurs Educ Pract 2013;3:1–12.
53. Forse RA, Bramble JD, McQuillan R. Team training can improve operating room performance. Surgery 2011;150:771–8.
54. Paige JT, Kozmenko V, Yang T, et al. Attitudinal changes resulting from repetitive training of operating room personnel using high-fidelity simulation at the point of care. Am Surg 2009;75:584–91.

# Simulation and Faculty Development

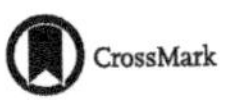

David A. Rogers, MD, MHPE[a,*], Dawn Taylor Peterson, PhD[b], Brent A. Ponce, MD[c], Marjorie Lee White, MD, MPPM, MA[d], John R. Porterfield Jr, MD, MSPH[e]

**KEYWORDS**

• Faculty • Teaching • Learning • Leading • Innovation

**KEY POINTS**

- Practicing surgeons will be increasingly exposed to simulation as learners in their own professional development; they have unique features as learners that have rarely been investigated.
- A faculty development program designed to prepare surgeons to teach using simulation should emphasize the unique role that debriefing plays in this instructional method.
- A team is required for a surgical simulation program to reach its full potential; the surgical faculty member who leads this team must have a full range of leadership competencies.
- Technological innovation allows for the development of a patient-specific simulation; this creates possibility of a role for simulation in the development of new surgical procedures.
- Practicing new procedures with simulation allows the possibility of mitigating the performance curve associated with the adoption of a new surgical procedure so that innovation can occur while patient care, quality, and safety are maintained.

## INTRODUCTION

A traditional interpretation of faculty development might suggest that this topic only interests full-time academic surgeons. However, faculty development has been recently defined as "...all activities health professionals pursue to improve their knowledge,

[a] Division of Pediatric Surgery, Department of Surgery, University of Alabama School of Medicine, FOT 1207, 1720 2nd Avenue South, Birmingham, AL 35294, USA; [b] Department of Pediatrics, Office of Interprofessional Simulation, University of Alabama School of Medicine, 1600 7th Avenue South, CPP1, Suite 102, Birmingham, AL 35233, USA; [c] Division of Orthopaedic Surgery, Department of Surgery, University of Alabama School of Medicine, 1313 13th Street South, Suite 203, Birmingham, AL 35205, USA; [d] Division of Emergency Medicine, Department of Pediatrics, University of Alabama School of Medicine, 1600 7th Avenue South CPPI 110, Birmingham, AL 35233, USA; [e] Division of Gastrointestinal Surgery, Department of Surgery, University of Alabama School of Medicine, KB 428, 1720 2nd Avenue South, Birmingham, AL 35294, USA

* Corresponding author.

*E-mail address:* darogers@uab.edu

Surg Clin N Am 95 (2015) 729–737

http://dx.doi.org/10.1016/j.suc.2015.03.004 surgical.theclinics.com skills, and behaviors as teachers and educators, leaders and managers, and researchers and scholars…"[1] Therefore, faculty development is a topic relevant to all surgeons, if only for their own professional development. There has been a tremendous surge of interest in simulation in surgical and medical education with an emphasis on new possibilities created by technological innovations; the focus has often been on the simulator. A more inclusive definition of simulation is that it is the "…the technique of imitating the behavior of some situation or process by means of a suitably analogous situation or apparatus, especially for the purpose of study or personnel training."[2] Therefore, simulation is an instructional method that encompasses much more than the technology of the simulator. One simple yet elegant example of using simulation for faculty development involves training actors to behave as medical students so that faculty can learn microteaching, a type of clinical instruction.[3]

The richness of the possible interaction between surgical faculty and simulation can be illustrated by examining the dynamics of a fictional scenario. An experienced surgeon serves as the Chief of Surgery at her hospital and has a vision of improving patient outcomes by enhancing teamwork in the operating room. She takes an interprofessional team to a course that is designed to equip participants to develop their own programs designed to improve teamwork. The course involves the use of simulation and the curriculum includes information about how to most effectively use simulation in the local educational program. This faculty member is simultaneously functioning as a leader and a learner and aspires to be a teacher and local educational innovator. The utility of simulation for each of these roles will be examined but this case serves as a reminder that these individual roles exist in some combination in faculty members who are interacting with simulation for the purpose of developing themselves or others.

## FACULTY AS LEARNERS

Given the continuous innovation that has occurred in surgery, a surgical faculty member must constantly seek new knowledge and skills to maintain competency.[4] Most personal professional development occurs during formal courses. Simulation has become a common feature of these types of courses. The surgical faculty learner can expect to encounter some variant of this instructional method in this setting.[5] It is difficult to imagine that a surgeon learner would be satisfied with a technical skills professional development course that did not involve a practical or simulated element. This expectation is supported by a substantial quantity of literature showing that simulation is effective for the purpose of teaching procedure skills and that there is transfer of skills to the analogous operative setting.[6–10] Regulators have recognized the value of simulation in teaching technical skills and have recently required training, with the demonstration of proficiency, in a simulated environment before the practitioner is credentialed to perform the actual procedure.[11] Simulation training is also being explored for robotic surgery with the goal of increasing proficiency and reducing the occurrence of adverse events.[12]

A type of learning uniquely relevant to a surgical faculty member is performing a procedure in a simulated environment immediately before the performance of the actual procedure. This is akin to a musician rehearsing a piece immediately before a performance.[13,14] The technique of simulating an event immediately before the actual performance has been used for entire teams with the results that unanticipated problems were identified and individual team member responsibilities were clarified.[15]

In addition to technical skills training, faculty members will increasingly be learners in simulated environments while seeking new team leadership or nontechnical skills.

These skills are critically important for optimizing team work in the operating room.[16–19] A case for financial support for this kind of training can be made from the growing appreciation that improved proficiency improves patient safety with an associated reduction in malpractice premiums.[20,21] Simulation-based training programs are also being developed for surgical teams that predominately work outside of the operating room.[22]

## FACULTY AS TEACHERS

Although faculty members are increasingly open to this possibility, they may bring a set of expectations of the use of simulation based on traditional instructional methods that do not exploit the experiential learning possibilities associated with simulation.[23] Therefore, it is useful to review the unique features of simulation contrasted with other forms of instruction commonly used in medical education.[24] A related part of this teacher development activity is to educate the surgical teacher about the most appropriate use of simulation. A recent examination of this issue suggests that simulation is particularly effective when used for the instruction of procedural skills, patient communication, and decision-making.[25]

A useful instructional development framework for enhancing the use of simulation by faculty teachers is one of planning, piloting, and debriefing.

Planning involves the careful consideration of the logistics of the simulation and assuring that the educational objectives are properly related to the learning outcome. The clinical experience level of the learner should be considered[26] with the goal of creating a simulation that is challenging enough for learners to be engaged yet not so difficult as to be overwhelming.[27] Even with proper planning, surgical teachers need to be prepared that the learner's performance may suggest new educational objectives during the course of the simulation and should be prepared to recognize and address these needs.[26]

Piloting involves conducting the proposed simulation session using learners similar to the target learners. This approach allows faculty to explore any pitfalls or unintended consequences before introducing the actual learners to the simulation. It also gives teaching faculty the chance to become familiar with the specific type of equipment used in the actual simulation. The pilot session should be thought of as a rehearsal session that allows faculty to make final adjustments to the simulation before the target learners become involved.[27]

Debriefing involves a systematic review of the simulated performance and is a key feature of simulation as an instructional method.[28–30] Quality debriefing begins with a prebriefing designed to prepare participants for the simulation. Learners often feel vulnerable and scrutinized during simulation experiences. The more information learners are given about the expectations and logistical details of the scenario, the more comfortable they will feel participating in the experience. Faculty should strive to establish a safe learning environment in which learners feel comfortable making mistakes and discussing their decision-making practices during the debriefing. Part of establishing a safe learning environment is informing learners that a debriefing or learning conversation will occur following the simulation that will allow an exploration of the rationale that learners used to make decisions and take specific actions. Learners should be prebriefed before every simulation regardless of whether the focus is on procedural skills or teamwork and communication. A thorough prebriefing will lay the foundation for an effective simulation to occur and for learners to feel comfortable participating in the experience.[31]

The amount of time available for the debriefing session will help determine the debriefing model that faculty use for each specific simulation session. One effective model of debriefing is the plus-delta model of debriefing in which learners are encouraged to discuss what went well during the simulation (ie, plus) and what they believe needs to be changed (ie, delta). Reviewing the positive features of performance helps to create an open and receptive learning climate. Additionally, the preferred stance for the faculty teacher is to facilitate active reflection of the learner group.[26] After hearing learners' reactions, most of the discussion should focus on understanding the actions that were taken during the simulation and providing reinforcing feedback for correct actions, as well as corrective feedback and remedial plans for errors. At this point, general concepts can be discussed and applied to actual clinical care situations.

Another aspect of preparing surgical faculty members to teach using simulation is to understand fundamentals of performance assessment. Validity is the psychometric quality of a test that shows the extent to which it truly measures the performance.[32] It is important for a surgical teacher to use validated tests to evaluate performance and to demand evidence of validity when the measurement system is a feature of a simulator.

## FACULTY AS LEADERS

Many surgical simulation centers were developed in response to mandates that residency training programs have a dedicated space for technical skills instruction. This mandate was sometimes addressed by the identification of a small space stocked with basic supplies and, in some but not all cases, a modest formal curriculum.[33] Other surgical faculty more quickly grasped the potential that simulation offered to improve surgical education. These individuals developed a vision that promoted excellence in the use of simulation in surgical education.[34] These standards included all of the elements of an appropriately developed curriculum.[35,36]

In additional to having an educational vision about the use of simulation, a surgeon-leader must identify and manage resources. Funding is a key resource that requires creative leadership.[37,38] Several surgical programs have been recipients of large gifts from grateful patients and strong believers in the need for such centers. These gifts have often been used to build the physical structures and provide an initial investment to sustain the center for a period of time. However, this is rarely enough to remain on the leading edge. Financial resources must be pooled from every available source. Directors must aggressively seek out grant opportunities sponsored by federal and state governments, associations, and industry. In addition, surgical simulation centers can often generate significant income from partnering with industry in their research, development, and training initiatives.

The existing research suggests that a properly trained nonsurgeon instructor can achieve the same educational outcomes as a surgeon faculty teacher for some skills.[39] This suggests that a contemporary simulation center should be led by a team. This is particularly true given the demands associated with creatively seeking and managing the financial resources that are required to maintain a simulation center. Only a few surgeons have sufficient business expertise to manage this aspect of the program. This team-based leadership approach requires the surgical faculty members to have a full range of leadership competencies to optimally manage a team.[40]

Interprofessional education is currently receiving considerable attention in surgical education[25] and the surgeon leader of a simulation center will need the skills to develop and cultivate strategic relationships with other professionals to develop and sustain this type of programming. In some respects, this type of leadership is more nuanced than being the designated leader of the team because it involves cultural differences between the different professions and perhaps an element of politics.

## FACULTY AS INNOVATORS

Simulation is an important mechanism whereby surgical faculty may innovate. Technological advancements have allowed for innovation in the use of simulation to enhance surgical care. Virtual reality involves the use of a computer to generate a 3-dimensional image or environment that allows an individual to interact in a seemingly real or physical way. Advancements in graphics, hardware, and software have enabled simulators to offer high-fidelity renderings of anatomy and associated surgical procedures. These technological advancements have been combined with imaging processing software to allow for the creation of patient-specific simulations through the incorporation of computed tomography or MRI data into the simulator.[41] This makes possible a unique simulation created for a specific patient that allows for planning or practice.[42,43] These same technological advances allow the combination of virtual and real-world elements into what is sometimes referred to as augmented reality.

Technological advancements have also made possible incorporating augmented reality into simulation. Augmented reality involves the use of technology to allow a superimposed composite image that is a combination of real-world and computer-generated images.[44] It may also be referred to as blended, mixed, or dual reality. It is different from virtual reality because the user is interacting with the actual environment instead of being immersed in a completely artificial environment. Having a superimposed image to direct a learner in a virtual simulation environment may improve contextual understanding for decision-making, teamwork, and prioritization of tasks. Learning is endorsed as being more authentic by providing students a more personalized learning experience.[45] The technology now exists that allows surgical teachers to be virtually present in the visual field of a surgeon performing a procedure on an actual patient or a physical simulator.[46] This combination of technologies could solve some of the practical barriers that have limited mentoring and allow it to be a more significant part of technical skills continuing education.

In addition to incorporating technological simulations to improve patient care, a faculty member can innovate educationally with the result of producing education scholarship. This scholarship can range from applied research designed to answer practical concerns about the usefulness of simulation for a particular purpose to more theoretic considerations that address fundamental aspects of learning in a simulated environment. The scholarship related to simulation has exploded. A surgeon aspiring to innovate in simulation education would be well served to comprehend the state of understanding through one of several programs focused on simulation; for instance, the certification program for health care simulation educators developed by the Society for Simulation in Healthcare (http://www.ssih.org/Certification/CHSE). A recent survey of thought leaders in surgical simulation has clarified the gaps that exist in the current understanding of this instructional method that should be examined in future investigations.[47]

## SUMMARY

Surgical faculty members take on multiple roles as they interact with simulation. Often these roles can change during the course of the interaction or can occur in varied combination simultaneously. Simulation will continue to emerge as an instructional method. Additional research is needed to determine how simulation can be most effectively used for the development of surgical faculty and other learners.

The surgeon learner is rarely the subject of educational investigation.[48] Assumptions about the appropriateness and utility of simulation for teaching this group must be inferred from research done using surgical residents or novices as subjects. Surgical faculty have unique features that affect their learning in a simulated environment. For example, surgical faculty may have considerable experience with a particular surgical technique and this experience might either enhance or interfere with the acquisition of a new technical skill in a simulated environment. A goal of continuing surgical education should be to mitigate or eliminate the performance or learning curve that occurs when a surgeon is mastering a new skill.[49] Surgical faculty members would seem to be the ideal subject group for study of this important quality issue because they are likely to perform a procedure in a simulated environment and then perform the same procedure with an actual patient. Determining the features that optimize this transfer would prove extremely valuable in improving patient safety. Clearly, surgeons have all of the cognitive and physical changes associated with aging and yet there is tremendous individual variation in those changes.[50] Both training and periodic evaluation in clinical simulation should be explored as a way to allow older surgeons to continue to contribute through an active practice if they choose to do so.

The suggestions for optimal teaching using simulation are largely drawn from experiences outside of surgery although the concept of briefing and debriefing should be familiar to most surgeons given their use in operating room teaching.[51] The use of briefing and other features specifically related to the use of simulation in instruction needs to be better defined to allow optimal faculty development programs to be created.

The original leaders in surgical simulation were visionary in recognizing the potential of simulation. Now simulation centers are common. Leadership challenges have evolved so that leadership involves maintaining a vision, building and leading teams, and identifying and managing resources. Leadership of a simulation center requires the ability to develop strategic partnerships for the purpose of gaining access to financial resources and conducting the multi-institutional studies that will likely constitute the next phase of scholarship. Additional investigation is needed to completely define what competencies the next generation of simulation center leaders must possess.

Innovation continuously occurs in surgery and in surgical education. Simulation now allows the possibility of creating a totally new procedure, including one designed for a specific patient. Perhaps this model of technical innovation will replace the current methods with the possibility of accelerating innovation while improving patient safety. This new use could be adapted to the development of novel surgical instrumentation and, therefore, avoid some of the workplace-associated injuries that surgeons have incurred using the current generation of instruments.[52]

## REFERENCES

1. Steinert Y, editor. Faculty development: core concepts and principles. In: Faculty development in the health professions. A focus on research and practice. New York: Springer; 2013. p. 3–25.
2. Bradley P. The history of simulation in medical education and possible future directions. Med Educ 2006;40(3):254–62.
3. Gelula MH, Yudkowsky R. Using standardised students in faculty development workshops to improve clinical teaching skills. Med Educ 2003;37(7):621–9.
4. Freischlag JA, Kibbe MR. The Evolution of Surgery: the Story of "Two Poems". JAMA 2014;312(17):1737–8.
5. Davis D, Fordis M, Colburn L, et al. Academic CMS in the U.S. and Canada: the 2010 AAMC/SACME Harrison survey. Society for Academic Continuing Medical Education. Washington, DC: Association of American Medical Colleges; 2011.

6. Aggarwal R, Ward J, Balasundaram I, et al. Proving the effectiveness of virtual reality simulation for training in laparoscopic surgery. Ann Surg 2007;246(5):771–9.
7. Ahlberg G, Enochsson L, Gallagher AG, et al. Proficiency-based virtual reality training significantly reduces the error rate for residents during their first 10 laparoscopic cholecystectomies. Am J Surg 2007;193(6):797–804.
8. Cook DA, Hatal R, Brydges R, et al. Technology-enhanced simulation for health professions education: a systematic review and meta-analysis. JAMA 2011; 306(9):978–88.
9. Fann JI, Caffarelli AD, Georgette G, et al. Improvement in coronary anastomosis with cardiac surgery simulation. J Thorac Cardiovasc Surg 2008;136(6):1486–91.
10. Seymour NE, Gallagher AG, Roman SA, et al. Virtual reality training improves operating room performance: results of a randomized, double-blinded study. Ann Surg 2002;236(4):458–64.
11. Gallagher AG, Cates CU. Approval of virtual reality training for carotid stenting: what this means for procedural-based medicine. JAMA 2004;292(24):3024–6.
12. Bahler CD, Sundaram CP. Training in robotic surgery: simulators, surgery and credentialing. Urol Clin North Am 2014;41(4):581–9.
13. Brunner WC, Korndorffer JR Jr, Sierra R, et al. Laparoscopic virtual reality training: are 30 repetitions enough? J Surg Res 2004;122(2):150–6.
14. Cates CU, Patel AD, Nicholson WJ. Use of virtual reality simulation for mission rehearsal for carotid stenting. JAMA 2007;297(3):265–6.
15. Simpao AF, Wong R, Ferrara TJ, et al. From simulation to separation surgery: a tale of two twins. Anesthesiology 2014;120(1):110.
16. Arora S, Miskovic D, Hull L, et al. Self vs. expert assessment of technical and non-technical skills in high fidelity simulation. Am J Surg 2011;202:500–6.
17. Barach P, Johson J, Ahmad A, et al. A prospective observational study of human factors, adverse events and patient outcomes in surgery for pediatric cardiac disease. J Thorac Cardiovasc Surg 2008;136(6):1422–8.
18. Hull L, Arora S, Symons NR, et al. Training faculty in nontechnical skill assessment: national guidelines on program requirements. Ann Surg 2013;258(2):370–5.
19. Yule S, Flin R, Paterson Brown S, et al. Non-technical skills for surgeons in the operating room: a review of the literature. Surgery 2006;139(2):140–9.
20. Arriaga AF, Gawande AA, Raemer DB, et al. Pilot testing of a model for insurer-driven, large-scale multicenter simulation training for operating room teams. Ann Surg 2014;259(3):403–10.
21. Cumin D, Boyd MJ, Webster CS, et al. A systematic review of simulation for multidisciplinary team training in operating rooms. Simul Healthc 2013;8(3):171–9.
22. Doumouras AG, Keshet I, Nathens AB, et al. Trauma Non-Technical Training (TNT-2): the development, piloting and multilevel assessment of a simulation-based, interprofessional curriculum for team-based trauma resuscitation. Can J Surg 2014;57(5):354–5.
23. Kim S, Dunkin BJ, Paige JT, et al. What is the future of training in surgery? Needs assessment of national stakeholders. Surgery 2014;156(3):707–17.
24. Krueger PM, Neutens J, Bienstock J, et al. To the point: reviews in medical education teaching techniques. Am J Obstet Gynecol 2004;191(2):408–11.
25. Seymour NE, Cooper JB, Farley DR, et al. Best practices in interprofessional education and training in surgery: experiences from American College of Surgeons-Accredited Education Institutes. Surgery 2013;154(1):1–12.
26. Motola I, Devine LA, Chung HS, et al. Simulation in healthcare education: a best evidence practical guide. AMEE Guide No. 82. Med Teach 2013;35(10): e1511–30.

27. Bath J, Lawrence PF. Twelve tips for developing and implementing an effective surgical simulation programme. Med Teach 2012;34(3):192–7.
28. Rudolph JW, Simon R, Dufresne RL, et al. There's no such thing as "nonjudgmental" debriefing: a theory and method for debriefing with good judgment. Simul Healthc 2006;1(1):49–55.
29. Rudolph JW, Simon R, Raemer DB, et al. Debriefing as formative assessment: closing performance gaps in medical education. Acad Emerg Med 2008; 15(11):1010–6.
30. Rudolph JW, Simon R, Rivard P, et al. Debriefing with good judgment: combining rigorous feedback with genuine inquiry. Anesthesiol Clin 2007;25(2):361–76.
31. Rudolph JW, Raemer DB, Simon R. Establishing a safe container for learning in simulation: the role of the presimulation briefing. Simul Healthc 2014;9(6):339–49.
32. Korndorffer JR Jr, Kasten SJ, Downing SM. A call for the utilization of consensus standards in the surgical education literature. Am J Surg 2010;199(1):99–104.
33. Scott DJ, Cendan JC, Pugh CM, et al. The changing face of surgical education: Simulation as the new paradigm. J Surg Res 2008;147(2):189–93.
34. Friedell ML. Starting a simulation and skills laboratory: what do I need and what do I want? J Surg Educ 2010;67(2):112–21.
35. Scott DJ, Dunnington GL. The new ACS/APDS skills curriculum: moving the learning curve out of the operating room. J Gastrointest Surg 2008;12(2):213–21.
36. Sachdeva AK, Pellegrini CK, Johnson KA. Support for simulation-based surgical education through American College of Surgeons–accredited education institutes. World J Surg 2008;32(2):196–207.
37. Danzer E, Dumon K, Kolb G, et al. What is the cost associated with implementation and maintenance of an ACS/APDS-based surgical skills curriculum? J Surg Educ 2011;68(6):519–25.
38. Haluck RS, Satava RM, Fried G, et al. Establishing a simulation center for surgical skills: what to do and how to do it. Surg Endosc 2007;21(7):1223–32.
39. Kim MJ, Boehler ML, Ketchum JK, et al. Skills coaches as part of the educational team: a randomized controlled trial of teaching of a basic surgical skill in the laboratory setting. Am J Surg 2010;199(1):94–8.
40. Wiseman L, McKeown G. Multipliers: how the best leaders make everyone smarter. New York: Harper Collins; 2010. e-books.
41. Willaert WI, Aggarwal R, Van Herzeele I, et al. Recent advances in medical simulation: patient-specific virtual reality simulation. World J Surg 2012;36(7): 1703–12.
42. Sadiq SK, Mazzeo MD, Zasada SJ, et al. Patient-specific simulation as a basis for clinical decision-making. Philos Trans A Math Phys Eng Sci 2008;366(1878): 3199–219.
43. Sierra R, Dimaio SP, Wada J, et al. Patient specific simulation and navigation of ventriculoscopic interventions. Stud Health Technol Inform 2007;125:433–5.
44. Lahanas V, Loukas C, Smailis N, et al. A novel augmented reality simulator for skills assessment in minimal invasive surgery. Surg Endosc 2014. http://dx.doi.org/10.1007/s00464-014-3930-y.
45. Zhu E, Hadadgar A, Masiello I, et al. Augmented reality in healthcare education: an integrative review. PeerJ 2014;2:e469 eCollection 2014.
46. Lindeque BG, Ponce BA, Menendez ME, et al. Emerging technology in surgical education: combining real-time augmented reality and wearable computing devices. Orthopedics 2014;37(11):751–7.
47. Stefanidis D, Sevdalis N, Paige J, et al. Simulation in surgery: what's needed next? Ann Surg 2014. http://dx.doi.org/10.1097/SLA.0000000000000826.

48. Rogers DA. The role of simulation in surgical continuing medical education. Semin Colon Rectal Surg 2008;19(2):108–14.
49. Rogers DA, Elstein AS, Bordage G. Improving continuing medical education for surgical techniques: applying the lessons learned in the first decade of minimal access surgery. Ann Surg 2001;233(2):159–66.
50. Drag LL, Bieliauskas LA, Langenecker SA, et al. Cognitive functioning, retirement status, and age: results from the Cognitive Changes and Retirement among Senior Surgeons study. J Am Coll Surg 2010;211(3):303–7.
51. Roberts NK, Williams RG, Kim MJ, et al. The briefing, intraoperative teaching, debriefing model for teaching in the operating room. J Am Coll Surg 2009;208(2):299–303.
52. Reyes DA, Tang B, Cuschieri AA. Minimal access surgery (MAS)-related surgeon morbidity syndromes. Surg Endosc 2006;20(1):1–13.

48. Rogers DA. The role of simulation in surgical continuing medical education. Semin Colon Rectal Surg 2008;19(2):108–14.
49. Rogers DA, Elstein AS, Bordage G. Improving continuing medical education for surgical techniques: applying the lessons learned in the first decade of minimal access surgery. Ann Surg 2001;233(2):159–66.
50. Drag LL, Bieliauskas LA, Langenecker SA, et al. Cognitive functioning, retirement status, and age: results from the Cognitive Changes and Retirement among Senior Surgeons study. J Am Coll Surg 2010;211(3):303–7.
51. Roberts NK, Williams RG, Kim MJ, et al. The briefing, intraoperative teaching, debriefing model for teaching in the operating room. J Am Coll Surg 2009;208(2):299–303.
52. Reeves DA, Tang B, Cuschieri AA. Minimal access surgery (MAS)-related surgeon morbidity syndromes. Surg Endosc 2006;20(1):1–13.

# The Evolving Role of Simulation in Teaching Surgery in Undergraduate Medical Education

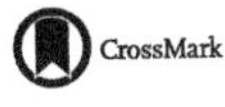

Robert D. Acton, MD

**KEYWORDS**

- Surgical simulation • Medical student • Education • Standardized patient
- Entrustable professional activity

**KEY POINTS**

- SBT has emerged as an effective training tool in undergraduate medical education (UME) in response to increasing volumes of knowledge, skills, and attitudes (KSA) that students must acquire and patient safety concerns resulting from medical students learning and practicing on actual patients.
- SBT is already used in select high-stakes assessments of medical students, such as the United States Medical Licensing Exam Step 2 Clinical Skills, and validity evidence for additional applications of SBT for formative and summative assessments is growing.
- Simulation has become the preferred method for teaching and training of several national medical student surgical education initiatives.

## INTRODUCTION

Simulation-based training (SBT) has long been employed by surgeons to teach their craft to residents and students. For example, surgical educators have frequently incorporated basic technical skills task simulators and animate laboratories into the educational curricula of medical students to teach basic operative skills and procedures.[1] Over the last 10 years, however, they have made a concerted effort to develop organized SBT curricula with assessments to teach and evaluate the cognitive, technical, and decision-making skills of students to enhance education and patient care.[2] These changes in undergraduate medical education (UME) are an attempt to meet the evolving need for continued education of medical students under the current demands of time, medical knowledge, quality, and patient safety.[2,3]

Division of Pediatric Surgery, Department of Surgery, University of Minnesota, East Building, MB505, 2450 Riverside Avenue South, Minneapolis, MN 55454, USA
*E-mail address:* Acton002@umn.edu

Surg Clin N Am 95 (2015) 739–750
http://dx.doi.org/10.1016/j.suc.2015.04.001
**surgical.theclinics.com**
0039-6109/15/$ – see front matter 

This article discusses the demands and drivers on undergraduate surgical education, the history of SBT for students, types of simulators commonly used in current curricula, and 3 major national efforts incorporating SBT at the UME level:

1. The American College of Surgeons/Association for Surgical Education (ACS/ASE) medical student simulation-based surgical skills curriculum[4]
2. The American College of Surgeons/Association of Program Directors in Surgery/Association for Surgical Education (ACS/APDS/ASE) resident preparatory curriculum[5]
3. The Association of American Medical Colleges (AAMC) core entrustable professional activities (EPAs) for medical students[6]

## BRIEF HISTORY OF SIMULATION

SBT has been utilized for hundreds of years in both medical and surgical education.[7] Recent efforts by surgical educators have focused on a systematic and concerted effort toward using such training to efficiently transfer information to and assess a surgical learner.[8] Very early simulators in the 14th to 17th centuries were clay figurines used to teach acupuncture points and meridians. Later in the 18th century, life-sized wax human models, the forerunners of today's current plastic models, were used to teach anatomy. One of the earliest SBT curricula can be traced to 18th century Italy and the development of obstetric simulators to educate midwives in order to lower the incidence of birth mortality. Giovanni Antonio Galli, a surgeon in Bologna, designed a birthing simulator and required students to demonstrate the delivery of a child while blindfolded. Galli's development of an SBT curriculum thus incorporated key educational principles used today: performance of a needs assessment, matching the teaching method to the skill desired, and development of an assessment tool to verify learning. The idea of SBT for midwives was expanded nationally in France in 1759 to address the decline in the population of rural France. Louis XV commissioned Angelique Marguerite Le Boursier du Coudray to teach midwifery across France to save infant lives during birth. Simulation continued to be used within obstetrics but was not uniformly accepted as the standard. By the time of the Flexner report in the United States, obstetric simulators were more accepted, and several medical schools were condemned, because their obstetric simulators were in such disrepair.[7]

Interestingly, the first SBT specific to surgeons can be traced to Sushruta, an Indian scholar from approximately the fourth century to the sixth century BC. His Sanskrit-language text was translated in 1907 and contains descriptions and lessons for students to practice inserting their knives and tools into natural objects mimicking body parts. Students were also asked to practice the art of bandaging specific body parts on full-sized linen dolls. The text describes several other simulated models such as using vegetables to practice cutting, excision on leather pouches or animal bladders filled with fluid, and cauterization of pieces of meat.[7]

With the development of anesthesia and the aseptic technique leading to a boom in the field of surgery, surgical SBT evolved throughout the 19th and 20th centuries with better models to teach specific procedures such as hernia repair, intubation, and ocular surgery. Some of the simulators were hybrids with both artificial and human parts.[7] In addition, cadaveric and animate animal models became more commonplace. Living anesthetized pigs were often used throughout the latter half of the 20th century to teach medical students and surgical residents operative skills in a simulated environment. This practice was largely abandoned in the beginning part of the 21st century secondary to the associated regulatory cost and pressure to use inanimate models; recent pressure to return to this model has been noted, however, because of the extreme realism that is possible with animate models.[1,9] SBT, therefore, has been part and parcel of surgical education from the earliest times. The recent focus on it has been in large part due to drivers that have altered the way surgery is taught, as discussed in the next section.

## DRIVERS ON SURGICAL UNDERGRADUATE MEDICAL EDUCATION

The last 10 years have seen significant changes in UME, and these changes have required surgical educators to adapt their approach to education.[2] Important drivers of these changes include 4 important trends in health care and education:

1. The ever-increasing amount of new medical knowledge that students are expected to learn[2,10]
2. Changes in patient safety, quality, and expectations on surgical faculty[9,11]
3. Work hour limitations and loss of surgical teams[10,11]
4. A move toward competency-based education and the creation of entrustable professional activities.[6]

SBT, and more specifically, SBT with assessment appears to be an answer to these changes. With simulation, the skills being taught and learned can be uncoupled from the stress of the clinical environment, to improve learning and cognition for the student/novice learner.[12–14]

For the last century, surgical educators have modeled William Halsted's classic model of surgical education that was developed and implemented at John Hopkins and spread across North America. Although this surgical training model was not directly intended for medical students, it had a strong impact on their education. Students were traditionally embedded for 8 to 12 weeks onto a surgical service, where they would receive a significant amount of their education from the surgical faculty and resident house staff, observing/participating in the operating room and caring for patients on the ward. Through this experience, students were expected to learn the knowledge, skills, and attitudes (KSAs) needed for efficient patient care.[15–17] The only real change seemed to be the ever-increasing amount of knowledge that a student was expected to learn, whether formally or informally. This Halstedian paradigm began to change dramatically in 2003 when the Accreditation Council for Graduate Medical Education (ACGME) implemented an 80-hour work hour restriction on residencies; many medical schools followed suit for the students.[15] This action was largely in response to a growing trend of increased public awareness of patient safety and quality with greater societal expectations around care, dating from the Libby Zion case in New York State in 1984.[16] Surgical Departments and educators worked to adjust call schedules for residents to remain compliant to work hour limitations with a concomitant increase in faculty obligations to be ever more present for surgical cases and clinical care. An unforeseen consequence of implementing these changes was the relegation of medical student education to a secondary level.[15] Traditionally surgical teams were larger and composed of a chief resident, junior residents, interns, and medical students, and they would be on-call every second to third night. Residents were responsible for fewer patients at any 1 time, with more residents on-call any one night. These teams were cohesive units, and education would take place during down times and was often focused on the teaching of the interns and students by the older residents. As work hour restrictions were implemented, the first casualty was the surgical team structure. In order to make the work hour numbers fit and reduce call nights, many programs combined the number of services that residents were responsible for at night, added physician assistants, or created night float rotations. These measures impeded education in the surgical team, and programs had to become more specific and creative about how and when they were teaching.[18] The only constant throughout this evolution was the number hours in the day. As the old surgical adage states, "They can do anything to me on call, but they can't turn back time." Thus, fewer of these hours were available for teaching in the ready-made small groups oriented around a traditional surgery service.

Educators realized that medical student education was suffering, and reports described that graduating students were not prepared to begin the duties of residency.[6,15] The Halstedian teaching days of "see one, do one, teach one" were over. Society now expected students to know how to do it and not practice on their loved ones. Educators needed an efficient method of teaching and assessing the information and skill that was being taught.[19,20] This teaching method also needed to be delivered in a universal, reproducible, and relatively inexpensive manner in order to be adopted in a widespread manner in UME.[17] SBT became such a teaching method, since it provided a safe environment for a student to fail, practice, and learn before a patient encounter.[10,13]

## TYPES OF SIMULATORS

Simulators can be divided into multiple classification schemes such as animate/inanimate, virtual/real, or partial task/procedural. These classifications can be combined to describe the various characteristics of a simulator, such as an inanimate porcine partial task trainer (a pig's foot model to teach suturing). A simulator, however, does not in and of itself constitute a curriculum. It is but 1 tool and it must be properly paired with the learning objectives of what is being taught and valid assessment and feedback for the learner. In UME, many types are currently employed (**Table 1**). A synopsis of key types of simulations and simulators follow:

### *Standardized Patients*

Standardized patients (SPs) have been used extensively in the UME setting, primarily for teaching physical diagnosis skills, typically around pelvic and ano-rectal exams.[21,22] An important contribution of SPs is the ability for them to participate in the assessment of and feedback to the student.[23] A down side is the expense and compensation for the professional patient. Hybrid simulation is a useful adaptation of the use of SPs, in which an SP is combined with an anatomic part task training model.[24] This set up permits for the demonstration of technical skills on the model that normally would not routinely be done with an SP, but it still incorporates the human interaction and allows the SP to assist in the assessment of and feedback to the student.[21,25] A recent adaptation to the classic SP is the incorporation of actors (ie, confederates, embedded educators) for teaching interprofessional and patient communication, teamwork and safety scenarios.[26,27]

### *Abstract Partial Task Trainers*

Abstract partial task trainers have great utility for teaching medical students key KSAs.[1] At this earlier phase of their medical education, they can be overwhelmed with information, impeding learning. Compartmentalizing the information or skill being taught through the use of part task trainers can increase the retention of the information.[28,29] The other advantage is that many of the part task simulation models can be produced inexpensively, which is an important consideration when considering expanding a curriculum across an entire medical school class. Many of the ACS/ASE medical student simulation-based surgical skills curriculum modules utilize partial task trainers (**Table 2**).[4]

**Table 1**
**Simulator classification**

| Simulator | Description | Uses | Cost |
|---|---|---|---|
| Abstract partial task trainers | Knot tying boards<br>Foam suture models<br>Simple laparoscopic box trainers | Teaching a repetitive simple task such at suturing, knot tying or pulling drains<br>Peg transfer for laparoscopy | $<br>Most are very inexpensive and reusable, or students can take them home to practice |
| Physical anatomic trainers | Silicone, plastic or foam replicas of humans or portions of humans | Teaching a complete procedure with multiple smaller steps – Foley, nasogastric tube, central line placement, intubation | $$-$$$<br>Commercially made products can get expensive for an entire school |
| Human simulators | Replicas of humans, may be computerized, may be simple or more complex | Team training, cardiopulmonary resuscitation, airway and intubation, codes | $-$$$$<br>Computerized Mannequins can be expensive and take training to run but are very realistic |
| Computer Based | Programmed clinical scenarios that can be repeated over and over | Very useful for teaching clinical decision making and pathways, allows for retesting across time and assessing knowledge acquisition | $-$$$<br>Initial purchase or writing of scenarios Subscription rates can build and increase |
| Standardized patients | Professional patients to volunteer students. Can assist with the assessment and ads realism | Physical examination skills, team training, immediate feedback | $-$$$<br>Professional patients can cost, volunteer students require training |
| Animate models | Live animals or food grade portions of animals | Performing complete operations or adding realism to tissue consistency for partial task trainers | $-$$$$$<br>Store bought models are reasonably priced, but live animal models are expensive due to housing, anesthesia, and disposal costs |
| Virtual anatomic trainers | Image-guided computer-assisted specific task trainers | Laparoscopic, endoscopic, and vascular procedures | $$$$<br>Initial purchase and maintenance and most procedures are beyond the need of a student |
| Virtual reality | Completely interactive computer- based environment | At the present time this option is not feasible for student education | $$$$$ - Very high upfront cost; hard to use with large student volumes |

**Table 2**
**American College of Surgeons/Association for Surgical Education medical student simulation-based surgical skills curriculum**

| Skill Level | Skills |
|---|---|
| Year 1 | • Abdominal examination<br>• Basic vascular examination<br>• Breast examination<br>• Digital rectal examination<br>• Female pelvic examination<br>• Male groin and genital examination<br>• Universal precautions<br>• Venipuncture and peripheral intravenous fluid administration |
| Year 2 | • Basic airway management<br>• Communication—history and physical and case presentation<br>• Foley bladder catheterization<br>• Intermediate vascular examination<br>• Nasogastric tubes<br>• Sterile technique—gloving and gowning<br>• Surgical drains—care and removal |
| Year 3 | • Arterial puncture and blood gas<br>• Basic knot tying<br>• Basic suturing<br>• Central venous line insertion<br>• Communication—during codes and safe and effective handoffs<br>• Intermediate airway<br>• Intraosseous intravenous fluid administration<br>• Local anesthetics<br>• Paracentesis<br>• Thoracentesis |

*Adapted from* American College of Surgeons. Medical student simulation-based surgical skills curriculum. 2013. Available at: http://MedStudentSimSkills.facs.org.

## *Animal Models*

Animal models can be useful for teaching medical students, primarily as partial task trainers in which food grade portions of animals are utilized for teaching a very specific task, such as using pigs feet for teaching suturing, portions of beef ribs as chest tube insertion models, or pig aorta for vascular training.[30] Whole live animal models are very expensive and best used for resident education or as part of a specific exposure of students to surgery for the purpose of increasing interest in the career or as a specific educational need.[9]

## *Virtual Anatomic Trainers*

Virtual anatomic trainers mostly represent specific task trainers with a computer interface for teaching operative skills, complete operations, or procedures.[31,32] These simulators include laparoscopic, endoscopic, and vascular trainers.[33,34] Students can achieve the skills needed to complete the procedures on such trainers to the level of a resident in a reasonable timeframe.[30] The larger question is not can a medical student learn the skills to complete a task, but whether he or she needs to learn the advance procedures simulated by the trainers and whether he or she can learn the decision making behind the procedure. Skill laboratories utilizing and exposing students to these trainers have demonstrated an ability to increase a student's interest in a surgical profession.[35–39]

## DEVELOPING SIMULATION-BASED TRAINING CURRICULA

When developing an SBT curriculum for medical students, a needs assessment of what the educator wants the student to learn is required with the decision of whether the knowledge or skill can be assessed.[1] Development should not start with the thought, "We have this nice simulator, let us have the students use it." To become a surgeon takes the development of knowledge, technical skill, and judgment, and the proper use of simulation can help to achieve this goal.[13,40] Research has demonstrated that the skills learned in the simulation laboratories are transferable to clinical practice and speed education.[40] For a novice learner, such as a medical student, assessment and feedback are the keys to their learning.[41] They can be overwhelmed with information and may not have the ability to multitask while learning. Utilizing and following existing national curricula that have been developed to teach surgical skills at the UME level will provide a major advantage in this arena.[29]

## ASSOCIATION OF AMERICAN MEDICAL COLLEGES CORE ENTRUSTABLE PROFESSIONAL ACTIVITIES FOR ENTERING RESIDENCY

In August of 2014, the AAMC released the Core EPAs for Entering Residency.[6] These EPAs are a list of 13 qualities or activities that are considered essential of all students finishing medical school (**Box 1**). This work was in response to concerns by program directors, primarily surgical, that students completing medical school were not ready to assume the duties required of a starting postgraduate year 1 resident.[15,42–44] It also came on the heels of the Milestone Project, which was initiated in 2013 by the Accreditation Council for Graduate Medical Education in partnership with the American Board of Medical Specialties. In the same year, the ACS/ASE medical student simulation-based surgical skills curriculum was also released, which is a modular skills curriculum, teaching most of the EPAs released by the AAMC. Assessing students based on the EPAs is a logical step toward a competency-based UME. Of note, the EPAs

**Box 1**
**Association of American Medical Colleges core entrustable professional activities for entering residency**

EPA 1. Gather a history and perform a physical examination

EPA 2. Prioritizing a differential diagnosis following a clinical encounter

EPA 3. Recommend and interpret common diagnostic and screening test

EPA 4. Enter and discuss orders and prescriptions

EPA 5. Document a clinical encounter in the medical record

EPA 6. Provide and oral presentation of a clinical encounter

EPA 7. Form clinical questions and retrieve evidence to advance patient care

EPA 8. Give or receive a patient handover to transition care responsibility

EPA 9. Collaborate as a member of an interprofessional team

EPA 10. Recognize a patient requiring urgent or emergent care and initiate evaluation and management

EPA 11. Obtain informed consent for test and/or procedures

EPA 12. Perform general procedures of a physician

EPA 13. Identify system failures and contribute to a culture of safety and improvement do not directly address medical knowledge, but a student's ability to use the knowledge he or she has acquired to make and act on decisions. Although the AAMC EPAs do not list specific SBT activities, they form the basis for building an SBT curriculum as key learning objectives that should be attained.

## AMERICAN COLLEGE OF SURGEONS/ASSOCIATION FOR SURGICAL EDUCATION MEDICAL STUDENT SIMULATION-BASED SURGICAL SKILLS CURRICULUM

In 2009 and 2010, leaders in surgical education within the ASE and ACS began to talk about a way to improve the education and apparent skill degradation within medical students rotating on surgical clerkships. A project modeled on the APDS Resident Curriculum was begun within the ASE Simulation Committee. Shortly after this beginning, a decision was made to form a Steering Committee composed of members of both the ACS and ASE. This Steering Committee worked in collaboration with the ASE Assessment Committee to perform a needs assessment and developed a list of 25 important surgically related skills and activities felt to be critical to all physicians.[45] Over the next 3 years, the modules were authored, peer reviewed, edited, published and released at Surgical Education Week in 2013. The curriculum was awarded the ASE Innovation in Surgical Education Award in 2014. At the current time, the curriculum is being used based on visits to the host site, and the Steering Committee is conducting a secondary project with 17 medical schools that are incorporating 3 modules into their curriculum for early adoption and feedback on usability of the models and assessment forms. Two of the modules were trialed in a large group format as part of the Medical Student program at the 2014 ACS Clinical Congress. Overall, feedback was good on the basic suturing and knot tying modules. The goal is to have this curriculum be a living curriculum that is constantly improving and meeting the needs of students and educators. The curriculum is available with an American College of Surgeons logon on the Division of Education webpage or at http://MedStudentSimSkills.facs.org.

## AMERICAN COLLEGE OF SURGEONS/ASSOCIATION OF PROGRAM DIRECTORS IN SURGERY/ASSOCIATION FOR SURGICAL EDUCATION RESIDENT PREPARATION CURRICULUM

Another curriculum for medical students that incorporates simulation is the ACS/APDS/ASE resident preparation curriculum. This curriculum came from an identified need that students were not entering surgical residency prepared to assume the responsibilities and tasks required.[42–44,46] Surgical educators worked to create an in time curriculum to challenge students and enable them to learn the KSAs and decision-making skills required to be an effective intern on day one.[18,47] Early research on using a boot camp showed that first-year residents who participated in a boot camp outperformed their nonboot camp peers in most categories for roughly the first 3 to 6 months of their training. The resident preparation curriculum is not designed to replace the medical knowledge that should be learned during a year 3 or year 4 surgery clerkship or subinternship.[44,47,48] The critical components of the resident preparation curriculum are listed in **Box 2**. This curriculum was piloted at over 25 medical schools in 2013 and 49 schools in 2014 and will be available to all schools in 2015.[5] The value of this preparatory curriculum was made evident by the issuance of a joint statement of its utility and need by the American Board of Surgery, ACS, APDS, and ASE. Such support signals that it will likely become the norm and expectation of program directors in general surgery residencies and that it could be adopted by other specialties.[46]

**Box 2**
**American College of Surgeons/Association of Program Directors in Surgery/Association for Surgical Education resident prep curriculum, critical content**

1. Being a first responder for critically ill or unstable patients
2. Emergency procedures (ventilation)
3. Common electrolyte abnormalities
4. Management of common and urgent perioperative conditions
5. Interpreting radiographs
6. Operative anatomy
7. Responding to pages from nurses
8. Handoffs
9. Difficult patients
10. Communication

*Adapted from* American College of Surgeons. ACS/APDS/ASE resident prep curriculum. Available at: https://www.facs.org/education/program/resident-prep.

## SUMMARY

Surgical SBT over the last 10 years has gone from being used by a few educators teaching traditional skills to a main focus of surgical education. Simulation has always been used to teach surgical skills, but the technique is rapidly becoming the standard for early surgical education. Key SBT benefits include its ability to compartmentalize education and combine immediate assessment and feedback, all in an effort to accelerate KSA acquisition for the young learner. SBT value is demonstrated in its being adopted in multiple national medical student surgical educational initiatives.

## REFERENCES

1. Acton RD, Chipman JG, Gilkeson J, et al. Synthesis versus imitation: evaluation of a medical student simulation curriculum via objective structured assessment of technical skill. J Surg Educ 2010;67(3):173–8.
2. Sachdeva AK. Establishment of American College of Surgeons-accredited Education Institutes: the dawn of a new era in surgical education and training. J Surg Educ 2010;67(4):249–50.
3. Zevin B, Aggarwal R, Grantcharov TP. Surgical simulation in 2013: why is it still not the standard in surgical training? J Am Coll Surg 2014;218(2):294–301.
4. American College of Surgeons/Association for Surgical Education. ACS/ASE medical student simulation-based surgical skills curriculum. 2013. Available at: http://MedStudentSimSkills.facs.org. Accessed November 27, 2014.
5. American College of Surgeons/Association of Program Directors in Surgery/Association for Surgical Education. ACS/APDS/ASE resident preparatory curriculum. 2014. Available at: http://www.facs.org/education/program/resident-prep. Accessed November 27, 2014.
6. Association of American Medical Colleges. AAMC core entrustable professional activities for medical students, curriculum developers guide. 2014. Available at: https://members.aamc.org/eweb/upload/Core%20EPA%20Curriculum%20Dev%20Guide.pdf.

7. Owen H. Early use of simulation in medical education. Simul Healthc 2012;7(2):102–16.
8. Agha RA, Fowler AJ. The validity of surgical simulation. Can J Surg 2014;57(4):226–7.
9. Drosdeck J, Carraro E, Arnold M, et al. Porcine wet lab improves surgical skills in third year medical students. J Surg Res 2013;184(1):19–25.
10. Buckley CE, Kavanagh DO, Traynor O, et al. Is the skillset obtained in surgical simulation transferable to the operating theatre? Am J Surg 2014;207(1):146–57.
11. Scott DJ, Pugh CM, Ritter EM, et al. New directions in simulation-based surgical education and training: validation and transfer of surgical skills, use of nonsurgeons as faculty, use of simulation to screen and select surgery residents, and long-term follow-up of learners. Surgery 2011;149(6):735–44.
12. Kahol K, Ashby A, Smith M, et al. Quantitative evaluation of retention of surgical skills learned in simulation. J Surg Educ 2010;67(6):421–6.
13. Kolozsvari NO, Feldman LS, Vassiliou MC, et al. Sim one, do one, teach one: considerations in designing training curricula for surgical simulation. J Surg Educ 2011;68(5):421–7.
14. Schlickum M, Hedman L, Enochsson L, et al. Surgical simulation tasks challenge visual working memory and visual-spatial ability differently. World J Surg 2011;35(4):710–5.
15. Brennan MF, Debas HT. Surgical education in the United States: portents for change. Ann Surg 2004;240(4):565–72.
16. DuCoin C. Second-place essay–revolution: five-year general surgery residency: reform or revolution? Bull Am Coll Surg 2014;99(11):20–2.
17. Pucher PH, Darzi A, Aggarwal R. Development of an evidence-based curriculum for training of ward-based surgical care. Am J Surg 2014;207(2):213–7.
18. Tocco N, Brunsvold M, Kabbani L, et al. Innovation in internship preparation: an operative anatomy course increases senior medical students' knowledge and confidence. Am J Surg 2013;206(2):269–79.
19. Mollo EA, Reinke CE, Nelson C, et al. The simulated ward: ideal for training clinical clerks in an era of patient safety. J Surg Res 2012;177(1):e1–6.
20. Tjiam IM, Schout BM, Hendrikx AJ, et al. Designing simulator-based training: an approach integrating cognitive task analysis and four-component instructional design. Med Teach 2012;34(10):e698–707.
21. Balkissoon R, Blossfield K, Salud L, et al. Lost in translation: unfolding medical students' misconceptions of how to perform a clinical digital rectal examination. Am J Surg 2009;197(4):525–32.
22. Sachdeva AK, Wolfson PJ, Blair PG, et al. Impact of a standardized patient intervention to teach breast and abdominal examination skills to third-year medical students at two institutions. Am J Surg 1997;173(4):320–5.
23. Wehbe-Janek H, Song J, Shabahang M. An evaluation of the usefulness of the standardized patient methodology in the assessment of surgery residents' communication skills. J Surg Educ 2011;68(3):172–7.
24. Cahan MA, Larkin AC, Starr S, et al. A human factors curriculum for surgical clerkship students. Arch Surg 2010;145(12):1151–7.
25. Isenberg GA, Berg KW, Veloski JA, et al. Evaluation of the use of patient-focused simulation for student assessment in a surgery clerkship. Am J Surg 2011;201(6):835–40.
26. Meier AH, Boehler ML, McDowell CM, et al. A surgical simulation curriculum for senior medical students based on TeamSTEPPS. Arch Surg 2012;147(8):761–6.

27. Ponton-Carss A, Hutchison C, Violato C. Assessment of communication, professionalism, and surgical skills in an objective structured performance-related examination (OSPRE): a psychometric study. Am J Surg 2011;202(4):433–40.
28. Dubrowski A, Brydges R, Satterthwaite L, et al. Do not teach me while I am working! Am J Surg 2012;203(2):253–7.
29. Patel V, Aggarwal R, Osinibi E, et al. Operating room introduction for the novice. Am J Surg 2012;203(2):266–75.
30. Nesbitt JC, St Julien J, Absi TS, et al. Tissue-based coronary surgery simulation: medical student deliberate practice can achieve equivalency to senior surgery residents. J Thorac Cardiovasc Surg 2013;145(6):1453–8 [discussion: 1458–9].
31. Bjurstrom JM, Konge L, Lehnert P, et al. Simulation-based training for thoracoscopy. Simul Healthc 2013;8(5):317–23.
32. Harrysson I, Hull L, Sevdalis N, et al. Development of a knowledge, skills, and attitudes framework for training in laparoscopic cholecystectomy. Am J Surg 2014;207(5):790–6.
33. Gormley GJ, McGlade K, Thomson C, et al. A virtual surgery in general practice: evaluation of a novel undergraduate virtual patient learning package. Med Teach 2011;33(10):e522–7.
34. Nguyen T, Braga LH, Hoogenes J, et al. Commercial video laparoscopic trainers versus less expensive, simple laparoscopic trainers: a systematic review and meta-analysis. J Urol 2013;190(3):894–9.
35. Antiel RM, Thompson SM, Camp CL, et al. Attracting students to surgical careers: preclinical surgical experience. J Surg Educ 2012;69(3):301–5.
36. Bernholt DL, Garzon-Muvdi J, LaPorte DM, et al. A survey of current policy and practice of surgical exposure for preclerkship medical students at American medical institutions. Am J Surg 2013;206(3):433–8.
37. Lee JT, Qiu M, Teshome M, et al. The utility of endovascular simulation to improve technical performance and stimulate continued interest of preclinical medical students in vascular surgery. J Surg Educ 2009;66(6):367–73.
38. Selden NR, Origitano TC, Hadjipanayis C, et al. Model-based simulation for early neurosurgical learners. Neurosurgery 2013;73(Suppl 1):15–24.
39. Tesche LJ, Feins RH, Dedmon MM, et al. Simulation experience enhances medical students' interest in cardiothoracic surgery. Ann Thorac Surg 2010;90(6):1967–73 [discussion: 1973–4].
40. Friedell ML. Starting a simulation and skills laboratory: what do I need and what do I want? J Surg Educ 2010;67(2):112–21.
41. Graziano SC. Randomized surgical training for medical students: resident versus peer-led teaching. Am J Obstet Gynecol 2011;204(6):542.e1–4.
42. Lyss-Lerman P, Teherani A, Aagaard E, et al. What training is needed in the fourth year of medical school? Views of residency program directors. Acad Med 2009;84(7):823–9.
43. Naylor RA, Hollett LA, Castellvi A, et al. Preparing medical students to enter surgery residencies. Am J Surg 2010;199(1):105–9.
44. Okusanya OT, Kornfield ZN, Reinke CE, et al. The effect and durability of a pre-graduation boot cAMP on the confidence of senior medical student entering surgical residencies. J Surg Educ 2012;69(4):536–43.
45. Glass CC, Acton RD, Blair PG, et al. American College of Surgeons/Association for Surgical Education medical student simulation-based surgical skills curriculum needs assessment. Am J Surg 2014;207(2):165–9.

46. American Board of Surgery, American College of Surgeons, Association of Program Directors in Surgery, et al. Statement on surgical preresidency preparatory courses. Surgery 2014;156(5):1059–60.
47. Antonoff MB, Swanson JA, Green CA, et al. The significant impact of a competency-based preparatory course for senior medical students entering surgical residency. Acad Med 2012;87(3):308–19.
48. Fernandez GL, Page DW, Coe NP, et al. Boot cAMP: educational outcomes after 4 successive years of preparatory simulation-based training at onset of internship. J Surg Educ 2012;69(2):242–8.

# Using Simulation in Interprofessional Education

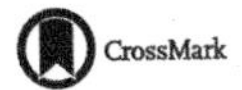

John T. Paige, MD[a,*], Deborah D. Garbee, PhD, APRN, ACNS-BC[b], Kimberly M. Brown, MD[c], Jose D. Rojas, RT, PhD[d]

**KEYWORDS**

- Simulation • Interprofessional education • Team training • Skills acquisition
- Operating room • Surgical education

**KEY POINTS**

- Interprofessional education (IPE) involves participants from 2 or more health professions learning interactively (ie, with, from, and about each other).
- The 4 major interprofessional competency domains are (1) values/ethics for interprofessional practice, (2) roles/responsibilities, (3) interprofessional communication, and (4) teams and teamwork.
- IPE is needed in surgical education because current teamwork is less than ideal.
- IPE has been shown to have positive impacts on professional practice and health outcomes in the clinical realm, and it gives participants the necessary surgical knowledge, skills, and attitudes (KSAs) for collaborative practice.
- Simulation-based training (SBT) is especially conducive to IPE-based activities because of its experiential nature.
- Challenges to implementing IPE can include issues related to logistics, curriculum, and teaching, but solutions exist to help overcome them and succeed in implementation.

## INTRODUCTION

In today's increasingly complex, ever-changing health care system in which the medical knowledge base is doubling at ever-shorter time intervals (ie, from 50 years in 1950

[a] Department of Surgery, LSU Health New Orleans School of Medicine, 1542 Tulane Avenue, Room 734, New Orleans, LA 70112, USA; [b] Department of Graduate Nursing Education, LSU Health New Orleans School of Nursing, 533 Bolivar Street, Room 4A21, New Orleans, LA 70112, USA; [c] Department of Surgery, University of Texas Medical Branch, 301 University Boulevard, Galveston, TX 77555-0737, USA; [d] Department of Respiratory Care, University of Texas Medical Branch, 301 University Boulevard, Galveston, TX 77555-1146, USA
* Corresponding author.
*E-mail address:* jpaige@lsuhsc.edu

Surg Clin N Am 95 (2015) 751–766
http://dx.doi.org/10.1016/j.suc.2015.04.004
0039-6109/15/$ – see front matter 

to 3.5 years in 2010 to a projected 73 days in 2020),[1–4] the physician's role has transformed from the sole practitioner overseeing all aspects of a patient's care to the leader of a team of health care professionals, each contributing their expertise in their scope of practice to help patients on their journey to health. This situation is especially true for surgeons who, thanks to advances in critical care, surgical equipment and techniques, pharmacology, anesthesia, and physical and occupational therapy, are now taking care of more and more challenging patients. As such, the contemporary surgeon must act more like a collaborative team coach than the autonomous captain of a ship. These changing requirements of leadership needed for the ever-evolving health care industry have prompted national organizations to recognize the importance of interprofessional interaction in patient care and to promote more interprofessional training and education. For example, the Institute of Medicine (IOM) made the ability to work in interprofessional teams one of its new core competencies for health care professionals in its seminal work entitled *Health Professions Education: A Bridge to Quality*.[5] This early call for more interprofessional teamwork has been followed by their work entitled *Redesigning Continuing Education in Health Professions* in which the IOM called for transforming continuing education into an interprofessional endeavor focusing on professional development.[3] Thus, interprofessional collaborative practice is now recognized as a critical component of modern day health care, and other prominent health care organizations and associations have begun defining key competencies and requirements for effective care.[6] The need, therefore, for effective IPE using well-designed curricula has become an imperative.

SBT is a powerful educational tool permitting the acquisition of KSAs at both the individual- and team-based level in a safe, nonthreatening learning environment at no risk to a patient.[1] As such, it is an ideal format for bringing together learners from different health care professions in IPE activities at the undergraduate medical education, graduate medical education, and continuing professional development levels. This article looks at the use of SBT for surgical IPE. First, it defines IPE and discusses key competencies and trends related to it. Next, it demonstrates the need for such education by reviewing the less-than-ideal state of teamwork in the surgical environment and interventions to improve it. Third, it reviews representative examples of IPE interventions that have been attempted and their impact. Finally, it discusses key barriers to implementation of simulation-based IPE and potential solutions through a review of one institution's experience in conducting such training.

## INTERPROFESSIONAL EDUCATION: DEFINITIONS AND TRENDS

IPE has taken on increasing importance among health professions educators in their curriculum development and implementation. For example, the Louisiana State University (LSU) Health New Orleans Health Sciences Center, like other health sciences centers, has made IPE the centerpiece of its Quality Enhancement Plan (QEP) for its most recent Southern Association of Colleges and Schools reaccreditation application. Nationally, this increased emphasis on IPE is reflected in the aforementioned IOM reports[3,5] and in the creation of the Interprofessional Education Collaborative (IPEC) in 2009 by 6 prominent national education associations of schools of health professions (ie, the American Association of Colleges of Nurses, the American Association of Colleges of Osteopathic Medicine, the American Association of Colleges of Pharmacy, the American Dental Education Association, the Association of American Medical Colleges, and the Association of Schools and Programs of Public Health) with the stated purpose "to promote and encourage constituent efforts that would advance substantive interprofessional learning experiences to help prepare future health professionals for enhanced team-based care of patients and improved population health outcomes."[7] Even the World Health Organization (WHO) has addressed the topic of IPE with its 2010 work entitled *Framework for Action on Interprofessional Education & Collaborative Practice*.[8]

Clearly, expanding IPE in all the health professions has become a top priority at both national and international levels. This increased attention brings up a pertinent question: what exactly is meant by IPE? (ie, how does one define IPE?). In 2005, D'Amour and Oandasan first promoted the concept of interprofessionality as "the process by which professionals reflect on and develop ways of practicing that provides an integrated and cohesive answer to the needs of the client [read patient]/family/population."[9] The investigators argued that such interprofessionality required "continuous interaction and knowledge sharing between professionals, organized to solve or explore a variety of education and care issues all while seeking to optimize the patient's participation."[9] From the outset, therefore, IPE and interprofessional collaborative practice have been seen as activities that are inherently patient centered in character.

Since this initial definition of interprofessionality, several definitions of IPE have been posited to help clarify what it means and to inform curriculum development and implementation. Reeves and colleagues[2] have defined IPE as "any type of educational training, teaching, or learning session in which two or more health and social care professions are learning interactively." Although useful, this definition does not explicitly detail what is meant by learning interactively. The WHO definition addresses this issue by defining IPE as "[w]hen students from two or more professions learn about, from, and with each other to enable effective collaboration and improve health outcomes."[8]

Thus, IPE has 3 key aspects of interactive learning. Students not only learn with one another but also learn from one another and about each other during an IPE activity. Didactic lectures bringing together students from different professions, therefore, are not in and of themselves sufficient for making an IPE activity. These lectures must be accompanied by opportunities for those students to learn about what the other professions do and to learn from each other. Owing to their inherently interactive and experiential quality, small group discussions and SBT are excellent modalities for this tripartite form of learning. For the WHO, such interactive learning helps prepare students for interprofessional collaborative team-based practice, helping to end the current fragmented nature of health systems.[8]

In 2011, an IPEC-sponsored expert panel published *Core Competencies for Interprofessional Collaborative Practice: Report of an Expert Panel*[6] in which it defined the key competency domains for effective interprofessional collaborative practice among different health professionals. The report differentiated interprofessional collaborative competencies from individual-based professional competencies and common professional competencies in an attempt to demonstrate the at times complementary and confrontational nature of interaction between various professions and the need for collaborative interaction (**Fig. 1**).[6] In addition, it identified the desired underlying principles for these interprofessional collaborative competencies and delineated the need for their creation (**Fig. 2**).[6] Finally, it defined 4 interprofessional collaborative domains with corresponding general and specific competencies (**Fig. 3**).[6] This comprehensive effort aimed at promoting IPE in order to prepare students from all professions to "deliberatively work together" to create a safer, more patient-centered and community-oriented health care system.[6] The IPEC, a US-based organization, is not alone, however, in creating a framework for interprofessional competencies. Such work was actually first untaken in the United Kingdom, and both Canada and Australia have also developed their own versions.[10]

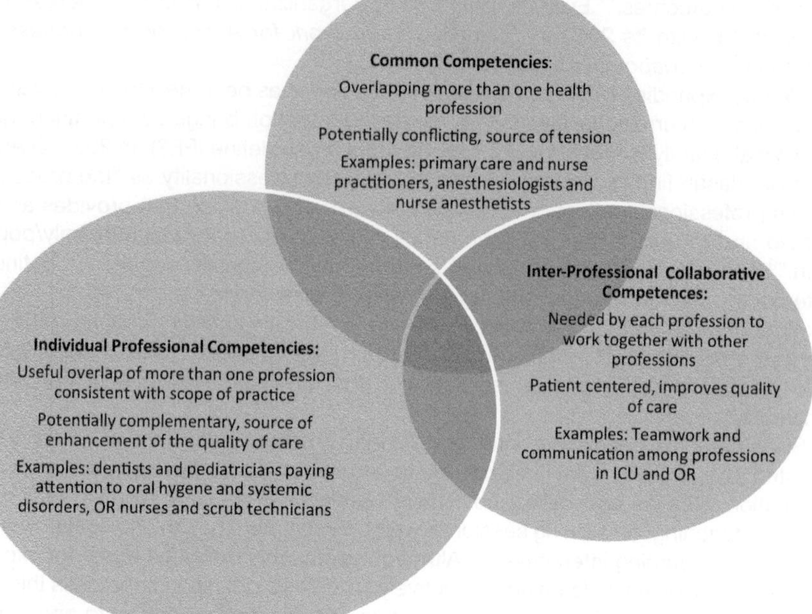


**Fig. 1.** Common, individual professional, and interprofessional collaborative competencies in health care. ICU, intensive care unit; OR, operating room. (*Adapted from* Interprofessional Education Collaborative Expert Panel. Core competencies for interprofessional collaborative practice: report of an expert panel. Washington, DC: Interprofessional Education Collaborative; 2011.)

## TEAMWORK IN THE OPERATING ROOM? WHY INTERPROFESSIONAL EDUCATION IS NEEDED IN SURGICAL PRACTICE

The value of IPE is nowhere more apparent than within the operating room (OR) itself where team dynamics continue to be less than ideal. More often than not, the modern day OR is home to the silo mentality[11] in which multiprofessional interaction is favored over true interprofessional teamwork.[12] This situation fosters a form of tribalism among the various health care professions working in the OR.[13] These attitudes are passed onto and adopted by students who rotate through the environment through the so-called hidden curriculum, thereby perpetuating a team structure characterized more as a team of experts than an expert team.[14]

The flaws in team interaction that result from this toxic OR culture have been known for quite some time and are well documented in the literature.[15] These flaws include a striking lack of communication,[16–18] role confusion,[19,20] heightened tension,[21] and ineffective teamwork[22] stemming from divergent leadership styles,[23] differing perceptions of the quality of professional collaboration,[24,25] less-than-ideal interpersonal skills among the professions,[26] and rigid, unwanted hierarchical structures.[27,28] All these issues combine to impact negatively the surgical care of the patient in the OR, leading to increased technical errors,[29,30] disruptions,[31] distractions,[32] decreased patient safety,[32,33] and increased morbidity and mortality.[34]

Of particular note, surgeons themselves are remarkably oblivious to these issues related to team dynamics, largely due to their privileged status and their traditional

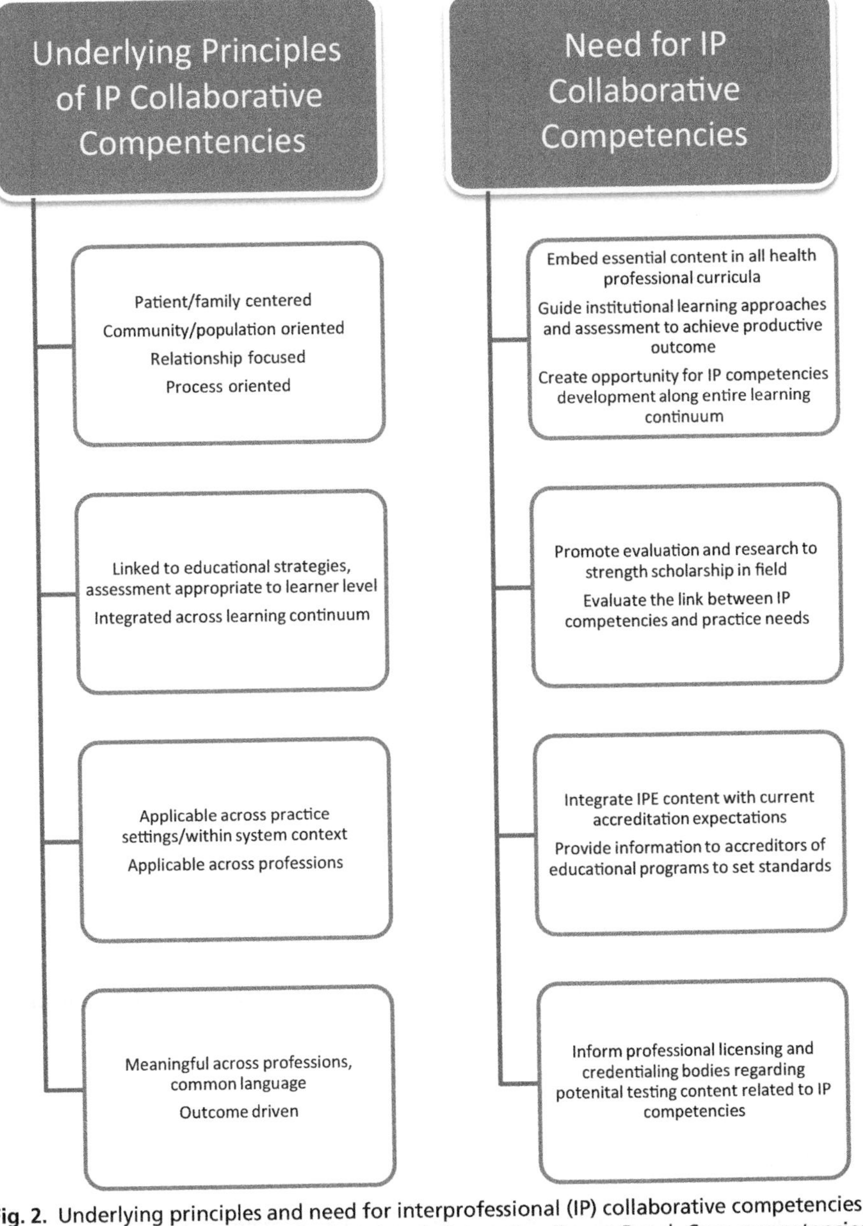


**Fig. 2.** Underlying principles and need for interprofessional (IP) collaborative competencies. (*Adapted from* Interprofessional Education Collaborative Expert Panel. Core competencies for interprofessional collaborative practice: report of an expert panel. Washington, DC: Interprofessional Education Collaborative; 2011.)

position as captain of the ship. For example, they are quite content with the current hierarchical structure.[28] In addition, they consistently give high ratings to the perceived quality of teamwork with other professions in the OR,[24] and, like other professionals in the OR, they tend to overestimate their own performance as team members.[35,36]

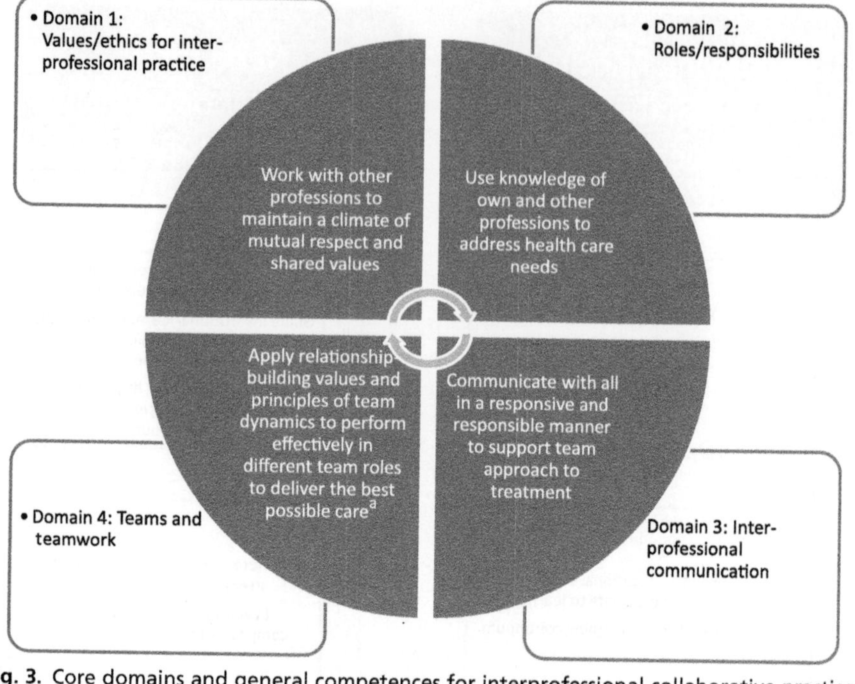


**Fig. 3.** Core domains and general competences for interprofessional collaborative practice. [a] Patient centered, safe, timely, efficient, effective, and equitable. (*Adapted from* Interprofessional Education Collaborative Expert Panel. Core competencies for interprofessional collaborative practice: report of an expert panel. Washington, DC: Interprofessional Education Collaborative; 2011.)

Unfortunately, these issues related to team dynamics extend beyond the OR itself, impacting preoperative and postoperative care. For example, surgical ward and intensive care unit (ICU) nurses are surprisingly unclear of the roles and responsibilities of surgical residents.[37] Information transfer and communication failures occur through the entire continuum of the surgical care of a patient, most commonly during the preprocedural teamwork and postoperative handover phases.[38] Such failures are even apparent between surgical residents and attending surgeons in the management of critical patient events,[39] and they have a negative impact on patient care.[36,40,41]

Clearly, ineffective communication is an endemic problem in the surgical care of the patient, and it can manifest itself in many guises. Information can be misunderstood, not heard, or given at the inappropriate time (ie, too soon or too late).[42] In addition, it can cause confusion or be delivered in an ambiguous manner, leading to a hint-and-hope situation (ie, the initiator of the communication hinting at a problem without explicitly stating the concern and hoping that the true meaning of the communication will be discerned by the recipient).[42] Fortunately, the need for its improvement, both at the team and patient level, is acknowledged by national stakeholders in the surgical care of the patient.[43]

Several teaching and training modalities are available for improving teamwork along the entire continuum of the surgical care of the patient. Briefings/huddles,[44] checklists [eg, team strategies and tools to enhance performance and patient safety (TeamSTEPPS)],[45] team training programs (eg, TeamSTEPPS),[46] and SBT[47] have all been successfully used to enhance teamwork, reduce malpractice rates, and impact positively process and outcome measures related to surgical patient care. IPE is yet another strategy that can help create highly reliable surgical teams.

## INTERPROFESSIONAL EDUCATION INTERVENTIONS IN THE LITERATURE: EFFECTIVENESS AND REPRESENTATIVE SIMULATION-BASED EXAMPLES

One reason for the increasing focus and attention on developing and implementing IPE-based curricula is their potentially far-reaching impact on the health care system. George Thibault of the Josiah Macy, Jr. Foundation sees IPE as a useful tool to help achieve the Institute for Healthcare Improvement's triple aim of improving patient care, improving health outcomes, and creating more efficient and affordable systems of care.[48] This view is supported in part by a series of systematic reviews[49–51] published by The Cochrane Collaboration, which looked at the effectiveness of IPE on health outcomes over the course of a decade. From a dearth of quality studies and strong evidence in 2001,[49] the IPE literature has grown to demonstrate its effectiveness in several different clinical settings (**Table 1**).[50,51] In addition, an earlier Best Evidence in Medical Education guide on interprofessional education found that IPE was well received by learners and aided in them acquiring the necessary knowledge and skills needed for collaborative working, but it seemed to have less of an impact on other service delivery team members' attitudes and perceptions.[52] Other investigators have also found evidence of a reduction in errors[53,54] and less stereotyping[55] as a result of IPE interventions. Adequately trained faculty and staff are necessary, however, in order to achieve successful outcomes related to IPE activities.[52]

The immersive, experiential nature of SBT lends itself to IPE-based activities at all stages of professional development. In addition, simulation-based IPE activities have been shown to enhance interprofessional competencies among prelicensure students,[56] improve students' team-based attitudes[57–60] and perceptions of collaboration,[59,61–65] and enhance students' team-based performance.[66–69] In surgery, IPE-based SBT has been used to train students, residents, and practitioners in the OR,[15,69,70] postoperative,[71,72] and trauma settings.[73–75] For example, both student OR teams[69] and trainee OR teams[70] have undergone SBT and demonstrated improved team-based performance. In addition, cardiac surgery teams[71] and trauma

**Table 1**
**Effectiveness of IPE on clinical practice and health care outcomes**

| Clinical Setting/Patient Population | Positive Findings |
|---|---|
| Emergency Department | Improved culture<br>Improved patient satisfaction<br>Improved collaborative team behavior<br>Reduced error rate of teams |
| Domestic Violence Victims | Improved management of care delivered |
| Mental Health | Improved competencies related to delivery of patient care |
| Diabetic Patients | Improved delivery of patient care |
| Operating Room | Improved collaborative team behavior |

*Data from* Reeves S, Zwarenstein M, Goldman J, et al. Interprofessional education: effects on professional practice and health care outcomes. Cochrane Database Syst Rev 2008;(1):CD002213; and Reeves S, Perrier L, Goldman J, et al. Interprofessional education: effects on professional practice and healthcare outcomes (update). Cochrane Database Syst Rev 2013;(3):CD002213.

teams[73] have demonstrated improvement in the perception of team performance and actual clinical performance, respectively. Finally, the American College of Surgeons (ACS) Accredited Education Institutes have described several best practice examples of IPE-based SBT, including the development of an interprofessional macrosystem simulation for testing a new facility, team training programs for the OR and in obstetrics, an IPE collaborative curriculum between nursing and medical schools, and a standardized training program to recognize deteriorating patients.[76] These examples demonstrate that IPE benefits are as apparent in surgical training and education as in health care overall.

## CHALLENGES AND SOLUTIONS TO IMPLEMENTING SIMULATION-BASED INTERPROFESSIONAL EDUCATION

Clearly, much has already been accomplished related to the use of simulation-based IPE in surgical education with positive impacts. Such accomplishments are even more impressive given the unique barriers and challenges to implementation that IPE-based activities present. Trying to bring together a diverse group of learners with different agendas, schedules, attitudes, perceptions, and talents can be daunting and can lead to a premature end of an IPE endeavor before it even starts. Knowing how to approach such issues is critical to achieve a successful implementation and ensure success.

Challenges to implementing an IPE-based activity can seem myriad initially. A recent systematic review,[77] however, classified commonly encountered barriers/challenges in IPE-based activities into 10 broad categories and suggested potential solutions: curriculum, leadership, resources, attitudes and stereotypes, students' characteristics, IPE concept, teaching, enthusiasm, profession jargons, and accreditation (**Table 2**).[77] Another systematic review[78] on IPE in prelicensure allied health identified power and status differentials among professions, time constraints, limited student knowledge regarding their professional role, and issues of placement of the IPE in the curriculum as barriers to effectiveness. Finally, an IOM publication on IPE for collaboration[48] enumerated the following 5 main categories of barriers to IPE implementation:

1. Logistical challenges (ie, matching learners, having adequate space)
2. Curriculum content (ie, finding suitable topic, having appropriate content, combating the hidden curriculum)
3. Culture (ie, entrenched views and attitudes)
4. Leadership (ie, lack of support, lack of champion)
5. Faculty development (ie, need to prepare faculty to teach IPE)

This publication identified the following 6 solutions to address these issues:

1. Support and leadership from top administrators
2. Extensive planning
3. Distributed IPE experiences throughout the educational experience
4. Avoiding IPE as end in itself (ie, make it accomplish something worthwhile and beneficial)
5. Use of new technologies to implement
6. Major commitment from faculty

How do such barriers and solutions apply to implementing simulation-based IPE? The authors' experiences have demonstrated similar themes and solutions related to IPE activities using SBT. At the LSU Health New Orleans Health Sciences Center,

**Table 2**
**Commonly encountered barriers/challenges to IPE implementation and possible solutions**

| Category | Issues | Solutions |
| --- | --- | --- |
| Curriculum | Integration into existing academic framework, scheduling, timing, content, rigidity of curriculum | Involve faculty and students in curriculum development, make IPE part of existing core curricula, involve leadership in addressing time and scheduling issues, create flexible curricula, obtain feedback from students and faculty |
| Leadership | Lack of or weak leadership | Identify and promote champions of IPE to lead endeavor, create institutional agreements for sustainability, have IPE committee to help with planning |
| Resources | Funding, distance, infrastructure | Integrate IPE into existing curricula to decrease costs, promote positive results to gain funding/support, use existing infrastructure, keep class size small, use Web-designed IPE |
| Attitudes and stereotypes | Negative faculty- and student-held beliefs and attitudes toward other professions, institutional barriers between different professional schools | Institute faculty development programs; involve professional organizations, deans, and faculty leaders to break down organizational/institutional barriers; identify own biases as faculty |
| Students' characteristics | Different learning needs and funds of knowledge, backgrounds, diverse populations | Address different learning needs and diversity, use problem-based learning |
| IPE concept | Implementation based on institution and thus different, lack of standardized conception of IPE, unclear expectations | Create clear curriculum integrated into calendar year, address misconceptions quickly, explain IPE goals |
| Teaching | Large classes, differing skills and knowledge among faculty of different professions, lack of background knowledge of students | Provide faculty development related to IPE teaching, encourage adequate preparation by faculty, ensure that student backgrounds are known to faculty |
| Enthusiasm | Students and faculty not engaged because IPE came from "above"; loss of interest at administrative level | Create incentives for students and faculty, promote continual training of faculty to keep involvement, involve deans/institutional leaders |
| Profession jargons | Unfamiliar jargon used by different professions | Explain jargon/terms to students and faculty beforehand, provide printed material explaining important terms |
| Accreditation | Lack of existence of a body to accredit IPE courses | Set regional or national accreditation bodies for IPE |

*Adapted from* Sunguya BF, Hinthong W, Jimba M, et al. Interprofessional education for whom? — challenges and lessons learned from its implementation in developed countries and their application to developing countries: a systematic review. PLoS One 2014;9(5):e96724.

the major barriers encountered to implementation of IPE activities within the prelicensure curricula of the Schools of Nursing and Medicine fell under 3 main categories: logistics, curriculum, and support. Each of these categories contained a 3-fold list of challenges. From a logistic standpoint, faculty availability, student scheduling, and student numbers were all major issues. First, incorporating the proper faculty into the sessions was difficult, given their time and scheduling constraints. For example, the computer-based mannequin programmer and operator did not have any free time for a new course in his very busy schedule of third year medical student training sessions on the surgery, medicine, and pediatrics clerkships. To help solve this issue, the interprofessional training was incorporated into the preexisting third year surgery clerkship simulation sessions, which focused on trauma resuscitation, an ideal setting to discuss teamwork. Second, the student schedules in the 2 schools did not overlap. The School of Nursing is semester based in which classes are held from late August to early December in the fall and mid-January to late April in the spring, whereas the School of Medicine schedule for third year students runs year-round and is divided into 4 major blocks. Team training sessions could only be scheduled when the School of Nursing was in session, preventing all the medical students from undergoing the IPE. Attempts are currently underway to expand the IPE to other clerkship training sessions, but they have run into issues of finding faculty within those specialties to assist with the debriefing. Third, the sheer size of School of Nursing classes, which consist of 2 a year, made it hard to include all the students in the initial sessions. To address this problem, simultaneous sessions were held in 2 separate simulation rooms starting in the second year, allowing all nursing students to be scheduled.

Curriculum challenges focused on learners, content, and teaching approaches. From a learner standpoint, determining the ideal ratio of students to optimize learning was important. Having a minimum of 2 from each profession helped to prevent feelings of isolation, and limiting total size to 5 to 6 participants allowed for full participation. Also, determining the appropriate level of student to match the content of the trauma resuscitation was essential. Thus, senior undergraduate nursing students taking intensive care were selected to be matched with the third year surgery clerkship students because the topics of burn management and trauma care were taught to them during the semester. This matching helped increase trust, because the nursing students who had gotten their lectures on the topics often knew more regarding management than the medical students who were getting the information for the first time. Finally, structuring the debriefing to address both the learning objectives related to medical knowledge and patient care aspects of trauma and burn resuscitation as well as teamwork within a very tight time window was difficult. Typically, the care management issues were reviewed first, and then they were tied to how to accomplish them more effectively as a team.

Institutional support issues included funding, faculty time, and administrative patronage. Funding and protected faculty time were in part achieved through applying for and being awarded small in-house Educational Enhancement Grants through the LSU Health New Orleans Academy for the Advancement of Educational Scholarship. For example, the third year medical student and senior undergraduate nursing student training was started as a result of 2011–2012 awarded project entitled Team Training of Inter-Professional Students. These grants paid for disposable supplies for the training and data input. In addition, they were structured to require department head agreement to support the faculty time needed to complete the project. They were a major incentive to complete the project within the timeline submitted and promoted dissemination of findings. Finally, ensuring institutional and stakeholder support was critical. Thus, face-to-face time with course directors was undertaken to "sell" incorporation of the IPE into the existing curricula to ensure cooperation with logistics. In addition, "managing up" was used by announcing victories to help demonstrate worth to the institution.

At the University of Texas Medical Branch (UTMB), as in many institutions, the impetus to accelerate ongoing efforts to integrate IPE into the curricula of medical, nursing, Physician Assistant, Respiratory Therapy (RT), Physical Therapy and Occupational Therapy programs came from the QEP for its Southern Association of Colleges and Schools reaccreditation application. Many programs at UTMB have students rotating at clinically remote sites, further complicating the logistics of offering IPE experiences to all students in a given school or program. Rather than adopting single experiences for all students, UTMB has addressed the challenges of logistics by incorporating IPE into multiple training and education activities, many of which involve SBT. Second year medical students have a 2-week mini-mester in which they are able to choose from a variety of options, many of which offer an early exposure to specialties, or subspecialties within departments. This experience offers an earlier opportunity to try on potential career options than the usual M3 or M4 clinical rotations. Embedded within many of the 2-week curricula are IPE experiences; the surgery mini-mester engages students with students from the RT program in an interactive problem-based learning activity using simulated ventilated patients. In the Respiratory Simulation Lab, small groups of RT and medical students rotate through stations depicting different clinical problems requiring action—adjusting ventilator setting based on interpretation of arterial blood gasses, troubleshooting a high peak airway pressure alarm, and making appropriate ventilator changes in a patient with poor compliance. At the completion of the workshop, students fill out peer assessments based on the competencies identified in the IPEC *Core Competencies for Interprofessional Collaborative Practice* document.[6]

Another example of surgical IPE involves the Prep for Surgical Internship elective, which is offered in collaboration with The ACS/Association of Program Directors in Surgery/Association for Surgical Education Resident Preparatory Curriculum. In this workshop, M4 students work with senior RT students in a more advanced series of clinical problem-solving stations involving human patient simulators connected to ventilators and an active lung simulator. Along with faculty facilitators, who are ICU physicians and respiratory therapists, students collaboratively initiate mechanical ventilation and determine ventilator settings for a simulated patient arriving in the ICU from a long OR case; they initiate a wean from mechanical ventilation trial and interpret blood gasses and weaning parameters to decide if the patient should be extubated. Students troubleshoot a low minute ventilation alarm in a patient who recently underwent lung resection. Again, as part of the workshop, they evaluate their small group peers on IPE competencies and receive feedback on their own performance as assessed by peers.

These IPE experiences are very well rated by participating students and faculty. Ongoing challenges include support for the labor- and resource-intensive SBT activities and incorporating IPE into enough activities so that all students are adequately trained. In addition, interprofessional practice competencies are not currently part of any summative assessments.

## SUMMARY

IPE involves bringing together 2 or more health profession students to learn with, from, and about each other. Core interprofessional competencies have been described and fall into 4 major domains: (1) values/ethics for interprofessional practice, (2) roles/responsibilities, (3) interprofessional communication, and (4) teams and teamwork. The need for IPE in surgery is highlighted by the fact that teamwork is currently less than ideal, negatively impacting patient care. IPE has demonstrated effectiveness in improving professional practice and health outcomes. SBT is an ideal methodology for IPE given its safe, experiential nature. Implementing IPE presents unique challenges related to bringing together learners from different professions, which can be overcome by following solutions that others have successfully used.

## REFERENCES


1. Beaubien JM, Baker DP. The use of simulation for training teamwork skills in health care: how low can you go? Qual Saf Health Care 2004;13:51–6.
2. Reeves S, Rice K, Conn LG, et al. Interprofessional interaction, negotiation and non-negotiation on general internal medicine wards. J Interprof Care 2009; 23(6):633–45.
3. IOM (Institute of Medicine). Redesigning continuing education in the health professions. Washington, DC: The National Academies Press; 2010.
4. Densen P. Challenges and opportunities facing medical education. Trans Am Clin Climatol Assoc 2011;122:48–58.
5. Greiner AC, Knebel E, editors. Health professions education: a bridge to quality. Washington, DC: Institute of Medicine, National Academies Press; 2003.
6. Interprofessional Education Collaborative Expert Panel. Core competencies for interprofessional collaborative practice: report of an expert panel. Washington, DC: Interprofessional Education Collaborative; 2011.
7. Inter-Professional Education Collaborative. About IPEC. Available at: https://ipecollaborative.org/About_IPEC.html. Accessed February 3, 2015.
8. World Health Organization (WHO). Framework for action on interprofessional education & collaborative practice. Geneva (Switzerland): World Health Organization; 2010. Available at: http://whqlibdoc.who.int/hq/2010/WHO_HRH_HPN_10.3_eng.pdf. Accessed February 3, 2015.
9. D'Amour D, Oandasan I. Interprofessionality as the field of interprofessional practice and interprofessional education: An emerging concept. J Interprof Care 2005;19(Supp1 1):8–10.
10. Thistlethwaite JE, Forman D, Matthews LR, et al. Competencies and frameworks in interprofessional education: a comparative analysis. Acad Med 2014;89(6): 869–75.
11. Bleakley A. You are who I say you are: the rhetorical construction of identity in the operating theatre. J Workplace Learn 2006;18(7–8):414–25.
12. Bleakley A, Boyden J, Hobbs A, et al. Improving teamwork climate in operating theatres: the shift from multiprofessionalism to interprofessionalism. J Interprof Care 2006;20(5):461–70.
13. Gillespie BM, Chaboyer W, Wallis M, et al. Why isn't 'time out' being implemented? An exploratory study. Qual Saf Health Care 2010;19:103–6.
14. Burke CS, Salas E, Wilson-Donnelly K, et al. How to turn a team of experts into an expert medical team: guidance from the aviation and military communities. Qual Saf Health Care 2004;13(Suppl 1):i96–104.
15. Paige JT. Surgical team training: promoting high reliability with nontechnical skills. Surg Clin North Am 2010;90(3):569–81.
16. Lingard L, Espin S, Whyte S, et al. Communication failures in the operating room: an observational classification of recurrent types and effects. Qual Saf Health Care 2004;13:330–4.

17. Halverson AL, Casey JT, Andersson J, et al. Communication failure in the operating room. Surgery 2011;149(3):305–10.
18. Sevdalis N, Wong HW, Arora S, et al. Quantitative analysis of intraoperative communication in open and laparoscopic surgery. Surg Endosc 2012;26(10): 2931–8.
19. Lingard L, Reznick R, DeVito I, et al. Forming professional identities on the health care team: discursive constructions of the 'other' in the operating room. Med Educ 2002;36:728–34.
20. Flin R, Yule S, McKenzie L, et al. Attitudes to teamwork and safety in the operating theatre. Surgeon 2006;4:145–51.
21. Lingard L, Garwood S, Poenaru D. Tensions influencing operating room team function: does institutional context make a difference? Med Educ 2004;38:691–9.
22. Sexton JB, Thomas EJ, Helmreich RL. Error, stress, and teamwork in medicine and aviation: cross sectional surveys. BMJ 2000;320:745–9.
23. McDonald R, Waring J, Harrison S, et al. Rules and guidelines in clinical practice: a qualitative study in operating theatres of doctors' and nurses' views. Qual Saf Health Care 2005;14:290–4.
24. Makary MA, Sexton JB, Freischlag JA, et al. Operating room teamwork among physicians and nurses: teamwork in the eye of the beholder. J Am Coll Surg 2006;202:746–52.
25. Carney BT, West P, Neily J, et al. Differences in nurse and surgeon perceptions of teamwork: implications for use of a briefing checklist in the OR. AORN J 2010;91: 722–9.
26. Nestel D, Kidd JM. Nurses' perceptions and experiences of communication in the operating theatre: a focus group interview. BMC Nurs 2006;5:1.
27. Helmrich RL, Davies JM. Team performance in the operating room. In: Bogner MS, editor. Human error in medicine. Hillside (NJ): Erlbaum; 1994. p. 225–53.
28. Undre S, Sevdalis N, Healy AN, et al. Teamwork in the operating theatre: cohesion or confusion? J Eval Clin Pract 2006;12:182–9.
29. Mishra A, Catchpole K, Dale T, et al. The influence of non-technical performance on technical outcome in laparoscopic cholecystectomy. Surg Endosc 2008;22(1): 68–73.
30. Hull L, Arora S, Aggarwal R, et al. The impact of nontechnical skills on technical performance in surgery: a systematic review. J Am Coll Surg 2012;214:214–30.
31. Rosenstein AH, O'Daniel M. Impact and implications of disruptive behavior in the perioperative arena. J Am Coll Surg 2006;203:96–105.
32. Sevdalis N, Undre S, McDermott J, et al. Impact of intraoperative distractions on patient safety: a prospective descriptive study using validated instruments. World J Surg 2014;38(4):751–8.
33. Christian CK, Gustafson ML, Roth EM, et al. A prospective study of patient safety in the operating room. Surgery 2006;139:159–73.
34. Mazzocco K, Petitti DB, Fong KT, et al. Surgical team behaviors and patient outcomes. Am J Surg 2009;197:678–85.
35. Paige JT, Aaron DL, Yang T, et al. Implementation of a preoperative briefing protocol improves accuracy of teamwork assessment in the operating room. Am Surg 2008;74:817–23.
36. Moorthy K, Munz Y, Adams S, et al. Self-assessment of performance among surgical trainees during simulated procedures in a simulated operating theater. Am J Surg 2006;192:114–8.
37. Schlitzkus LL, Agle SC, McNally MM, et al. What do surgical nurses know about surgical residents? J Surg Educ 2009;66(6):383–91.

38. Nagpal K, Vats A, Ahmed K, et al. An evaluation of information transfer through the continuum of surgical care: a feasibility study. Ann Surg 2010;252(2):402–7.
39. ElBardissi AW, Regenbogen SE, Greenberg CC, et al. Communication practices on 4 Harvard surgical services: a surgical safety collaborative. Ann Surg 2009; 250(6):861–5.
40. Nagpal K, Vats A, Lamb B, et al. Information transfer and communication in surgery: a systematic review. Ann Surg 2010;252(2):225–39.
41. Symons NR, Almoudaris AM, Nagpal K, et al. An observational study of the frequency, severity, and etiology of failures in postoperative care after major elective general surgery. Ann Surg 2013;257(1):1–5.
42. Yule S, Paterson-Brown S. Surgeons' non-technical skills. Surg Clin North Am 2012;92(1):37–50.
43. Kim S, Dunkin BJ, Paige JT, et al. What is the future of training in surgery? Needs assessment of national stakeholders. Surgery 2014;156(3):707–17.
44. Paige JT, Aaron DL, Yang T, et al. Improved operating room teamwork via SAFETY prep: a rural community hospital's experience. World J Surg 2009;33(6):1181–7.
45. Haynes AB, Weiser TG, Berry WR, et al, Safe Surgery Saves Lives Study Group. A surgical safety checklist to reduce morbidity and mortality in a global population. N Engl J Med 2009;360(5):491–9.
46. Armour Forse R, Bramble JD, McQuillan R. Team training can improve operating room performance. Surgery 2011;150(4):771–8.
47. Arriaga AF, Gawande AA, Raemer DB, et al, Harvard Surgical Safety Collaborative. Pilot testing of a model for insurer-driven, large-scale multicenter simulation training for operating room teams. Ann Surg 2014;259(3):403–10.
48. IOM (Institute of Medicine). Interprofessional education for collaboration: learning how to improve health from interprofessional models across the continuum of education to practice: workshop summary. Washington, DC: The National Academies Press; 2013.
49. Zwarenstein M, Reeves S, Barr H, et al. Interprofessional education: effects on professional practice and health care outcomes. Cochrane Database Syst Rev 2001;(1):CD002213.
50. Reeves S, Zwarenstein M, Goldman J, et al. Interprofessional education: effects on professional practice and health care outcomes. Cochrane Database Syst Rev 2008;(1):CD002213.
51. Reeves S, Perrier L, Goldman J, et al. Interprofessional education: effects on professional practice and healthcare outcomes (update). Cochrane Database Syst Rev 2013;(3):CD002213.
52. Hammick M, Freeth D, Koppel I, et al. A best evidence systematic review of interprofessional education: BEME Guide no. 9. Med Teach 2007;29(8):735–51.
53. Barr H, Freeth D, Hammick M, et al. The evidence base and recommendations for interprofessional education in health and social care. J Interprof Care 2006;20:75–8.
54. Thistlethwaite J, Moran M, World Health Organization Study Group on Interprofessional Education and Collaborative Practice. Learning outcomes for interprofessional education (IPE): literature review and synthesis. J Interprof Care 2010;24:503–13.
55. Ateah CA, Snow W, Wener P, et al. Stereotyping as a barrier to collaboration: Does interprofessional education make a difference? Nurse Educ Today 2011; 31:208–13.
56. Murdoch NL, Bottorff JL, McCullough D. Simulation education approaches to enhance collaborative healthcare: a best practices review. Int J Nurs Educ Scholarsh 2014;10.

57. Hobgood C, Sherwood G, Frush K, et al. Teamwork training with nursing and medical students: does method matter? Results of an interinstitutional, interdisciplinary collaboration. Qual Saf Health Care 2010;19(6):e25.
58. Stewart M, Kennedy N, Cuene-Grandidier H. Undergraduate interprofessional education using high-fidelity paediatric simulation. Clin Teach 2010;7:90–6.
59. Sigalet E, Donnon T, Grant V. Undergraduate students' perceptions of and attitudes toward a simulation-based interprofessional curriculum. Simul Healthc 2012;7:353–8.
60. Brock D, Abu-Rish E, Chiu CR, et al. Interprofessional education in team communication: working together to improve patient safety. BMJ Qual Saf 2013;22:414–23.
61. Whelan JJ, Spencer JF, Rooney K. A 'RIPPER' project: advancing rural interprofessional health education at the University of Tasmania. Rural Remote Health 2008;8:1017.
62. Dillon PM, Noble KA, Kaplan L. Simulation as a means to foster collaborative interdisciplinary education. Nurs Educ Perspect 2009;30:87–90.
63. Reese CE, Jeffries PR, Engum SA. Learning together: simulation to develop nursing and medical student collaboration. Nurs Educ Perspect 2011;31:33–7.
64. Vyas D, McCulloh R, Dyer C, et al. An interprofessional course using human patient simulation to teach patient safety and teamwork skills. Am J Pharm Educ 2012;76:71.
65. Liaw SY, Zhou WT, Lau TC, et al. An interprofessional communication training using simulation to enhance safe care for a deteriorating patient. Nurse Educ Today 2014;34(2):259–64.
66. Jankoukas TS, Haidet KK, Hupcey JE, et al. Targeted crisis resource management training improves performance among randomized nursing and medical students. Simul Healthc 2011;6:316–26.
67. Garbee DD, Paige JT, Bonanno L, et al. Effectiveness of teamwork and communication education using an interprofessional high-fidelity human patient simulation critical care code. J Nurs Educ Pract 2013;3:1–12.
68. Sigalet E, Donnon T, Cheng A, et al. Development of a team performance scale to assess undergraduate health professionals. Acad Med 2013;88(7):989–96.
69. Paige JT, Garbee DD, Kozmenko V, et al. Getting a head start: high-fidelity, simulation-based operating room team training of interprofessional students. J Am Coll Surg 2014;218(1):140–9.
70. Boet S, Bould MD, Sharma B, et al. Within-team debriefing versus instructor-led debriefing for simulation-based education: a randomized controlled trial. Ann Surg 2013;258(1):53–8.
71. Stevens LM, Cooper JB, Raemer DB, et al. Educational program in crisis management for cardiac surgery teams including high realism simulation. J Thorac Cardiovasc Surg 2012;144(1):17–24.
72. Paull DE, Deleeuw LD, Wolk S, et al. The effect of simulation-based crew resource management training on measurable teamwork and communication among interprofessional teams caring for postoperative patients. J Contin Educ Nurs 2013;44(11):516–24.
73. Capella J, Smith S, Philp A, et al. Teamwork training improves the clinical care of trauma patients. J Surg Educ 2010;67(6):439–43.
74. Ziesmann MT, Widder S, Park J, et al. S.T.A.R.T.T.: development of a national, multidisciplinary trauma crisis resource management curriculum-results from the pilot course. J Trauma Acute Care Surg 2013;75(5):753–8.

75. Doumouras AG, Keshet I, Nathens AB, et al. Trauma Non-Technical Training (TNT-2): the development, piloting and multilevel assessment of a simulation-based, interprofessional curriculum for team-based trauma resuscitation. Can J Surg 2014;57(5):354–5.
76. Seymour NE, Cooper JB, Farley DR, et al. Best practices in interprofessional education and training in surgery: experiences from American College of Surgeons-Accredited Education Institutes. Surgery 2013;154(1):1–12.
77. Sunguya BF, Hinthong W, Jimba M, et al. Interprofessional education for whom? — challenges and lessons learned from its implementation in developed countries and their application to developing countries: a systematic review. PLoS One 2014;9(5):e96724.
78. Olson R, Bialocerkowski A. Interprofessional education in allied health: a systematic review. Med Educ 2014;48:236–46.

# Current Status of Simulation-Based Training in Graduate Medical Education

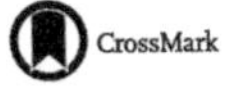

Ross E. Willis, PhD*, Kent R. Van Sickle, MD

**KEYWORDS**

- Simulation • Technical skills • Proficiency-based training • Virtual reality
- Nontechnical skills

**KEY POINTS**

- The use of simulation in Graduate Medical Education (GME) has changed significantly in the past decade; this has been largely due to advances in technology and a fundamental shift in the principles and delivery of medical education.
- New requirements and mandates by governing bodies and accreditation organizations in GME have influenced the adoption of simulation.
- The most common application of simulation in GME is in technical skills. However, simulation can also be used to teach nontechnical skills.
- Simulation has become a cornerstone in the delivery of surgical education; several national curricula have been established and are based on integrating simulation into the educational curricula.
- The field of simulation in health care continues to grow; local, state, and national organizations and consortia have been established and are creating networks to foster research and collaborative efforts.

## INTRODUCTION

The role of simulation in the current environment of GME has experienced a substantial transformation during the past decade. There has been a major paradigm shift in the format of medical teaching, highlighted by the incorporation of problem-based learning into the curricula of medical schools.[1] GME has likewise shifted, from the traditional apprenticeship model to more directed clinical skills training.[2] Concurrently, the nature of health care delivery in the United States has changed substantially during

---

Disclosures: K.R. Van Sickle, MD: Covidien (speaking, teaching, honoraria); Intuitive Surgical (speaking, teaching, honoraria).
Department of Surgery, University of Texas Health Science Center at San Antonio, 7703 Floyd Curl Drive, MC 7737, San Antonio, TX 78229, USA
* Corresponding author.
*E-mail address:* willisr@uthscsa.edu

Surg Clin N Am 95 (2015) 767–779
http://dx.doi.org/10.1016/j.suc.2015.04.009 **surgical.theclinics.com**
0039-6109/15/$ – see front matter 

the same period, particularly affecting resident supervision and autonomy. These changes have created gaps in training, and the use of simulation has been expanded to help bridge these gaps. The accessibility and fidelity of simulation have clearly benefited from the technological advances of the Digital Age and will continue to grow in the future.

Simulation has long been used in various fields of medicine.[3,4] Advocates of simulation-based training in medical education posit that patient safety is improved when residents practice on simulators before performing procedures and operations on actual patients. There is a growing body of research that confirms the benefits of simulation-based training in terms of skill development and transfer of these skills to actual patients.[5–14]

Perhaps one of the most significant studies demonstrating the effectiveness of simulation-based training involved using a virtual reality (VR) platform (the Minimally Invasive Surgery Trainer—Virtual Reality, or MIST-VR) to train junior residents' basic technical skills, followed by operative performance assessment of a laparoscopic cholecystectomy.[5] This study was known as the VR to OR study; strict training criteria were established by experienced minimally invasive surgeons, and operative performance assessment was done by a blinded, 2-reviewer method comparing VR-trained to control subjects. This study was one of the first to demonstrate that a simulation-based training curriculum in an inanimate skills laboratory translated into improved performance in a real-world operating room environment.

## MANDATES

Empirical data showing the benefit of simulation-based training coupled with recent fundamental changes in the delivery of GME and the implementation of various mandates for the inclusion of simulation-based training into surgical residency programs have accelerated the application of simulation in today's training curricula.

In 2006, members of the Residency Review Committee for Surgery (RRC-S) voted unanimously to require simulation training in surgery residency programs.[15] Programs were given 2 years to incorporate simulation-based skills education into their residency training curricula, with the understanding that these requirements could be met with low-tech simulators (eg, laparoscopic box trainers).[15]

In 2009, the American Board of Surgery (ABS) required all surgeons seeking board certification to have successfully passed the Fundamentals of Laparoscopic Surgery (FLS) examination. The FLS examination comprises 2 sections, a multiple choice examination that assesses basic knowledge of laparoscopic surgery and a manual skills examination that assesses technical performance on 5 exercises using inanimate objects placed in a laparoscopic box trainer.

Recently, the ABS mandated completion of the Flexible Endoscopy Curriculum (FEC) as a requirement for all general surgery residents graduating in the 2017–18 academic year and beyond. The FEC is designed to provide general surgery training programs with a stepwise, milestone-based curriculum that includes both didactic and hands-on training. On the successful completion of the FEC, a general surgery resident should possess the knowledge and skill to be a surgical endoscopist with the ability to provide endoscopic services to patients in any clinical setting. The FEC culminates in passing the Fundamentals of Endoscopic Surgery (FES) certification examination to be eligible to take the ABS certifying examination. The FES examination comprises 2 sections: A multiple-choice knowledge test and a technical skills examination on 5 exercises using the GI Mentor II (Simbionix USA, Cleveland, OH, USA) endoscopy simulator.

Also under development by the Society of American Gastrointestinal and Endoscopic Surgeons (SAGES) is the Fundamentals of Robotic Surgery (FRS). With a focus specifically on robotic surgery, this platform is equivalent to FLS and FES and has both knowledge and skills components in the program. FRS is expected to be formally released within the next 12 to 24 months, and it is unclear at this time whether it will become a mandatory training or credentialing requirement for robotic privileges. Given the success and impact of FLS and the inclusion of FES as a new mandate, however, it would seem likely.

## PREPARING MEDICAL STUDENTS FOR RESIDENCY

Surgery residents often begin internship with a widely variable fund of knowledge and technical skills.[16] Many institutions have implemented preparatory curricula, often colloquially referred to as boot camps, for senior medical students who are interested in pursuing surgery residencies or for first-year surgery residents.

Numerous boot camps have been reported in the literature and include low-fidelity simulation models to teach knot tying and suturing,[17–23] airway management,[19,20,22–24] central venous catheterization,[17,18,20–24] chest tubes,[17,18,20–24] and basic laparoscopy skills.[17–21,23] Higher-fidelity simulation models have been used to teach basic endoscopy skills[22] and resuscitation management.[19,24,25] Software-based simulators have been used to teach arrhythmia recognition[20,25] and patient management scenarios.[26] Standardized patients and nurses have been called upon to simulate nursing pages that interns frequently encounter.[18,19] Human cadavers have been used to teach anatomy.[17,19,22,23] These studies have demonstrated immediate increases in self-reported comfort and confidence,[17,19,22–24] technical skills,[17,20,21,23] and knowledge.[18,20,23,26]

As evident by the number of existing boot camps, preparatory curricula for medical students pursuing general surgery residencies are widely variable in terms of content, duration, and timing of deployment. In 2014, members of the American College of Surgeons (ACS) and Association for Surgical Education (ASE) conducted a survey of clerkship directors and medical students to identify gaps in medical students' knowledge and skills needed for surgery clerkships and residency.[27] The needs analysis resulted in a list of topics that are recommended for inclusion in the first 3 years of the medical school curriculum (**Table 1**). The curriculum is freely available on the ACS Web site at https://www.facs.org/education/program/simulation-based.

In addition to a standardized curriculum to be included in the first 3 years of medical school, a collaborative effort among the ACS, ASE, and Association of Program Directors in Surgery (APDS) is developing a resident preparatory curriculum that can be used to standardize content delivered in boot camps to fourth-year medical students who will be entering surgical residencies. The curriculum is currently being pilot tested at several institutions and will be freely available in the spring of 2015 (https://www.facs.org/education/program/resident-prep).

## NATIONAL SURGERY RESIDENT SKILLS CURRICULUM

Following the RRC-S mandate that all surgery residency programs "must include simulation and skills laboratories" (program requirement II.D.2), the ACS and the APDS released the Surgery Resident Skills Curriculum in 2007. The goals of the curriculum were to synchronize curriculum development efforts, share curricula with training programs, and standardize simulation-based training efforts among residency programs.[28] The ACS/APDS Surgery Resident Skills Curriculum was released in 3 phases, with the first phase introduced in 2007. Phases 1 and 2 focus on acquiring

**Table 1**
**ACS/ASE simulation-based training curriculum for years 1 to 3 of medical school**

| Year 1 Modules | Year 2 Modules | Year 3 Modules |
|---|---|---|
| Abdominal Examination | Basic Airway Management | Arterial Puncture and Blood Gas |
| Basic Vascular Examination | Communication—History and Physical, and Case Presentation | Basic Knot Tying |
| Breast Examination | Foley Bladder Catheterization | Basic Suturing |
| Digital Rectal Examination | Intermediate Vascular Examination | Central Venous Line Insertion |
| Female Pelvic Examination | Nasogastric Tubes | Communication—During Codes, and Safe and Effective Handoffs |
| Male Groin and Genital Examination | Sterile Technique—Gloving and Gowning | Intermediate Airway |
| Universal Precautions | Surgical Drains—Care and Removal | Intraosseous IV |
| Venipuncture and Peripheral IV | — | Local Anesthetics |
| — | — | Paracentesis |
| — | — | Thoracentesis |

*Abbreviation:* IV, intravenous.

*Data from* American College of Surgeons. Medical student simulation-based surgical skills curriculum. Available at: https://www.facs.org/education/program/simulation-based. Accessed May 5, 2014.

technical skills, whereas phase 3 focuses on nontechnical (ie, team-based) skills. A listing of the modules in each phase is presented in **Table 2**. The curriculum is freely available on the ACS Web site at https://www.facs.org/education/program/apds-resident.

## TECHNICAL SKILLS

One of the more significant changes in which technical skills are taught to surgery trainees has been the move away from the traditional time- or repetition-based methods in favor of proficiency-based training (PBT). PBT is based on the construct of deliberate practice,[29] which is defined as providing learners with specific goals and ample opportunities for immediate feedback after each practice trial. Previous research comparing time-, repetition-, and proficiency-based training protocols has shown that learners who practice according to the proficiency-based protocol achieve higher levels of performance with little variability among trainees, even when total training time and repetitions are held constant among these training protocols.[30]

Proficiency metrics have been established and validated for many surgical tasks, such as knot tying and suturing,[31,32] laparoscopic skills,[33] and endoscopic skills,[34] and continue to add to the growing body of data supporting the use of simulation-based training in GME.

### *Knot Tying and Suturing*

The University of Texas Southwestern developed a cost-effective, proficiency-based basic open knot tying and suturing curriculum in 2007[31,35] using inexpensive, commercially available, low-fidelity models. This curriculum comprises 12 core surgical skills, including instrument handling, various one- and two-handed knot-tying

**Table 2**
**ACS/APDS surgery resident skills curriculum**

| Phase 1 | Phase 2 | Phase 3 |
|---|---|---|
| 1. Asepsis and Instrument Identification | 1. Laparoscopic Ventral Hernia Repair | 1. Module for Faculty |
| 2. Knot Tying | 2. Laparoscopic Right Colon Resection | 2. Teamwork in the Trauma Bay |
| 3. Sutures and Suturing Techniques | 3. Laparoscopic Sigmoid Resection | 3. Postoperative Hypotension |
| 4. Tissue Handling, Dissection, and Wound Closure | 4. Open Right Colon Resection | 4. Laparoscopic Crisis |
| 5. Advanced Tissue Handling: Skin Grafts and Flaps | 5. Laparoscopic and Open Common Bile Duct Exploration | 5. The Preoperative Briefing |
| 6. Urethral and Suprapubic Catheterization | 6. Laparoscopic Ventral/ Incisional Hernia Repair | 6. Laparoscopic Troubleshooting |
| 7. Airway Management | 7. Laparoscopic Appendectomy | 7. Postoperative Pulmonary Embolus |
| 8. Chest Tube and Thoracentesis | 8. Porcine Laparoscopic Nissen Fundoplication Laboratory | 8. Postoperative MI (Cardiogenic Shock) |
| 9. Arterial and Venous Catheterization | 9. Sentinel Lymph Node Mapping and Axillary Lymph Node Dissection | 9. Latex Allergy Anaphylaxis |
| 10. Surgical Biopsy Techniques | 10. Open Repair of Inguinal and Femoral Hernias | 10. Patient Handoff |
| 11. Arterial Anastomosis | 11. Laparoscopic Inguinal Hernia Repair | 11. Retained Sponge on Postoperative Chest Radiograph |
| 12. Laparotomy Opening and Closure | 12. Laparoscopic/Open Splenectomy | |
| 13. Principles of Bone Fixation and Casting | 13. Laparoscopic and Open Cholecystectomy | |
| 14. Introduction to Inguinal Anatomy | 14. Peptic Ulcer Disease and Gastric Resections | |
| 15. Upper Endoscopy | 15. Thyroidectomy and Parathyroidectomy | |
| 16. Colonoscopy Techniques | | |
| 17. Basic Laparoscopic Skills | | |
| 18. Advanced laparoscopic Skills | | |
| 19. Hand-Sewn Gastrointestinal Anastomosis | | |
| 20. Stapled Anastomosis | | |

*Abbreviation:* MI, myocardial infarction.

*Data from* American College of Surgeons. ACS/APDS surgery resident skills curriculum. Available at: https://www.facs.org/education/program/apds-resident. Accessed May 5, 2014.

techniques, and several interrupted and continuous suturing exercises. Goova and colleagues[35] demonstrated educational benefit and construct validity. In 2013, they expanded on this curriculum and released a proficiency-based intermediate open knot tying and suturing curriculum[32] that includes more advanced knot-tying and suturing exercises. Since the inception of these curricula, several other institutions have implemented these curricula with similar results.[36,37]

### *Laparoscopic Skills*

Fried and colleagues[6] developed a series of 5 low-fidelity laparoscopic exercises performed in a standard box trainer. These skills were designed to provide basic practice on basic laparoscopic skills. The curriculum was shown to be correlated with intraoperative technical skills ratings during actual laparoscopic cholecystectomy procedures, and performance improvement was significantly related to the amount of practice on these skills. SAGES later adopted these 5 exercises in the FLS certification examination. Ritter and Scott[33] developed a proficiency-based curriculum for the 5 FLS exercises and demonstrated that residents who trained to proficiency using the established curriculum achieved a 100% pass rate on the manual skills portion of the FLS examination,[38] and these laparoscopic skills were retained at 1 year.[39]

### *Endoscopic Skills*

The Texas Association of Surgical Skills Laboratories consortium developed a PBT curriculum for basic flexible endoscopy skills using the GI Mentor II simulator.[34] Study participants showed significant improvements in objective flexible endoscopy skills, and the curriculum was found to be educationally useful and effective. Gomez and colleagues[14] used this curriculum with the addition of practice on 10 colon cases on the GI Mentor II simulator to show that flexible endoscopy skills transferred to the clinical environment.

### *Robotic Surgery Skills*

Dulan and colleagues[40] developed a proficiency-based robotic surgery curriculum comprising 9 inanimate exercises using physical models. The curriculum comprised 5 tasks derived from FLS exercises and 4 novel exercises specific to robotic surgery. The curriculum has demonstrated reliability, feasibility, and educational benefit,[41] as well as construct validity and workload.[42] Gomez and colleagues[43] developed a similar proficiency-based robotic curriculum comprising 7 of the VR exercises offered in the da Vinci Skills Simulator. Participants showed significant gain in skills, regardless of prior level of surgical training, suggesting that robotic skills are independent of prior surgical experience.

### *Central Venous Catheterization*

Simulation-based training has been shown to be an effective method for reducing bloodstream infections related to central venous catheterization.[44,45] Barsuk and colleagues[44] found that residents who engaged in deliberate practice with a central line simulator required fewer needle passes to place a central line and displayed higher levels of confidence than residents who learned to place central lines in situ. Cohen and colleagues[45] demonstrated that residents who engaged in deliberate practice with a central line manikin showed a significant reduction in bloodstream infections compared with residents who were not trained using deliberate practice or a simulator. This reduction in infections resulted in 14 fewer hospital days and a net annual savings of more than $700,000.

### *Advanced Surgical Skills for Exposure in Trauma*

The ACS Committee on Trauma established the Advanced Surgical Skills for Exposure in Trauma (ASSET) curriculum in 2005, which includes a standardized skills-based course designed to teach surgical exposure of vital structures. This 1-day course is targeted at senior residents and fellows and uses human cadavers to teach surgical exposure in the areas of neck, chest, abdomen and pelvis, and upper and lower extremities. Trainees completing the course have reported higher levels of self-confidence and self-efficacy in all body regions.[46,47]

### *Advanced Trauma Operative Management*

The Advanced Trauma Operative Management (ATOM) curriculum was developed to help residents and fellows gain experience with the operative management of penetrating trauma injuries.[48] The curriculum combines lecture materials and a 1-day porcine operative experience focusing on injuries to the small bowel, bladder, duodenum, kidney, spleen, diaphragm, stomach, pancreas, liver, inferior vena cava, and heart. Trainees completing the course have reported higher levels of confidence and have achieved significant gains in knowledge[48] that persist up to 6 months after course completion.[49]

### *Refreshing Technical Skills*

Another area in which simulation can be incorporated into the GME setting is preparing residents to return to the clinical training environment after completing research years. A study by Willis and colleagues[50] revealed that residents and faculty believe that nonclinical years have a slightly negative impact on technical skills and believe this decrement persists up to 4 months after returning to clinical training. Residents who completed a technical skills refresher curriculum comprising proficiency-based practice with inanimate simulation exercises and a 4-hour session performing surgical procedures on human cadavers reported higher levels of subjective comfort and decreased anxiety associated with returning to the clinical environment. Objective clinical evaluations revealed that residents who completed the technical skills refresher curriculum before returning to the clinical environment achieved higher technical skills ratings than residents who conducted research years but did not complete the refresher curriculum.

## NONTECHNICAL SKILLS

Nontechnical skills are generally defined as interpersonal, cognitive, and personal resource skills and include the following[51,52]:

- Communication and teamwork
- Decision making
- Situational awareness
- Leadership
- Seeking feedback
- Coping with stress
- Management of fatigue

Although technical skills are undoubtedly necessary for safe and effective patient care, breakdowns in nontechnical skills can be attributed to errors committed in surgery. Poor communication has been identified as a casual factor in 43% of surgical errors.[53] Thus, it is important for surgical educators to develop a deeper understanding of nontechnical skills, their application in the surgical environment, methods of assessment, and strategies for improving deficiencies.

Communication can take place in one-to-one situations (eg, having an end-of-life discussion with a patient's family) or team-based situations (eg, resuscitation activation). In the surgical environment, team-based communication focuses on ensuring that all team members have a shared mental model of the current status of events and future plans.

In 2009, the World Health Organization introduced the surgical checklist[54] that includes a surgical pause designed to improve communication before surgery and improve patient safety. Haynes and colleagues[54] showed significant decreases in patient deaths and inpatient complications after the checklist was implemented.

**Box 1**
**ISBAR**

*I*dentify: Who? Where?

*S*ituation: What is the problem?

*B*ackground: Relevant patient historical presentation

*A*ssessment: What is the assessment of the problem?

*R*ecommendation: What should be done?

Another model designed to enhance patient safety through safer communication and teamwork was developed by the Department of Defense and the Agency for Healthcare Research and Quality called Team Strategies and Tools to Enhance Performance and Patient Safety (Team STEPPS).[55] This model empowers all members of the health care team to play a role in patient safety. Team STEPPS proposes the use of callbacks (repeating orders to ensure that communication was properly received), the 2-challenge rule (requesting the information be reevaluated to ensure that orders were properly given), and pneumonic devices such as ISBAR (**Box 1**), CUSS (**Box 2**), and I PASS the BATON (**Box 3**) to enhance communication in stressful situations and during transitions in patient care.

### *Teaching and Assessing Nontechnical Skills*

Phase 3 of the ACS/APDS Surgery Resident Skills curriculum (see **Table 1**) is designed to provide methods of teaching teamwork and preoperative, intraoperative, and postoperative communication skills to residents. High-fidelity simulation has been used with resuscitation activations to enhance teamwork, leadership, and communication.[56,57]

The nontechnical skills for surgeons (NOTSS) project represents a novel teamwork assessment tool designed from the ground-up by surgical educators for use with surgical teams.[58] The NOTSS taxonomy is divided into 4 main categories, and each has associated elements (**Table 3**). The taxonomy was derived via cognitive task analysis with surgeons and written in surgical language in a way that suitably trained surgeons could observe, rate, and provide feedback on trainees' nontechnical skills. Yule and colleagues[58] have shown that surgeons who have been trained for 3 hours can provide valid and reliable ratings for social skills.

## EXPANSION OF NATIONAL AND LOCAL CONSORTIA

As simulation-based training gains acceptance in medical education and the costs of these simulators increase, several surgery residency training programs have devised ways to share equipment and curricula. In 2005, the ACS advocated a formal

**Box 2**
**CUSS**

*C*oncern and clarification: "I am concerned and need clarification."

*U*ncomfortable: "I am uncomfortable with this action."

*S*erious worry: "I am seriously worried with this action."

*S*top: "Please stop immediately so we can discuss."

**Box 3**
**I PASS the BATON**

*I*ntroduction: Introduce yourself and your role on the team

*P*atient: Give patient identifiers

*A*ssessment: Describe the patient's chief complaint, vital signs, and diagnosis

*S*ituation: Describe the patient's current status, including code status and recent changes

*S*afety: Provide the patient's critical laboratory values and reports

the

*B*ackground: Describe the patient's comorbidities and medications

*A*ctions: Outline which actions have been taken

*T*iming: Indicate the level of urgency

*O*wnership: Explain which health care team members are responsible for this patient

*N*ext: Describe what will happen next, anticipated changes, and contingency plans

accreditation for both basic and comprehensive educational institutes that were charged to advance patient safety through simulation.[59] The goals of the program are to:

1. Promote patient safety through the use simulation
2. Develop new education and technologies
3. Identify best practices
4. Promote research and collaboration among accredited education institutes

Accreditation requirements include space, personnel, curricula, and assessment. The ACS has now accredited 70 comprehensive and 12 focused institutes across the United States and in 9 additional countries.

Two examples of state-level collaborations include the Oregon Simulation Alliance (OSA) and the Texas Association of Surgical Skills Laboratories (TASSL). The OSA[60] is an interprofessional nonprofit organization 501(c)(3) that has created a statewide network of health care professionals and hospital systems, with a focus of improving quality in a multidisciplinary approach. The TASSL consortium was established in

**Table 3**
**NOTSS taxonomy**

| Category | Element |
|---|---|
| Situation awareness | Gathering information, understanding information, projecting and anticipating future state |
| Decision making | Considering options, selecting and communicating option, implementing and reviewing decisions |
| Leadership | Setting and maintaining standards, supporting others, coping with pressure |
| Communication and teamwork | Exchanging information, establishing shared understanding, coordinating team |

*From* Yule S, Flin R, Maran N, et al. Surgeons' non-technical skills in the operating room: reliability and testing of the NOTSS behavior rating system. World J Surg 2008;32:553; with permission.

2007 and comprises predominantly of surgeons and surgical educators and has a primary focus on surgical residency training with rotating annual meetings held at sponsoring academic institutions. Both consortia have governance structure and formal meetings and are freely accessible online: www.oregonsimulation.com, www.tassl.org. The TASSL group has published research in the use of simulation in multicenter settings for residents[34] and to evaluate competency in the FLS program among surgery faculty.[61]

## SUMMARY

During the past decade there has been a significant paradigm shift in surgical education. Regulatory agencies have implemented mandates for the inclusion of simulation-based training and assessment in GME. The current published literature continues to demonstrate how simulation-based training can effectively be used to teach technical and nontechnical skills to learners of all levels in GME. Many surgical societies have recognized the value of simulation, and with the growth of programs such as FLS, FES, ASSET, ATOM, and the ACS Surgical Education Institutes, the role of simulation in surgical education will continue to expand.

## REFERENCES


1. Neville AJ, Norman GR. PBL in the undergraduate MD program at McMaster University: three iterations in three decades. Acad Med 2007;82:370–4.
2. Maran NJ, Glavin RJ. Low- to high fidelity simulation: a continuum of medical education? Med Educ 2003;37(Suppl 1):22–8.
3. Peyre SE, Smink DS. Chapter 13: Simulation of open surgical skills. In: Tsuda ST, Scott DJ, Jones DB, editors. Textbook of simulation: skills and team training. Woodbury (CT): Cine-Med; 2012. p. 147–54.
4. Boyle DE, Guis JA. Tie and suture board. Surgery 1968;63:434–6.
5. Seymour NE, Gallagher AG, Roman SA, et al. Virtual reality training improves operating room performance: results of a randomized, double-blinded study. Ann Surg 2002;236:458–64.
6. Fried GM, Feldman LS, Vassiliou MC, et al. Proving the value of simulation in laparoscopic surgery. Ann Surg 2004;240:518–28.
7. Issenberg SB, McGaghie WC, Petrusa ER, et al. Features and uses of high-fidelity medical simulations that lead to effective learning: a BEME systematic review. Med Teach 2005;27:10–28.
8. Seymour NE. VR to OR: a review of the evidence that virtual reality simulation improves operating room performance. World J Surg 2008;32:182–8.
9. McGaghie WC, Issenberg SB, Cohen ER, et al. Does simulation-based medical education with deliberate practice yield better results than traditional clinical education? A meta-analytic comparative review of the evidence. Acad Med 2011;86:1–6.
10. Didwania A, McGaghie WC, Cohen ER, et al. Progress toward improving the quality of cardiac arrest medical team responses at an academic teaching hospital. J Grad Med Educ 2011;3:211–6.
11. Norman G, Dore K, Grierson L. The minimal relationship between simulation fidelity and transfer of learning. Med Educ 2012;46:636–47.
12. Gallagher AG, Seymour NE, Jordan-Black JA, et al. Prospective, randomized assessment of transfer of training (ToT) and transfer effectiveness ration (TER) of virtual reality simulation training for laparoscopic skill acquisition. Ann Surg 2013;257:1025–31.

13. Zendejas B, Brydges R, Hamstra SJ, et al. State of the evidence on simulation-based training for laparoscopic surgery: a systematic review. Ann Surg 2013;257:586–93.
14. Gomez PP, Willis RE, Van Sickle KR. Evaluation of two flexible endoscopy simulators and transfer of skills into clinical practice. J Surg Educ 2015;72(2):220–7.
15. Britt LD, Richardson JD. Residency Review Committee For Surgery: an update. Arch Surg 2007;142(6):573–5.
16. Lyss-Lerman P, Teherani A, Aagaard E, et al. What training is needed in the fourth year of medical school? Views of residency program directors. Acad Med 2009;84(7):823–9.
17. Brunt LM, Halpin VJ, Klingensmith ME, et al. Accelerated skills preparation and assessment for senior medical students entering surgical internship. J Am Coll Surg 2008;206:897–907.
18. Boehler ML, Rogers DA, Schwind CJ, et al. A senior elective designed to prepare medical students for surgical residency. Am J Surg 2004;187(6):695–7.
19. Esterl RM Jr, Henzi DL, Cohn SM. Senior medical student "Boot Camp": can result in increased self-confidence before starting surgery internships. Curr Surg 2006;63(4):264–8.
20. Fernandez GL, Page DW, Coe NP, et al. Boot camp: educational outcomes after 4 successive years of preparatory simulation-based training at onset of internship. J Surg Educ 2012;69:242–8.
21. Parent RJ, Plerhoples TA, Long EE, et al. Early, intermediate, and late effects of a surgical skills "boot camp" on an objective structured assessment of technical skills: a randomized controlled study. J Am Coll Surg 2010;210:984–9.
22. Peyre SE, Peyre CG, Sullivan ME, et al. A surgical skills elective can improve student confidence prior to internship. J Surg Res 2006;133(1):11–5.
23. Zeng W, Woodhouse J, Brunt M. Do preclinical background and clerkship experiences impact skills performance in an accelerated internship preparation course for senior medical students? Surgery 2010;148:768–77.
24. Okusanya OT, Kornfield ZN, Reinke CE, et al. The effect and durability of a pregraduation boot camp on the confidence of senior medical student entering surgical residencies. J Surg Educ 2012;69:536–43.
25. Antonoff MB, D'Cunha J. PGY-1 surgery preparatory course design: identification of key curricular components. J Surg Educ 2011;68:478–84.
26. Willis RE, Peterson RM, Dent DL. Usefulness of the American College of Surgeons' Fundamentals of Surgery Curriculum as a knowledge preparatory tool for incoming surgery interns. Am J Surg 2013;205:131–6.
27. Glass CC, Acton RD, Blair PG, et al. American College of Surgeons/Association for Surgical Education medical student simulation-based surgical skills curriculum needs assessment. Am J Surg 2014;207:165–9.
28. Scott DJ, Dunnington GL. The new ACS/APDS skills curriculum: moving the learning curve out of the operating room. J Gastrointest Surg 2008;12:213–21.
29. Ericsson KA, Krampe RT, Tesch-Romer C. The role of deliberate practice in the acquisition of expert performance. Psychol Rev 1993;3:363–406.
30. Willis RE, Richa J, Oppeltz R, et al. Comparing three pedagogical approaches to psychomotor skills acquisition. Am J Surg 2012;203:8–13.
31. Scott DJ, Goova MT, Tesfay ST. A cost-effective proficiency-based knot-tying and suturing curriculum for residency programs. J Surg Res 2007;141:7–15.
32. Mashaud LB, Arain NA, Hogg DC, et al. Development, validation and implementation of a cost-effective intermediate-level, proficiency-based knot-tying and suturing curriculum for surgery residents. J Surg Educ 2013;70:193–9.

33. Ritter EM, Scott DJ. Design of a proficiency-based skills training curriculum for the Fundamentals of Laparoscopic Surgery. Surg Innov 2007;14:107–12.
34. Van Sickle KR, Buck L, Willis R, et al. A multicenter, simulation-based skills training collaborative using shared GI Mentor II systems: results from the Texas Association of Surgical Skills Laboratories (TASSL) flexible endoscopy curriculum. Surg Endosc 2011;5(9):2980–6.
35. Goova MT, Hollett LA, Tesfay ST, et al. Implementation, construct validity, and benefit of a proficiency-based knot-tying and suturing curriculum. J Surg Educ 2008;65:309–15.
36. Brunsvold ME, Schmitz CC. Replicating an established open skills curriculum: are the same results obtained in a different setting? J Surg Educ 2014;71(6):e97–103.
37. Gomez PP, Willis RE, Schiffer BL, et al. External validation and evaluation of an intermediate proficiency-based knot-tying and suturing curriculum. J Surg Educ 2014;71(6):839–45.
38. Scott DJ, Ritter EM, Tesfay ST, et al. Certification pass rate of 100% for fundamentals of laparoscopic surgery skills after proficiency-based training. Surg Endosc 2008;22:1187–93.
39. Castellvi AO, Hollett LA, Minhajuddin A, et al. Maintaining proficiency after Fundamentals of Laparoscopic Surgery training: a 1-year analysis of skill retention for surgery residents. Surgery 2009;146:387–93.
40. Dulan G, Rege RV, Hogg DC, et al. Developing a comprehensive, proficiency-based training program for robotic surgery. Surgery 2012;152:477–88.
41. Arain NA, Dulan G, Hogg DC, et al. Comprehensive proficiency-based inanimate training for robotic surgery: reliability, feasibility, and educational benefit. Surg Endosc 2012;26:2740–5.
42. Dulan G, Rege RV, Hogg DC, et al. Proficiency-based training for robotic surgery: construct validity, workload, and expert levels for nine inanimate exercises. Surg Endosc 2012;26:1516–21.
43. Gomez PP, Willis RE, Van Sickle KR. Development of a virtual reality robotic surgical curriculum using the Da Vinci SI surgical system. Surg Endosc 2014. [Epub ahead of print].
44. Barsuk JH, McGaghie WC, Cohen ER, et al. Use of simulation-based mastery learning to improve the quality of central venous catheter placement in a medical intensive care unit. J Hosp Med 2009;4:397–403.
45. Cohen ER, Feinglass J, Barsuk JH, et al. Cost savings from reduced catheter-related bloodstream infection after simulation-based education for residents in a medical intensive care unit. Simul Healthc 2010;5:98–102.
46. Kuhls DA, Risucci DA, Bowyer MW, et al. Advanced surgical skills for exposure in trauma: a new surgical skills cadaver course for surgery residents and fellows. J Trauma Acute Care Surg 2013;74:664–70.
47. Bowyer MW, Kuhls DA, Haskin D, et al. Advanced surgical skills for exposure in trauma (ASSET): the first 25 courses. J Surg Res 2013;183:553–8.
48. Jacobs LM, Burns KJ, Kaban JM, et al. Development and evaluation of the advanced trauma operative management course. J Trauma 2003;55:471–9.
49. Jacobs LM, Burns KJ, Luk SS, et al. Follow-up survey of participants attending the advanced trauma operative management (ATOM) course. J Trauma 2005;58:1140–3.
50. Willis RE, Van Sickle KR, Peterson RM. Impact of non-clinical years on surgery residents' technical skills: evaluation of a technical skills refresher curriculum. Surg Sci 2013;4:131–4.

51. Yule S, Flin R, Paterson-Brown S, et al. Development of a rating system for surgeons' non-technical skills. Med Educ 2006;40:1098–104.
52. Hull L, Arora S, Aggarwal R, et al. The impact of nontechnical skills on technical performance in surgery: a systematic review. J Am Coll Surg 2012;214:214–30.
53. Gawande AA, Zinner MJ, Studdert DM, et al. Analysis of errors reported by surgeons at three teaching hospitals. Surgery 2003;133:614–21.
54. Haynes AB, Weiser TG, Berry WR, et al. A surgical safety checklist to reduce morbidity and mortality in a global population. N Engl J Med 2009;360:491–9.
55. King HB, Battles J, Baker DP, et al. TeamSTEPPS: team strategies and tools to enhance performance and patient safety. In: Henriksen K, Battles JB, Keyes MA, et al, editors. Advances in patient safety: new directions and alternative approaches. Performance and tools, vol. 3. Rockville (MD): Agency for Healthcare Research and Quality (US); 2008. p. 1–14.
56. Riley W, Davis S, Miller K, et al. Didactic and simulation nontechnical skills team training to improve perinatal patient outcomes in a community hospital. Jt Comm J Qual Patient Saf 2011;37:357–64.
57. Langdorf MI, Strom SL, Yang L, et al. High-fidelity simulation enhances ACLS training. Teach Learn Med 2014;26:266–73.
58. Yule S, Flin R, Maran N, et al. Surgeons' non-technical skills in the operating room: reliability and testing of the NOTSS behavior rating system. World J Surg 2008;32:548–56.
59. Jones DB. Foreword. In: Tsuda ST, Scott DJ, Jones DB, editors. Textbook of simulation: skills and team training. Woodbury (CT): Cine-Med; 2012. p. xvii–xviii.
60. Seropian MA, Driggers B, Taylor J, et al. The Oregon simulation experience: a statewide simulation network and alliance. Sim Healthc 2006;1:56–61.
61. Hafford ML, Van Sickle KR, Willis RE, et al. Ensuring competency: are fundamentals of laparoscopic surgery training and certification necessary for practicing surgeons and operating room personnel? Surg Endosc 2013;27:118–26.

# National Simulation-Based Training of Fellows

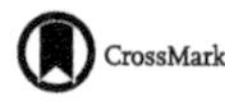


## The Vascular Surgery Example

Malachi G. Sheahan, MD[a,*], Cassidy Duran, MD[b], Jean Bismuth, MD[b]

**KEYWORDS**

• Simulation • Fellowship training • Vascular surgery • Boot camp • Assessment

**KEY POINTS**

- Vascular surgery trainers face many challenges in assuring graduates possess appropriate technical skills for open and endovascular procedures, including reduced work hours, rapidly evolving technology, and the need to teach complex but infrequently performed open surgical procedures.
- Using methods similar to general surgery technical skills assessments in laparoscopic and endoscopic surgery, vascular surgery educators developed a set of fundamental technical skills stations for purposes of training and assessment.
- Elements contributing to an effective simulation-based training course in vascular surgery include faculty-to-trainee ratios; large fresh cadaver component; emphasis on less commonly encountered procedures; and focused training, feedback, and assessment of trainees.

Surgical educators have experienced mounting pressure to train competent surgeons within the scope of decreasing work hours, increasing patient safety concerns, and mounting public scrutiny. Vascular surgery is no exception and, in fact, faces the additional challenges of a rapidly changing field in which new and evolving technologies have drastically affected the practice. The scope of disease once relegated entirely to open surgical management is shifting increasingly and exponentially toward endovascular interventions. The result is a field in which open operations are less often encountered by trainees and those circumstances requiring an open procedure now involve highly complex and challenging cases. Meanwhile, new endovascular technologies are coming to market constantly, requiring users to learn new skills (in training and beyond). The obvious answer to some educators is the use of simulation. Simulation-based technologies are useful for endovascular procedures in much the

[a] Department of Surgery, LSU Health Sciences Center, A1542 Tulane Avenue, New Orleans, LA 70112, USA; [b] Department of Surgery, Houston Methodist, 6565 Fannin Street, Houston, TX 77030, USA

* Corresponding author.

*E-mail address:* msheah@lsuhsc.edu

Surg Clin N Am 95 (2015) 781–790

http://dx.doi.org/10.1016/j.suc.2015.04.008 **surgical.theclinics.com**

0039-6109/15/$ – see front matter 

same way as they are for laparoscopy because the 3-dimensional to 2-dimensional conversion of both approaches leads to ease of developing high-fidelity images of anatomy. Open surgery, on the other hand, presents more challenges in the creation of high-fidelity, responsive simulations. Nonetheless, vascular surgery has obvious applications for simulation-based technology. The implementation of simulation-based training for surgical trainees has evolved rapidly in the past 20 years. Trainees, as well as vascular educators, increasingly support integration of simulation into the training paradigm. In a recent survey of current vascular surgery trainees, 86% of respondents reported a belief in the educational value of simulation-based training. Fifty-six percent of vascular surgery programs currently offer simulation-based training, most commonly in the form of peripheral endovascular simulators (70%), anastomotic models (58%), or endovascular aortic aneurysm repair models (53%). More than a third of current vascular fellows and senior residents (37%) have attended outside simulation-based courses.[1]

## ENDOVASCULAR SIMULATION

When it was first introduced, endovascular simulation was a largely industry-driven means of introducing interventionalists to new endovascular devices and techniques using virtual reality (VR) simulators. Carotid artery stenting was identified as a high-risk procedure with potentially devastating consequences for patients. VR simulators could help mediate good outcomes. To meet this need, VR simulation was developed to allow users to be trained on a safe platform. Similarly, to be approved for use of a device by industry, simulation-based practice was required for thoracic and abdominal endovascular repair. Several validation studies were published to demonstrate the utility of this approach. These studies confirmed that performance improved with standardized simulation-based practice.[2,3] Based in part on these findings, a 2005 consensus statement from the Society for Vascular Surgery, the American College of Cardiology, and the Society for Vascular Medicine and Biology encouraged the use of simulation-based training. The statement read, "In an effort to assist physicians with differing backgrounds and skills to reach a common benchmark of proficiency, metric-based simulation should be incorporated into training. This will provide skills acquisition in an objective manner, based on real-world situational experience."[4]

VR simulation for endovascular interventions was rapidly developed for the breadth of vascular interventions from aortic to mesenteric and lower extremity. Numerous studies evaluating validity and utility of endovascular simulation were carried out and, across the board, results supported the utility of endovascular simulation-based training. Participants improved their performance on the simulated procedures for aortic, renal, lower extremity, and carotid interventions as measured by global rating scales, procedural checklists, and procedural metrics (ie, task completion time, fluoroscopy time, contrast use).[5–7] In select studies, these improvements translated to skills demonstrated on a live animal model.[8,9] These encouraging findings have led the vascular surgery programs with adequate funding to make the large investment (>$200,000) in VR simulators. However, many programs simply cannot afford that expense, making standard implementation of VR simulation into the curriculum impractical.

## SIMULATION-BASED TRAINING FOR OPEN VASCULAR PROCEDURES AND TASKS

The earliest forms of vascular simulation-based training for surgical trainees came in the form of bench-top anastomotic models. Requiring only a stable platform, woven graft material, sutures, and basic instruments, structured, low-risk practice could be performed and it was shown to be useful (primarily for junior residents) in improving skill.[10,11] These simple models, however, failed to capture the interest of senior residents and fellows as well as faculty because their utility for mastery of the highly specialized skill required of a vascular surgeon was quite limited. Because work-hour reductions and growing endovascular options for traditionally open surgical techniques began to limit trainee exposure, a role for more complex vascular simulation models was presented. In response to growing concerns that trainees were simply not exposed to a sufficient volume of open surgical cases, high-fidelity, pulsatile flow models were developed to allow for a standardized training platform. These pulsatile flow and other open surgical models have been incorporated into courses to train vascular surgeons.

## SIMULATION-BASED TRAINING COURSES TO TEACH VASCULAR SURGICAL SKILLS

Vascular International, a school in Europe dedicated to providing supplementary training for vascular surgeons through short, intensive courses using hands-on skills training (for open and endovascular procedures), has been offering courses for more than 20 years. This model has been widely embraced in Europe, where work hours are limited to 48-hour weeks, as a means for trainees with insufficient operative exposure to gain experience. Furthermore, because training models vary widely throughout the European Union, these standardized teaching methods ensure some measure of homogeneity in training. These techniques of standardized training have proven to be superior to traditional techniques in a randomized study. The standardized group demonstrated improved technical scores (95% vs 75%) and global rating scores (84% vs 67%).[12] These short training courses have also been shown to improve technical performance and quality on carotid PATCH and open aortic repair.[13,14]

Following this model, weekend skills courses have been developed in the United States to address the needs and concerns of vascular faculty and trainees. Houston Methodist Hospital began hosting a 3-day boot camp with hands-on workshops and didactics 5 years ago. Collaboration between the vascular international group, US leaders in vascular surgery education, and industry vendors and VR simulation companies, has provided vascular surgery fellows with an opportunity to gain early experience with proven techniques in open and endovascular scenarios.[15] Currently, several state of the art simulation centers host similar courses throughout the year, including the Center for Advanced Medical Learning and Simulation in Tampa, the Louisiana State University Health New Orleans School of Medicine Learning Center, and the Methodist Institute for Training Innovation and Education in Houston. Likewise, major academic meetings offer hands-on courses to trainees that expose them to open surgical techniques as well as the latest technologies in endovascular interventions, helping them to gain familiarity with new devices and techniques in that realm. These include the Society for Vascular Surgery Annual Meeting, the Society for Clinical Vascular Surgery Top Gun competition, and the Everest Symposium.

## DEVELOPMENT OF FUNDAMENTALS OF VASCULAR AND ENDOVASCULAR SURGERY NATIONAL TRAINING SYMPOSIUM

Despite the demonstrable successes of the use of simulation for vascular training, it continues to be met with a considerable degree of skepticism. In large part, this resistance is due to the fragmented manner in which it has been developed and implemented. Although most vascular surgery trainees now have some exposure to simulation-based training, a lack of standardization and availability of simulation-based models for all trainees persists. Compounding the problem is a lack of a practical curriculum for implementation of simulation-based methodologies. At a minimum, the authors estimate that a major issue is the lack of structured performance assessment. We have boorishly thought that the only way to assess a trainee is by the current subjective manner, which has been in place since the advent of formal surgical education. The reality is that, along with new training paradigms and the ever evolving field of vascular surgery, it is time to consider what requisites comprise the essential skills for practicing vascular surgery. This idea is by no means a novel concept. It is adopted in general surgery with the Fundamentals of Laparoscopic Surgery and Fundamentals Endoscopic Surgery programs.

With this in mind, a working group representing the education committee for the association of program directors in vascular surgery began to determine the best approach for addressing these needs. Following the well-described path of our colleagues in general surgery, we first set out to define a basic skills set for both open and endovascular surgery. In the course of several months, this team of leaders agreed on a task list and developed models designed to test those skills. From this start, the concept of fundamentals of vascular and endovascular surgery was developed, which included models for Fundamentals of Vascular Surgery (FVS) and Fundamentals of Endovascular Surgery (FEVS).

The pilot program for open skill testing (FVS) occurred in October 2012. Twenty surgical trainees completed 3 vascular skill assessment models under the observation of 2 experienced assessors blinded to their training level. Models were designed to simulate an end-to-side (ES) anastomosis (**Fig. 1**) and a patch angioplasty (Patch) (**Fig. 2**). A third model required suturing around a clock-face (CF) design printed on patch material (**Fig. 3**). Accreditation Council for Graduate Medical Education log experience was recorded. Secondary evaluations of the finished models were then performed by 4 blinded assessors. Inter-rater reliability among the 7 assessors was high (Cronbach's $\alpha = 0.93$). Evaluations acquired by direct observation correlated well with participants' training level or experience for all 3 models (ES bivariate correlation coefficient [r] = 0.85, Patch r = 0.71, CF r = 0.82). Highest correlation with training level or experience was obtained with a combined score for each participant incorporating all observed ratings on each model (r = 0.93). Construct validity was demonstrated by each model's ability to discern junior (premedical to postgraduate year [PGY] 2) from senior (PGY 3–5) trainees (ES $P<.005$, Patch $P<.05$, CF $P<.001$). Internal consistency was confirmed for each participant on all 3 models (Cronbach's $\alpha = .89$).

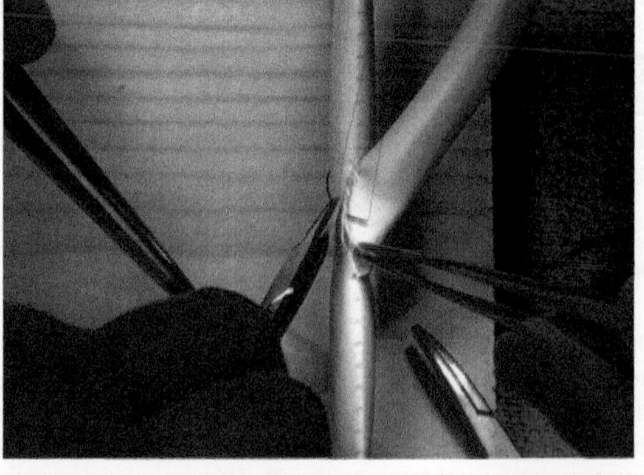

**Fig. 1.** The ES model. Trainees are given 20 minutes and a passive assistant to complete the task.

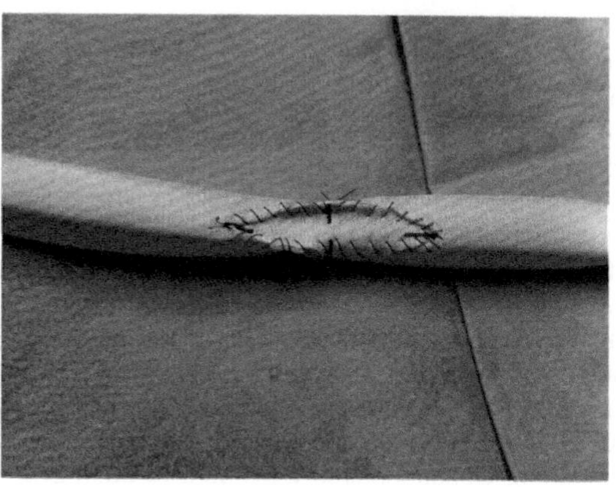

**Fig. 2.** The Patch Model as completed by a postgraduate year 2 vascular resident.

Finished product evaluation demonstrated fair to poor correlation with training level or experience (ES r = .54, Patch r = .53, CF r = .24). These results provided construct validity for 3 vascular skill assessment models. There are data that demonstrate that the most accurate assessments are obtained by direct observation with trained evaluators.[16]

Based on the success of this pilot project, the FEVS Symposium at Louisiana State University was first held in February 2013. Scholarships were given to 24 integrated vascular surgery residents from around the United States. The Symposium was held again the following year. The goals of the course were twofold:

1. For vascular surgery residents: With a faculty to resident ratio approaching 1:1, attendees spent 3 days receiving hands-on instruction in vascular techniques. Special emphasis was placed on procedures less commonly performed during residency such as open thoracoabdominal aortic approaches, subclavian or tibial vessel exposures, and complex endovascular procedures.
2. For program directors: Using vascular skill assessment models, the course faculty spent hours observing and grading each attendee. This feedback was provided directly back to the program director. These outside assessments of residents' skill are a unique and valuable resource for portfolio building, milestone development, and individualized simulation curriculum design.

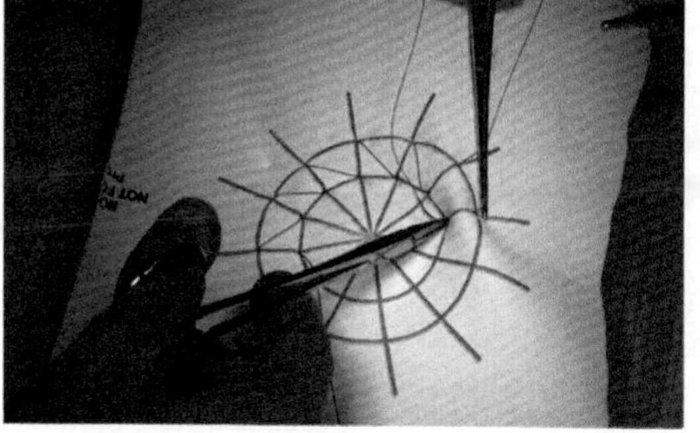

**Fig. 3.** The CF Model is designed to test radial suturing ability with a larger small half-circle needle. Trainees are given 5 minutes and a passive assistant to complete the task.

The course curriculum includes instruction (fresh cadaver laboratory, endovascular skill stations, open skill stations, didactics) and assessment (FVS, FEVS). There are also opportunities for simultaneous teaching and assessment, such as Suturing with the Experts (**Fig. 4**) and planning stations for endovascular aneurysm repair (EVAR) measurement. Course content has been adjusted based on attendee feedback; most notably, increasing the cadaver content, shortening the didactics, and providing more hands-on instruction and immediate feedback.

As a measure of educational effectiveness, all residents complete a before and after self-assessment of confidence in 9 vascular skills. Pooled results from the first 2 years demonstrate a statistically significant improvement in each proficiency, including performance of carotid stent ($P<.05$), thoracoabdominal aorta exposure ($P<.001$), and EVAR planning based on computed tomography angiography measurement ($P<.01$). All attendees (100%, 48/48) reported being either very or extremely satisfied with the education experience. Questionnaires were sent to each program director after the course and a 93% response (28/30) was achieved. All respondents reported being either very or extremely satisfied with the skill assessments generated by the course and 96% of the responders (27/28) thought the reports would be useful in helping the residency program address the attendees' strengths and weaknesses.[16]

From this experience, the authors consider the following components useful in creating a valuable vascular surgery simulation-based course:

1. High faculty-to-attendee ratio (minimum 1:2)
2. Low attendee-to-simulation station ratio (maximum 2:1)
3. Large fresh cadaver component
4. Emphasis on procedures rarely performed during residency
5. Limited didactics
6. Focused individual skill training and feedback to attendees
7. Focused individual skill assessment and feedback to program directors.

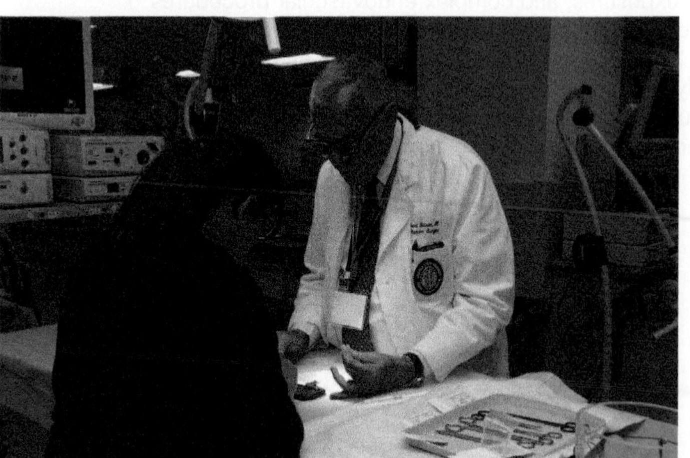

**Fig. 4.** The "Suturing with the Experts" session has obtained uniformly positive feedback from the attendees of the FEVS Symposium at Louisiana State University. Residents receive 60 minutes of one-on-one training with an experienced vascular surgeon. Instrument handling and suture technique are stressed.

The FEVS model was developed in both silicon and virtual-reality versions (**Fig. 5**). Twenty individuals (with a range of experience) performed 4 tasks on each model in 3 separate sessions. Tasks on the silicon model were performed under fluoroscopic guidance and electromagnetic tracking captured motion metrics for catheter tip position. Image processing captured tool tip position and motion on the virtual model. Performance was evaluated using a global rating scale, blinded video assessment of error metrics, and catheter tip movement and position. Motion analysis was based on derivations of speed and position that define proficiency of movement, including spectral arc length, duration of submovement, and number of submovements (**Fig. 6**).

Performance was significantly different between competent and noncompetent interventionalists for all 3 performance measures: motion metrics (see **Fig. 2**), error metrics, and global rating scale. The mean error metric score was 6.83 for noncompetent individuals and 2.51 for the more experienced group ($P<.0001$). Median global rating scores were 2.25 for the noncompetent group and 4.75 for the competent users ($P<.0001$).[16] The FEVS model successfully differentiated competent and noncompetent performance of fundamental endovascular skills based on a series of objective performance measures. Furthermore, it was successfully demonstrated that performance on an exact replica VR model correlated to performance on the physical model, further lending support to the validity of this platform. This model is now being proposed as a platform for skills testing for all trainees. Multi-institution trials of both models are planned for launch in 2015.

Despite the success of simulation-based training and assessment in vascular surgery, major shortcomings of simulation as a training tool remain. First, the assessment tools have been adapted from Resnik's Objective Structured Assessment of Technical

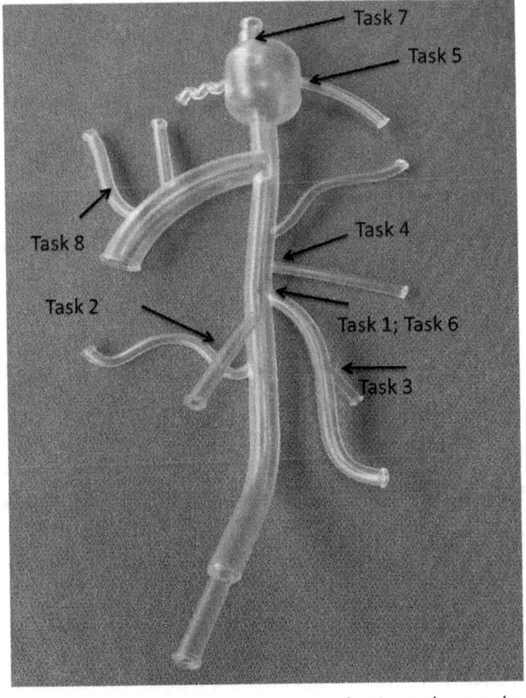


**Fig. 5.** The FEVS model with 8 tasks designed to test basic endovascular skill.

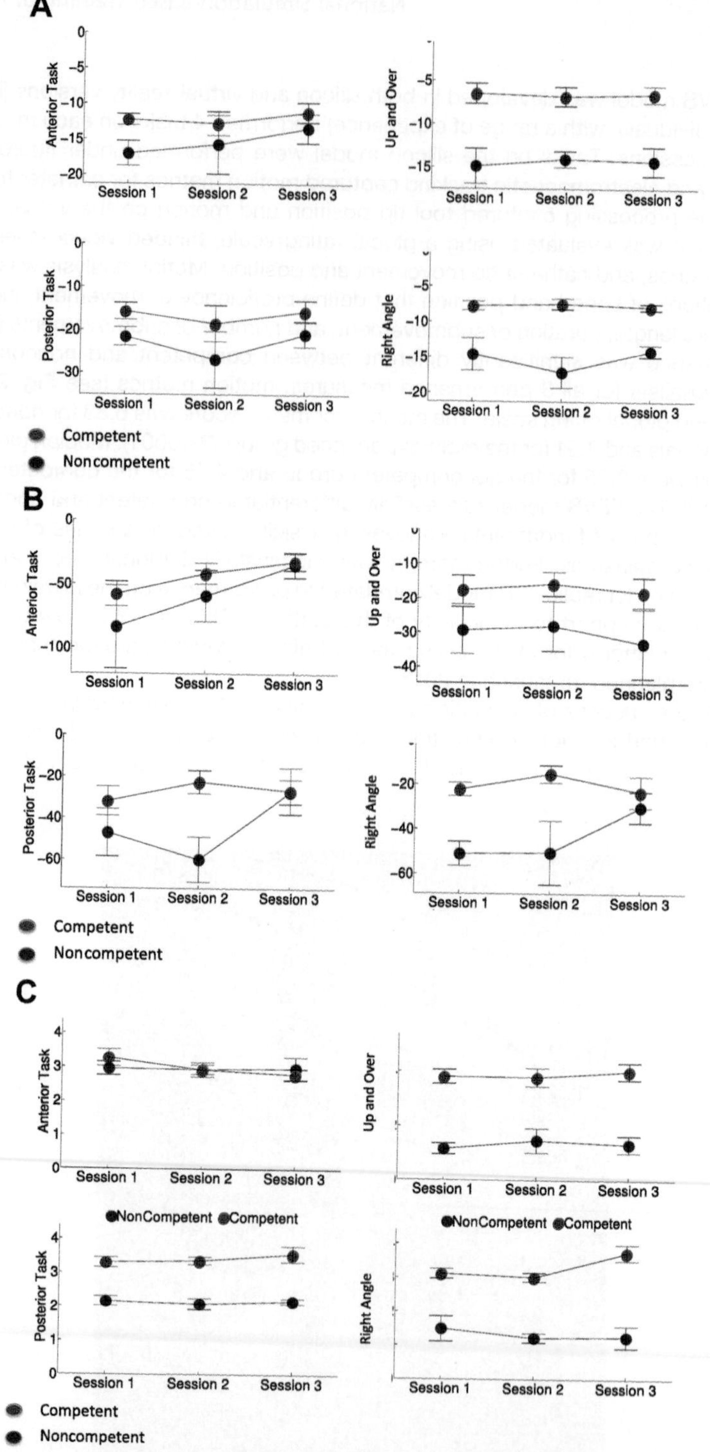


**Fig. 6.** Mean metric scores for competent (*red*) and noncompetent (*blue*) subjects performing fundamentals tasks. From analysis of variance; only nondimensional jerk did not show reliable difference between groups. (*A*) Spectral arc length. (*B*) Number of submovements. (*C*) Average submovement duration.

Skill model for evaluation of surgical skill without rigorous validation. A recently published review of studies assessing vascular surgical performance found that 84% pertained only to the simulated environment and that, although existing assessment tools may be relevant to individual technical skill acquisition, a generalizable tool has yet to be developed or validated, and practical assessment of resident readiness to operate remains elusive.[17] Houston Methodist Hospital has sought to meet this need with the validation of a Global Rating Assessment Device for Endovascular Skill in the live operating room setting. Clearly, however, further assessment tool development will be required to meet the need described by Mitchell and colleagues.[17] Cost has also posed a significant challenge to widespread access to vascular, especially endovascular, simulation-based platforms. At anticipated costs of less than $5000 for the endovascular and open vascular simulation models used in FVS and FEVS, these models are financially accessible to any educational program. In addition to a lack of valid and practical assessment tools, simulation for most users is viewed as an isolated tool without a well-described means of implementation. This means that, like simulation centers in general surgery, vascular simulators are often left largely unused due to constraints of faculty time and lack of curriculum for standard use.

Perhaps the largest obstacle facing the use of simulation-based training is skepticism about its ability to translate into operating room skill and measurable patient outcomes. To overcome this obstacle, the authors suggest that a working group supported by the vascular societies be identified to work through implementation, which includes development of testing, resolving cost issues, and addressing the question of identifying adequate assessors.

## SUMMARY

Much work has been done by vascular educators toward making the concept of fundamentals of vascular and endovascular surgery a reality. Having an efficient way of assessing the fundamental skills of trainees in vascular surgery has become a necessity, much like it has been for general surgery. Despite that most vascular surgery trainees now have some exposure to simulation-based training, there remains a lack of a practical curriculum for implementation. New training paradigms and the ever-evolving field of vascular surgery, mandate that educators identify and apply the requisites that comprise the essential skills for practicing vascular surgery.

## REFERENCES


1. Duran C, Bismuth J, Mitchell E. A nationwide survey of vascular surgery trainees reveals trends in operative experience, confidence, and attitudes about simulation. J Vasc Surg 2013;58:524–8.
2. Seymour NE, Gallagher AG, Roman SA, et al. Virtual reality training improves operating room performance: results of a randomized, double-blinded study. Ann Surg 2002;236:458–63 [discussion: 463–4].
3. Van Herzeele I, Aggarwal R, Neequaye S, et al. Experienced endovascular interventionalists objectively improve their skills by attending carotid artery stent training courses. Eur J Vasc Endovasc Surg 2008;35:541–50.
4. Rosenfield K, Babb JD, Cates CU, et al. Clinical competence statement on carotid stenting: training and credentialing for carotid stenting–multispecialty consensus recommendations: a report of the SCAI/SVMB/SVS Writing Committee to develop a clinical competence statement on carotid interventions. J Am Coll Cardiol 2005;45:165–74.

5. Dawson DL, Meyer J, Lee ES, et al. Training with simulation improves residents' endovascular procedure skills. J Vasc Surg 2007;45:149–54.
6. Van Herzeele I, Aggarwal R, Choong A, et al. Virtual reality simulation objectively differentiates level of carotid stent experience in experienced interventionalists. J Vasc Surg 2007;46:855–63.
7. Bech B, Lönn L, Falkenberg M, et al. Construct validity and reliability of structured assessment of endovascular expertise in a simulated setting. Eur J Vasc Endovasc Surg 2011;42:539–48.
8. Chaer RA, Derubertis BG, Lin SC, et al. Simulation improves resident performance in catheter-based intervention: results of a randomized, controlled study. Ann Surg 2006;244:343–52.
9. Dayal R, Faries PL, Lin SC, et al. Computer simulation as a component of catheter-based training. J Vasc Surg 2004;40:1112–7.
10. Anastakis DJ, Regehr G, Reznick RK, et al. Assessment of technical skills transfer from the bench training model to the human model. Am J Surg 1999;177:167–70.
11. Reznick R, Regehr G, MacRae H, et al. Testing technical skill via an innovative "bench station" examination. Am J Surg 1997;173:226–30.
12. Bath J, Lawrence P, Chandra A, et al. Standardization is superior to traditional methods of teaching open vascular simulation. J Vasc Surg 2011;53:229–34, 235.e1–2; [discussion: 234–5].
13. Duschek N, Assadian A, Lamont PM, et al. Simulator training on pulsatile vascular models significantly improves surgical skills and the quality of carotid patch plasty. J Vasc Surg 2013;57:1148–54.
14. Pandey V, Wolfe JH, Moorthy K, et al. Technical skills continue to improve beyond surgical training. J Vasc Surg 2006;43:539–45.
15. Bismuth J, Duran C, Donovan M, et al. The Cardiovascular Fellows Bootcamp. J Vasc Surg 2012;56:1155–61.e1.
16. Duran CA, Shames M, Bismuth J, et al. Validated assessment tool paves the way for standardized evaluation of trainees on anastomotic models. Ann Vasc Surg 2014;28:115–21.
17. Mitchell EL, Arora S, Moneta GL, et al. A systematic review of assessment of skill acquisition and operative competency in vascular surgical training. J Vasc Surg 2014;59:1440–55.

# Financing a Simulation Center

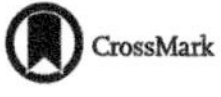

Shawn Tsuda, MD[a,*], Adnan Mohsin, BS[a], Daniel Jones, MD[b]

**KEYWORDS**

• Surgery • Simulation center • Skills laboratory • Education • Training • Finance • Costs • Funding

**KEY POINTS**

- Many avenues exist to attain funding for establishing surgical skills laboratories, with industry, hospital, and departmental funding being the most common.
- Industry funding or grants can provide substantial initial funding to start the operation; internal support, however, from the surgery department and hospital administration are essential for sustaining the laboratory.
- Collaboration with other medical departments and specialties, such as gynecology, urology, gastroenterology, nursing, and other allied health professions, is key for optimizing the utility of and amount of revenue generated by the laboratory.
- Budgeting factors for financing a laboratory should include both initial and maintenance costs, and acquisition of equipment is generally the most expensive capital investment. Costs for personnel, use of facility or laboratory space, supplies and consumables, and equipment maintenance are ongoing costs for maintaining the laboratory.

## INTRODUCTION

The operating room and the patients' bedside historically have been the foundation for surgical skills training. Although these environments continue to be important, concerns with learning efficiency and patient safety have shifted the training process to include simulation-based training in a structured environment. Teaching residents in a live patient setting increases operative time and costs.[1] As the importance of simulation-based training has been established across various medical and health professional disciplines, skills training laboratories have become a standard in surgery training programs. In 2008, the American College of Surgeons and Association of

[a] Department of Surgery, University of Nevada School of Medicine, 2040 West Charleston Boulevard, Las Vegas, NV 89102, USA; [b] Beth Israel Deaconess Medical Center, Harvard Medical School, Boston, MA, USA

* Corresponding author. Department of Surgery, University of Nevada School of Medicine, 2040 West Charleston Boulevard, Suite #601, Las Vegas, NV 89102.

*E-mail address:* stsuda@medicine.nevada.edu

Surg Clin N Am 95 (2015) 791–800
http://dx.doi.org/10.1016/j.suc.2015.03.002 **surgical.theclinics.com**
0039-6109/15/$ – see front matter 

Program Directors in Surgery developed a simulation-based surgical skills curriculum; this curriculum was followed by the Residency Review Committee for Surgery of the Accreditation Council for Graduate Medical Education mandating resident access to a skills laboratory.

Although laparoscopic skills training laboratories existed at the time of the reform, institutions without laboratories were forced to modify their program in order to remain compliant. Funding was reported as a major obstacle; establishing a surgical skills laboratory and adapting the training curriculum requires a significant amount of resources, including a physical location, equipment, and manpower.[2,3] A systematic approach, therefore, is necessary to secure the needed funds, optimize, and budget appropriately in order to build a first-rate training facility.

## OBTAINING FUNDING

After establishing a plan for a surgical skills training center, the next step is identifying appropriate funding sources. Finding funding is a critical, yet challenging step in developing a simulation center. Because most laboratories do not initially generate revenue, funding must be acquired from other sources. Numerous avenues for sourcing funds exist, including industry; the surgery department/health sciences center; hospitals; government at the federal, state, or local level; and philanthropic organizations (**Box 1**).

Industry sponsors are one of the most common sources of funding through educational partnerships or grants. According to a survey of training centers, 68% of laboratories have received funding from industry.[2] Funding opportunities are available from various companies, such as medical device, pharmaceutical, and medical education vendors. Successful funding from a granting agency, however, requires the skills laboratory to meet industry objectives. For example, the center may be asked to conduct specific training activities or use recommended equipment. Commitment to industry stipulations may lead to increased activities and may provide continued funding. Most industry funding, however, is provided for start-up or for a limited duration. In addition to cash grants, medical device companies are also able to donate equipment. These donations are valued similarly to cash, which would otherwise be used for equipment purchases. Equipment donations are more readily available and can result in considerable reductions in start-up costs.

**Box 1**
**Funding sources**

- Surgery department
- Medicine specialties
- Allied health disciplines
- Hospital
- Industry
- Medical school/health sciences center
- Alumni
- Community fundraising
- Government
- Research grants

Although industry sponsorship can provide a substantial amount of funding, support from the surgery department/health sciences center (ie, leadership at the home academic institution) is essential for the success of the operation. Faculty and administration buy-in are necessities. Beyond initial funding, the surgery department must remain committed for ongoing sustainability. After all, surgeons and surgery residents are generally the primary users of the laboratory. The simulation center provides a controlled environment where individuals can hone skills to attain competency or mastery without compromising patient safety. The skills laboratory is a training environment for residents as well as a place for continuing education and professional development for practicing surgeons (**Fig. 1**).

Other medical or allied health departments with concurrent interests are potential sources for support. Medical specialties, such as gastroenterology, gynecology, or urology, as well as allied health professionals, such as operating room technicians, nurses, and respective trainees, perform patient procedures or require simulation-based training that benefits from a simulation training center. A shared learning environment facilitates development of a diversified and comprehensive skills laboratory, enhancing the experience for all users. The more specialties and professions that get involved in the training center, the greater the revenue generated. In addition to cost sharing for the initial start-up and establishment of the center, collaboration also provides a strong foundation for ongoing contributions. Multi-departmental collaboration forges bonds and leads to the sharing of space, equipment, students (or users), or educational support. Surveys suggest that shared laboratory training programs are associated with larger space and increased variety and number of simulators, including video box trainers and virtual reality trainers.[2] Other benefits from a pooled commitment from different departments include maximization of faculty members and efforts to manage and oversee the laboratory.

When multiple departments or schools are involved in supporting the cost of such an endeavor, a memorandum of understanding (MOU) should be established. An MOU is a mutual agreement between multiple parties and outlines the utilization and payment strategies of the shared environment. A strong partnership with multiple

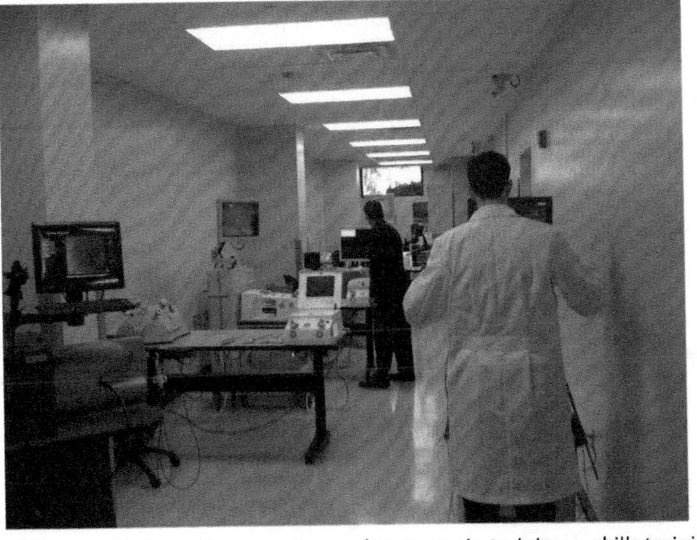

**Fig. 1.** In addition to the benefits to novices and surgeons in training, a skills training center allows practicing surgeons to rehearse skills and stay abreast of current techniques.

programs also increases the laboratory's competitive advantage when seeking grants from external sources.

Endorsement from local hospitals can provide supplementary funding. With a vested interest in improving patient safety, hospitals can save costs from shorter operations and fewer patient complications. These benefits outweigh the steep investment involved with establishing a training laboratory. Like partnerships with other medical departments and allied health disciplines, support from and collaboration with local hospitals will provide a stronger foundation for sustaining the laboratory.

Medical school tuition in the form of laboratory fees is another mode of funding. In addition to residents and practicing providers, medical students also benefit from access to a simulation-based skills laboratory. The growing belief in early education of basic surgical skills, including laparoscopy, has led to increased utilization of simulation-based training centers by medical students. Recently, the American College of Surgeons and the Association of Surgical Education established a Simulation-Based Surgical Skills Curriculum that is increasingly being adopted by medical schools. A recent survey of surgery programs indicated that 69% of laboratories are concurrently used by medical students.[3] In addition, the commitment to educational excellence increases the competitiveness and attractiveness of the medical school, serving as a recruiting tool to incoming medical students.

External support beyond laboratory users can be acquired from federal, state, or local government support or philanthropic donations from alumni, local community organizations, or private entities. Because the aim of charities is to benefit the public good, fundraising activities should emphasize how the community's reputation and overall health is enhanced by the presence of a simulation center within it. For example, the skills laboratory enhances education for current and future health care providers, thus improving the health care for the community. Government funding can also be secured for the laboratory; the election season for local government officials who share support of the laboratory is a strategic time to request funding.

Incremental funding can be acquired from continuing education course fees or research grants. For example, programs that offer certification can charge credentialing fees. For research, funds can be requested in the form of overhead and fringe costs when the laboratory space is used. Use or purchase of supplies for research activities also warrants budget line items. Simulation laboratories can charge fees for activities that use the space, equipment, and personnel for purposes aside from the intended surgical skills training and education. The fees will vary based on factors such as what facilities are available, the capacity for live-animal surgery, the geographic location, and the viable alternatives for a given desired activity.

## BUDGETING

Establishing a surgical skills laboratory requires a start-up and maintenance budget. The start-up budget is the initial financial plan for starting the skills laboratory through operation in its initial years. Included in this budget are personnel, physical space, materials, supplies, and training equipment, assuming facility space is already constructed (**Table 1**). Costs are derived from the curriculum and are estimated from the size of residency. Several programs have reported start-up costs as low as $100,000, whereas other laboratories cost up to several million dollars to establish. The average cost of a laboratory start-up is approximately $450,000.[4]

Beyond the start-up, a plan for ongoing support to sustain the laboratory should also be established. Compared with start-up, when most expenditure occurs, maintenance is generally less expensive, ranging from $12,000 to $300,000 annually.

**Table 1**
**Sample budget configuration for principal costs**

| Budget Items | Estimated Costs ($) |
|---|---|
| Simulation Equipment | |
| Fundamental of Laparoscopic Surgery Trainer Box | 4715 |
| GI-Mentor Endoscopy Simulator (Simbionix, Cleveland, OH) | 64,500 |
| MIST (Mentice, Gothenburg, Sweden) | 16,000–25,000 |
| LapSim Basic (Surgical Science, Minneapolis, MN) | 39,000 |
| Lap Mentor (Simbionix, Cleveland, OH) | 90,000 |
| Extended warranty | Varies per equipment |
| Operating Equipment and Materials | |
| Varies per curriculum | |
| Training laboratory computer | 400 |
| Television monitors | 200 |
| Portable video recording devices | 200 |
| Stapler reloads | 3000 |
| Suture | 3000 |
| Endoloops (Ethicon, Somerville, NJ) | 1000 |
| Task trainer disposables | 3000 |
| Animal part resections | 800 |
| FLS disposables | 800 |
| Building materials | 400 |
| Personnel Costs | Varies from part-time to 1.00 full-time equivalent |
| Facilities Expense | |
| Lease or rent | Varies per institution |
| Total | — |

*Abbreviation:* FLS, Fundamentals of Laparoscopic Surgery.

Recurring and maintenance costs include laboratory consumables, personnel, facility fee, and warranty support or upkeep for equipment.[4]

***Equipment and Supplies***

The initial investment is substantial as most of the capital expenditures occur during start-up. Capital expenses include major equipment, which is defined as property that has an acquisition cost greater than $5000 and has a service or utility life of 1 year or greater. Simulators and operating room equipment, such as laparoscopy towers, are examples of capital expenses. Simulators vary in price depending on the sophistication of technology. Almost all laboratories have box trainers, such as the Fundamentals of Laparoscopic Surgery (FLS) Box Trainer (Limbs & Things LTD, Savannah, GA) or Simulab Lap Trainer (Simulab Corporation, Seattle, WA). Although the number of trainers does not necessarily correlate with the size of the program, most laboratories have an average of 3 trainers.[2] Investment in box trainers is less costly initially; but it can require significant personnel commitment in the long-term, as optimal use of box trainers requires expert read-time feedback. Self-practice training methods, such as video tutorials, can offset manpower needs and its cost for training.

Virtual reality simulators are extremely expensive. Many training laboratories possess at least one virtual reality simulator. Examples of virtual reality simulators include MIST (Mentice, Gothenburg, Sweden), LapSim (Surgical Science, Minneapolis, MN), or Lap VR Mentor (Simbionix, Cleveland, OH). The advanced technology allows for self-directed training and self-assessment, saving both time and effort for training center personnel. In order to balance the costs of equipment and manpower, relying more on inexpensive low technology trainers in addition to a few virtual reality simulators may be cost-effective. Regardless of laparoscopic training methods, simulation laboratories that serve resident trainees should have the trainers and equipment to allow residents to practice for the FLS certification examination. Additionally, the ability to practice for Fundamentals of Endoscopic Surgery (FES) is recommended, because certification in FES is soon to become a requirement for graduating chiefs wanting to sit for the Qualifying Examination of the American Board of Surgery. With the steep capital investment in equipment, its maintenance should also be considered. Although limited warranties are typically available with the purchase of new apparatuses, the purchase of an extended warranty is recommended, given that replacement or repair of simulators is inevitable and can be expensive. These warranties can cost tens of thousands of dollars per annum, an expense that needs to be budgeted at the time of purchase.

The inventory of the training center also includes consumable materials and supplies necessary for conducting skills simulation training. These costs must also be included in the start-up budget. These items include sutures, absorbable clips, and stapler reloads. Other initial purchases that are necessary for administering skills modules include television monitors, portable video carts, camera lens, and laboratory manuals.

When constructing a budget for equipment or supplies, price quotes from different vendors should be obtained and negotiated accordingly. Although many of these products are available in bulk or prepackaged assortments, items should be purchased according to the needs of the curriculum, required tasks for training, and available resources. Unused items are wasteful over time. Establishing a relationship or rapport with hospitals and industry is also helpful and may also allow savings in costs and donations.

### *Salaries and Wages*

At a minimum, skills laboratories generally require one individual to run and manage activities (**Fig. 2**). Administrative duties include scheduling coordination of learners and inventory management. In addition, personnel must help with the set up/breakdown of training equipment, teaching courses, and evaluating trainees. Having an employed staff can help reduce the time commitment needed from faculty members, but faculty participation can never be eliminated. Although the initial stages may require little support from personnel, increased utilization over time requires at least one full-time employee. As demand increases, other full-time equivalents may need to be added to the staff. The budget must account for salaries and wages of all such personnel involved with the training center.

Determining who is best suited to staff a training center is an important and challenging task. The credentials needed depend on the curricula being taught and the learner groups being targeted. For example, a surgical technician knowledgeable with operating room (OR) instruments and equipment might be sufficient for a training center focusing mainly on teaching residents technical skills. A nurse educator may be required for a training center training multiple professions in both technical and

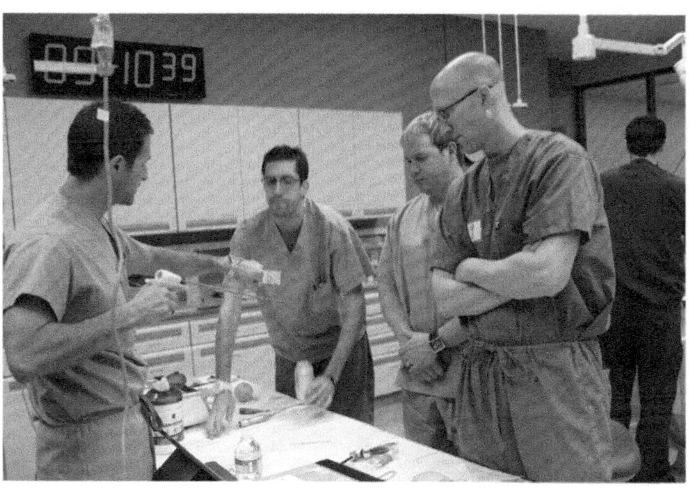

**Fig. 2.** Coordinators are necessary for the operation of the skills laboratory. Coordinators manage the laboratory and provide teaching assistance to reduce time commitments from faculty.

nontechnical skills. Larger centers may need to add a PhD educator to help with curriculum development and assessment, or a human factors expert may be recruited to help with research in teamwork or evaluation tool development. As different learner groups are added, more individuals may be hired to focus on a particular component of the training curriculum or type of learner.

### *Facilities*

Physical space dedicated for simulation-based training is necessary for establishing a simulation center. Assurance of space is more feasible and cost-effective by converting available space rather than constructing a new facility. Using space within or nearby hospitals is most convenient; converting unused operating rooms or an existing clinical classroom environment can potentially save costs. Conversely, institutions can elect to renovate or construct a new facility to leverage additional funding. At a minimum, 800 sq ft of space should be allocated for simulators, workstations, monitors, other patient care equipment, and supplies (**Fig. 3**). For budget preparation, the cost of the occupied space is listed as an ongoing cost. In a shared laboratory, facility fees can be divided among each collaborator. For example, the percentage of use by each department or specialty is used to determine the amount of funds that each contributes toward the use of facility, equipment, and materials.

## REPRESENTATIVE AND INNOVATIVE FUNDING AND REVENUE EXAMPLES

### *Funding Examples*

#### *Core laboratory model*

One funding solution used to address financing of a simulation-based skills training center is to treat it much like a core laboratory used to conduct bench research. Core laboratories are typically common resources housed within a health sciences center or school housing laboratory equipment and materials requiring large capital expenses that are essential to conduct key aspects of research. The cost to obtain the equipment is assumed by the larger health sciences center or school, and multiple

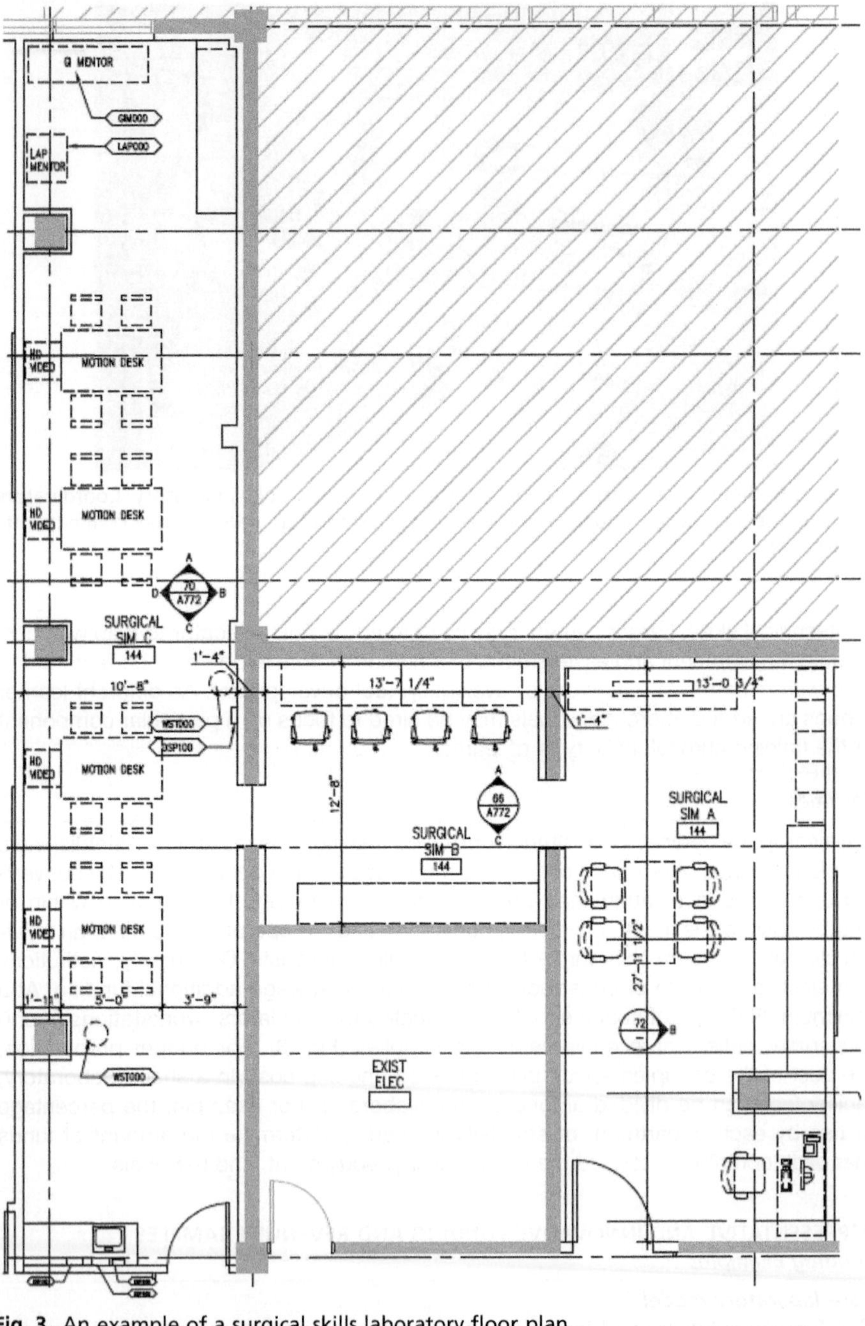


**Fig. 3.** An example of a surgical skills laboratory floor plan.

research groups share its use. In addition, the core laboratory becomes an in-kind institutional resource that allows groups to apply for larger federal and/or private grants. Thus, although the institution absorbs the initial cost, the core laboratory is a potential multiplier in terms of research grants.

A simulation center can serve much the same function. The space, simulation rooms, high-cost simulators, and other equipment can be housed within a school or health sciences center in lieu of a smaller department, allowing for its use across multiple specialties and professions. Use of the facility could be on a per-use basis or based on mission priorities for the institution. For example, a school of medicine might assume the cost for student-based training and education because it is considered part of the mission of the entity. Continuing professional development activities, on the other hand, may be permitted at a fixed or variable rate. With such a model, capital purchases tend to involve equipment and/or simulators with multi-specialty/profession applications, allowing for optimal utilization of resources.

#### *Pay-to-play model*

Another solution to funding a simulation-based skills training center is a pay-to-play model in which user groups assume part of the cost of running the center. Major participant specialties and/or professions may be assessed an annual tuition or fee. This amount might be evenly distributed among the specialties or prorated based on the number of residents/learners in each group. Alternatively, an additional charge based on learners per group might be assessed in order to cover disposables or the like. Major purchases of large-scale capital equipment would be supported through one or all of the user groups based on consensus building. This model ensures that all key user groups have so-called skin in the game, ensuring engagement in center-based decision making and purchases.

### *Innovative Revenue Examples*

#### *Partnering with malpractice insurance companies*

One potential revenue source for a skills training center is with malpractice insurance companies. These entities are continually looking for ways to reduce costs and payout amounts and, thus, could be willing to pay for training in certain high-risk procedures or in teamwork in order to lower risk. Such partnerships are particularly likely to occur in situations in which institutions or groups are self-insured, because the incentives benefit both the insurer and the institution. An example of such a revenue partnership is the Harvard CRICO funding of an OR team training project to determine its effectiveness in reducing occurrences.[5]

#### *Training at outside hospitals*

Another source of revenue for a training center is from training at outside hospitals. Thus, training is taken on the road in which center personnel travel to designated hospitals to perform technical, nontechnical, or combined technical/nontechnical skills training with hospital staff and physicians based on the needs of the institution. For this in situ training, the hospitals can pay the training center, providing revenue to offset costs of activities at the center itself. Central line placement instruction is an example of a skill-based training activity. Team-based training for low-frequency, high-risk events, such as emergency department delivery, is an example of combined technical/nontechnical training.

#### *Maintenance of certification programs*

MOC simulation-based training is already an established component of the American Board of Anesthesiology recertification program. The American Board of Surgery and other surgical specialty boards will no doubt follow suit within the short to midterm. These programs will likely be administered through regional or state-based training centers. Thus, surgeons will be continually searching for MOC courses for which the center can charge tuition to provide revenue.

## SUMMARY

Careful financial planning is imperative for establishing a skills laboratory. Support from the surgery department and hospital and collaborations with medical departments are essential for the initial foundation and sustenance of the laboratory. Endorsement can also be attained from external sources, such as industry sponsorship, donations, and miscellaneous activities. When budgeting, all expenses should be justifiable and attuned appropriately, and services should be charged appropriately to all laboratory users. Although initial costs can be substantial, prudent management of finances and proper use of resources will demonstrate how the benefits of a laboratory will outweigh the operational costs over time.

## REFERENCES

1. Babineau TJ, Becker J, Gibbons G, et al. The "cost" of operative training for surgical residents. Arch Surg 2004;139(4):366–9.
2. Gould JC. Building a laparoscopic surgical skills training laboratory: resources and support. JSLS 2006;10(3):293–6.
3. Kapadia MR, Darosa DA, Macrae HM, et al. Current assessment and future directions of surgical skills laboratories. J Surg Educ 2007;64(5):260–5.
4. Henry B, Clark P, Sudan R. Cost and logistics of implementing a tissue-based American College of Surgeons/Association of Program Directors in Surgery surgical skills curriculum for general surgery residents of all clinical years. Am J Surg 2014;207(2):201–8.
5. Arriaga AF, Gawande AA, Raemer DB, et al. Pilot testing of a model for insurer-driven, large-scale multicenter simulation training for operating room teams. Ann Surg 2014;259:403–10.

# Surgical Simulation Centers as Educational Homes for Practicing Surgeons

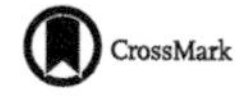

Brian J. Dunkin, MD

**KEYWORDS**

- Educational home • Practicing surgeons • Retooling

**KEY POINTS**

- The pace of change in surgery is unprecedented, requiring surgeons to retool more often during their careers.
- Technical performance of surgery impacts patient outcome more than process measures.
- Currently, there is no infrastructure to support the training of surgeons in practice.
- Practicing surgeons need an "educational home" where they can return to intermittently through their career to retool.

## INTRODUCTION

The pace of change in surgery today is unparalleled. Carl Langenbuch performed the first open cholecystectomy in 1882 and the operation was done without variation from his technique for more than 100 years.[1] However, in 1985, Eric Muhe performed the operation laparoscopically and within 5 years, the majority of cholecystectomies in Europe and the United States were being done laparoscopically.[2] More modern examples of this pace of change include robotic surgery, where the first robotically assisted prostatectomy was performed in the United States in 2000 and by 2006 the majority of operations were being performed this way, or the management of Barrett's esophagus with high-grade dysplasia, where the standard of care has transitioned from esophagectomy in 2009 to endoscopic radiofrequency ablation by 2011.

Richard Buckminster "Bucky" Fuller, an American neo-futurist, author, designer, and inventor, created the "Knowledge Doubling Curve." He noted that, in 1900, human knowledge doubled approximately every century. By the end of World War II, it was doubling every 25 years. By 2010, the doubling time decreased to 3 years and it is currently estimated that clinical knowledge doubles every 18 months (**Fig. 1**). This means that a surgeon entering practice at the age of 32

Department of Surgery, Houston Methodist Institute for Technology, Innovation, and Education (MITIE), 6550 Fannin Street, Suite 1661, Houston, TX 77030, USA
*E-mail address:* mitie@houstonmethodist.org

Surg Clin N Am 95 (2015) 801–812
http://dx.doi.org/10.1016/j.suc.2015.04.002 **surgical.theclinics.com**
0039-6109/15/$ – see front matter 

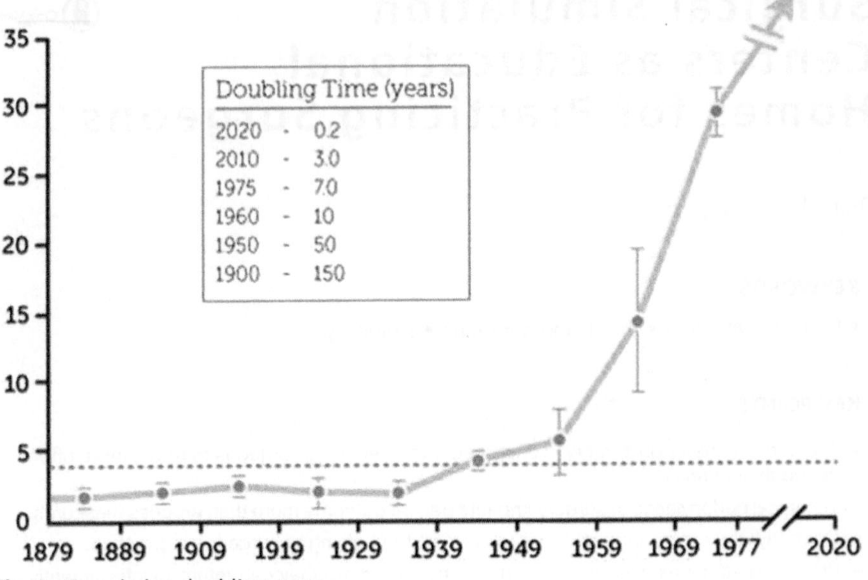


**Fig. 1.** Knowledge doubling curve.

will live through 22 doublings of clinical knowledge before he or she retires at the age of 65. This pace of change is putting increasing pressure on practicing surgeons to stay abreast of their field.

Rapid change leads to gaps in knowledge and skill for surgeons, which contributes to variability in the delivery of care. This variability increases cost while decreasing quality. The Institute of Medicine of the National Academies estimates that if all states in the United States could provide the quality of care provided by the highest performing states, there would have been 75,000 fewer deaths in 2005 and $210 billion saved in eliminating unnecessary services. In an age where US health care expenditures are exceeding 10% of the gross domestic product, controlling costs by reducing variability in care and providing value to patients is critical. Birkmeyer and colleagues[3] argue that variability in surgery patient outcomes are more directly related to surgeon skill and operative technique than to process measures. They asked 20 practicing bariatric surgeons to submit a video of one of their operations for independent review and compared the quality of operative technique with patient outcomes. The results demonstrated significant variability in technical skill, with 5 surgeons ranking in the bottom quartile, 10 in the middle, and 5 in the top. Compared with the top-quartile surgeons, the bottom quartile had higher complications rates and mortality with longer operations, higher rates of reoperation, and more readmissions.

Confronted with this rapid pace of change and a need to be remain technically proficient, practicing surgeons require an infrastructure that supports them throughout their decades of practice. This infrastructure should provide knowledge for the delivery of the most up-to-date and cost-effective treatment strategies as well as hands-on training with deliberate practice to ensure adequate technical proficiency. Ideally, surgeons would have a relationship with an "educational home" that provides to them the ongoing training they require in practice similar to what they had during residency training.

This article reviews the current state of education for practicing surgeons, describes the desired features of an educational home, and provides examples of how this home may function, who pays for it, and how it can be used to improve national health.

## CURRENT STATE OF TRAINING FOR PRACTICING SURGEONS

Over the last century, medical training in the United States has become among the best in the world. This was accomplished by creating a formalized infrastructure that includes accredited medical schools, postgraduate residencies and fellowships, and a robust board certification process. Unfortunately, once this training is complete, there is no formalized method of support for the continuing education of the practicing surgeon. As a result, surgeons are left to navigate an ad hoc world of limited training opportunities.

### *Maintenance of Certification*

Recently, the American Board of Surgery (ABS) has worked to encourage surgeons to stay current in their field by instituting a maintenance of certification (MOC) process. The ABS MOC contains 4 elements:

1. *Professional standing*. This requires maintaining a full and unrestricted medical license in the United States or Canada, holding hospital or surgical center privileges in good standing, and having favorable professional references.
2. *Lifelong learning and self-assessment*. Board-certified surgeons must demonstrate on-going learning by participating in at least 90 hours of continuing medical education (CME) category I activities relevant to their practice every 3 years. Sixty of these hours must include self-assessment, which is deemed to be a written examination about the CME material. A score of 75% or higher must be achieved on these examinations.
3. *Cognitive expertise*. Surgeons must successfully pass a recertification exam every 10 years.
4. *Evaluation of performance in practice*. This requires ongoing participation in a local, regional, or national outcomes registry or quality assessment program, either individually or through an institution.

Limitations to the MOC process include a lack of directive for topics that should be covered by surgeons during their CME study to maximize public health and an inability to measure technical skill. As a result, individual surgeons are left to study any topic of interest within their field to meet their CME requirements and to participate in hospital or national registries of patient outcomes that do not provide enough granular data to provide meaningful feedback on individual practice.

The MOC process does not address the needs of a practicing surgeon who wants to learn to use a new technology or technique and introduce it safely into his or her practice. To date, this has been addressed mainly by society-sponsored postgraduate courses or industry-sponsored training programs.

### *Postgraduate Courses*

Society-sponsored postgraduate hands-on training courses have become a common offering at the annual meeting of many surgical societies. These programs most often consist of a series of lectures by expert faculty followed by a hands-on training experience in a laboratory setting. Models used for this training range from inanimate to explant, animate, or cadaver. Because of the compressed time frame of these programs, open access to any level of practitioner, and high learner to faculty ratios, postgraduate courses are useful as an introduction to new techniques or technology, but not for successful and safe incorporation into practice.

One society is piloting a novel program to change the structure of its postgraduate courses into a longitudinal year-long training event. The Society of American Gastrointestinal and Endoscopic Surgeons (SAGES) has initiated a program called ADOPT. Beginning with the SAGES annual meeting in 2015, surgeons attending a postgraduate course on abdominal wall reconstruction will have the opportunity to go through the ADOPT training pathway, which uses the postgraduate course as the entry point into a year-long training initiative (**Fig. 2**). The postgraduate course itself has been restructured with faculty having to be trained specifically to teach in the hands-on laboratory. In the months after the course, surgeons have access to a series of webinars conducted by the postgraduate course expert faculty to support their attempts at procedural adoption. They then have the opportunity for another face-to-face faculty meeting at the American College of Surgeons (ACS) annual meeting in the fall of 2015, followed by more webinars. Efforts are also being made to include social media solutions to aid communication between learners and faculty and to offer regional hands-on refresher courses throughout the year. The program culminates with final follow-up at the SAGES 2016 annual meeting, where self-reported procedural adoption will be measured. This novel program may change the face of traditional postgraduate courses and lead to more meaningful procedural adoption.

### *Industry-Sponsored Training*

The most common procedural training programs available to surgeons are industry-sponsored courses. Medical device manufacturers are motivated to provide training on the correct use of their products to ensure safe use in practice. As surgical procedures have become more device dependent, industry has invested heavily in surgeon training. Most industry-sponsored training programs are "win–win" opportunities. Surgeons are given the opportunity to train on new devices and techniques with the cost offset by industry, and manufacturers are able to showcase their technology and ensure that it is used properly. In addition, many of the faculty used for these programs are widely recognized experts, adding to the credibility of the programs. Limitations of this training include the risk of bias to promote a manufacturer's products, potentially narrow focus on one technique or technology only, and a compressed time frame with

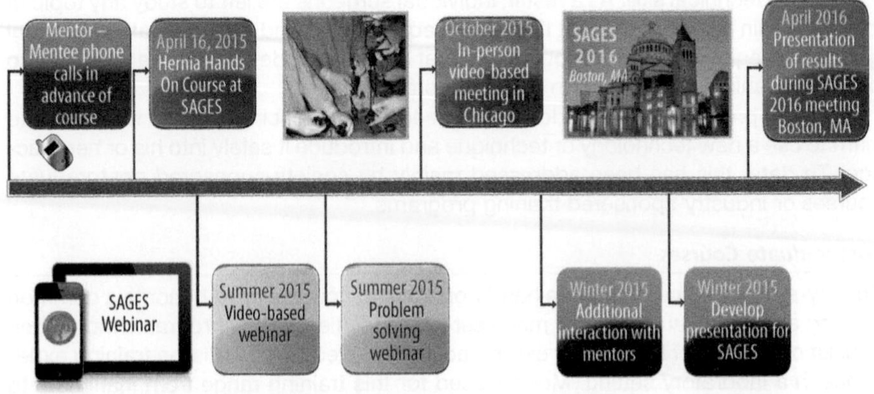


**Fig. 2.** Society of American Gastrointestinal and Endoscopic Surgeons (SAGES) project adopt timeline.

no metrics of procedural performance built into the curriculum. There are strict guidelines as to the structure of a category I CME program to avoid bias, but because these guidelines forbid industry from directly supporting a surgeon to attend a CME event, industry-sponsored courses usually occur outside of CME oversight.

## NEED FOR AN EDUCATIONAL HOME FOR SURGEONS

This ad hoc world of training opportunities for practicing surgeons speaks to a need to develop a national infrastructure for a distributed network of "educational homes." Bass and colleagues[4] in their review of surgical privileging and credentialing recognized this need and stated that, "A new infrastructure to support surgical training and technical retooling must be developed." They went on to say that, "Most surgeons in practice rely on a self-created program of self-study, skills acquisition, and review of their own surgical practice results," and that "No component of the health care industry considers procedural educational infrastructure to be 'its' problem with respect to facilities for training, provision of faculty for training, proctors, etc." Although the authors recognize that surgical societies, academic centers, and the surgical industries have tried to provide this important service, the facilities for technology training and retooling remain inadequate, inappropriately used, and very unevenly funded. Despite this, they conclude that, "No singular other investment could provide a more durable and substantial impact on the quality of surgical care."

### *Structure of an "Educational Home"*

So what should an educational home look like? To begin with, it should be a purpose-built facility for practicing surgeons who have specific educational needs that differ from medical students and residents. The physical structure should be large enough to service a significant number of surgeons and include environments to support cognitive, procedural, and team training. The cognitive learning environments should allow for interactive education using the latest in adult learning theory and provide for viewing of live cases with 2-way interaction. Practicing surgeons learn a great deal by observing experts during live cases (**Fig. 3**). The procedural learning environments

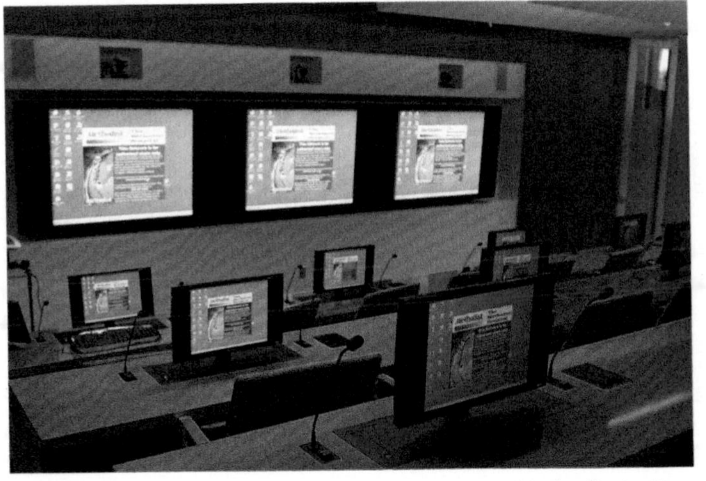

**Fig. 3.** Audiovisual suite for observing live surgery at Houston Methodist Institute for Technology, Innovation, and Education (MITIE).

must be able to accommodate all appropriate surgical training models, including inanimate or computer-based simulators, explants, live animals, and cadavers (**Fig. 4**). The fidelity of the model used for surgical training is more important for practicing surgeons than trainees because an experienced surgeon will not buy-in to working in an environment that he or she knows does not emulate the real world. Team training environments should be capable of recreating any part of the surgical care environment, including operating room, recovery room, intensive care unit, and the patient ward (**Fig. 5**). As surgery has evolved into a "team sport," these environments are critical for rehearsal by all members of the surgical team—surgeon, nurse, technician, anesthesiologist, and so on.

In addition to a physical structure, educational homes must have access to expert faculty who are trained to teach others, and curriculum design experts capable of creating meaningful educational experiences. These curricula should include measures of procedural performance that can be used for formative and summative feedback both in the hands-on training laboratory and in the real operating room. Finally, educational homes should be able to support surgeons when they return to their own institutions and begin traversing the early part of their learning curve for a new technique or technology. This support can be done with in-person mentoring or telementoring.

### *Telementoring*

Once a surgeon has completed hands-on training to learn a new technique or technology, they should be supported in their own operating room as they begin to provide this new offering to their patients. In-room mentoring has been used since the beginning of surgery for this effort. However, modern-day logistics make in-room mentoring difficult. There are not enough skilled mentors available to train large numbers of surgeons across a country the size of the United States and the lost revenue incurred for a

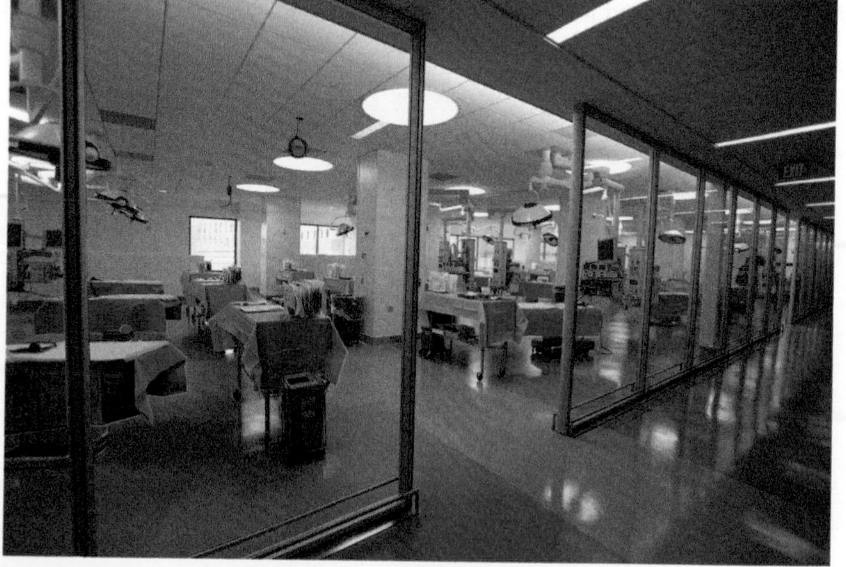


**Fig. 4.** Procedural training laboratory for rehearsing surgical procedures at Houston Methodist Institute for Technology, Innovation, and Education (MITIE).

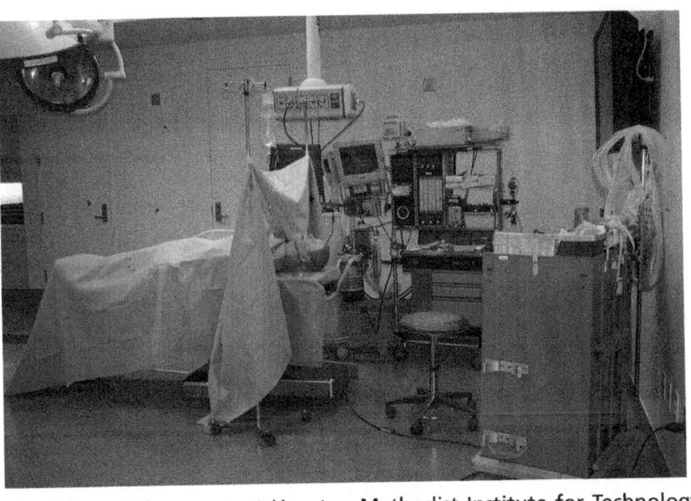

**Fig. 5.** Simulated operating room at Houston Methodist Institute for Technology, Innovation, and Education (MITIE).

mentor to be away from their own operating room is significant. In addition, legal and regulatory hurdles have become more complex, causing many expert mentors to abandon the practice.

Recently, audiovisual technology has evolved to the point of enabling a meaningful 2-way interaction into an operating room. Telementoring using this audiovisual technology could be used to develop a scalable mentoring program that minimizes the burden of expert mentors and makes them more readily available. The practice has been used successfully in a number of institutions around the world, but its widespread adoption in the United States has been limited by regulatory and legal barriers. Part of the problem is that telementoring has been lumped-in with telemedicine, the latter of which is regulated by state medical boards and prohibited across state lines. The SAGES Telementoring Task Force defines telementoring and differentiates it from telemedicine as follows:

> *Telemedicine is providing a service directly to a patient over distance. Telementoring is a quality initiative for the practicing surgeon and requires three essential elements: (1) An established relationship between the mentor and the mentee. This makes telementoring different from teleconsultation where there is not an established relationship prior to the event, or telemedicine which is the direct interaction between the patient and the expert. In telementoring the skills and knowledge of both mentor and mentee are understood through a relationship developed prior to the telementoring event. (2) Telementoring occurs within an educational framework. Both the mentor and mentee have worked together within this framework and been properly prepared for the mentoring experience. (3) Telementoring is done with a competent mentee. This means that the mentee is completely capable of managing the patient's disease as if the mentor were not there – just with a different technique or using a different technology. The mentoring session is to help adopt a new technique or technology into clinical practice, but always with a safe fall back plan if anyone is uncomfortable with how the procedure is progressing.*

This clear definition has been useful in overcoming institutional concerns about the liability involved with telementoring. It is also being used in an effort to persuade state medical boards to allow telementoring across state lines.

### *Distribution of Educational Homes*

Surgeons in the midst of a busy practice and rural surgeons who have no coverage support when they are absent cannot afford to be away from their practices for a significant period of time. As a result, a distributed network of training centers across the United States must be developed so that surgeons do not have to travel far from home to get the training they need. Comprehensive training centers in every state are not necessary to meet this need. Regional training centers strategically located across the country would be the most economical.

## DEVELOPMENTS IN CREATING SURGICAL EDUCATIONAL HOMES IN THE UNITED STATES

### *The American College of Surgeons Accredited Education Institutes*

In 2005 the ACS recognized the need for creating an infrastructure of institutes that could provide hands-on surgical training. It considered a centralized program versus a distributed one and decided that a distributed network would be best. It went on to set standards for programs and features an institute should have to be a valuable training center and created the Accredited Education Institute (AEI) program. The ACS AEIs are meant to educate and train practicing surgeons, surgical residents, medical students, and members of the surgical team using simulation-based education. The goal of the consortium is to promote patient safety through the use of simulation, develop new education and technologies, identify best practices, and promote research and collaboration among the institutes. There are 68 comprehensive and 11 focused ACS AEIs, most of which are in North America, but also spanning the globe.

Although the ACS-AEI consortium is a significant step in the creation of a national network of educational homes for surgeons, the majority of the institutes within the consortium focus primarily on medical student and resident training. In addition, the vision of centrally creating curricula arising from the needs of the surgical community and distributing those curricula through the AEIs is just now beginning to be realized.

### *The Lapco Model: An Example of a National Training Program for the Practicing Surgeon*

In 2006, the National Institute for Health and Care Excellence (NICE) in the United Kingdom reviewed existing data on the surgical management of colon cancer and the potential benefits of performing the procedure laparoscopically. Based on this review, NICE concluded that laparoscopic colon cancer surgery is at least equivalent to open surgery in oncologic outcomes, with less postoperative pain, shorter duration of hospital stay, and quicker return to full activity, and created a national mandate requiring all colorectal surgeons in the UK to offer laparoscopic surgery to their patients. To support this directive, a national training program to upskill surgeons in this technique called Lapco was implemented. In 2006, fewer than 5% of colorectal surgeons in England were performing laparoscopic colectomy. Today, it is 51% and climbing, saving the English health care system an estimated £18 million in direct costs alone. In the United States, fewer than 40% of colorectal operations are performed laparoscopically with great variability from hospital to hospital.

Surgeons who enrolled in the Lapco program were required to attend a hands-on training course at one of a number of approved training sites in the UK. The structure of these courses was not standardized. Afterward, they had in-room mentoring during live cases as they worked through their learning curve. One of the keys to the success of Lapco was a partnership with the department of surgery at the Imperial College in London to create validated metrics of procedural performance. This practice allowed for formative and summative assessment of the trainees who could not graduate from the program until blinded review of video recordings of their procedures met a minimum standard. Another critical element of the Lapco program was the development of a train-the-trainers course to teach experts how to mentor in the operating room. The Lapco train-the-trainers program developed a teaching methodology that fosters clear communication to minimize the need for an expert to take over the case while still maximizing patient safety.

One ACS AEI that is focused primarily on training practicing surgeons is working to "import" the Lapco training model into the United States and make it into a more scalable program. The Houston Methodist Institute for Technology, Innovation, and Education (MITIE) has partnered with the leadership of Lapco and the Imperial College to create a curriculum that shortens the learning curve for laparoscopic colectomy and uses telementoring instead of in-room mentoring (**Fig. 6**). The MITIE Lapco curriculum uses the same Lapco train-the-trainers program to teach faculty how to mentor in the operating room, but adapts it for telementoring. Interestingly, the Lapco communication technique, which emphasizes maintaining the independence of trainees in the operating room, is ideally suited for telementoring where a mentor is not physically present to take over the procedure. Unlike Lapco in the UK, MITIE Lapco developed a formalized hands-on training curriculum for trainees with a sophisticated structure that includes rigorous procedure rehearsal in a cadaver laboratory with multiple metrics of procedural competence. During the 4-day hands-on training, learners perform 6 cadaveric operations and are evaluated with 14 separate assessment tools while participating in 6 debriefing sessions. It is hoped that the increased rigor of the hands-on training will shorten the learning curve in the actual operating room.

During the MITIE Lapco cadaver training, learners and faculty progressed to being taught in the hands-on laboratory using the same telementoring platform they would use in their own operating room (**Fig. 7**). This familiarized all parties to the technology and allowed them to test its utility before using it in a live operating room. Upon completion of the hands-on training, the telementoring technology was installed in each of the learner's home institutions to support them through their learning curve. The performance of the trainee surgeons during each telementored case is evaluated with validated assessment forms to document progress. Like Lapco, they graduate from the program when blinded video review of their cases confirms that they have reached a minimum threshold of technical performance.

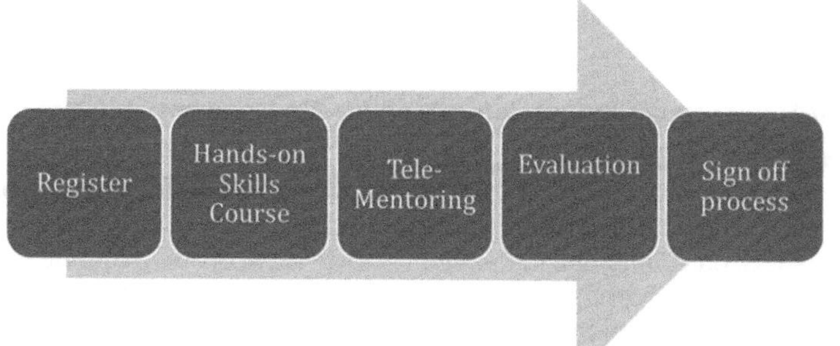


**Fig. 6.** Houston Methodist Institute for Technology, Innovation, and Education (MITIE)-Lapco curriculum pathway.

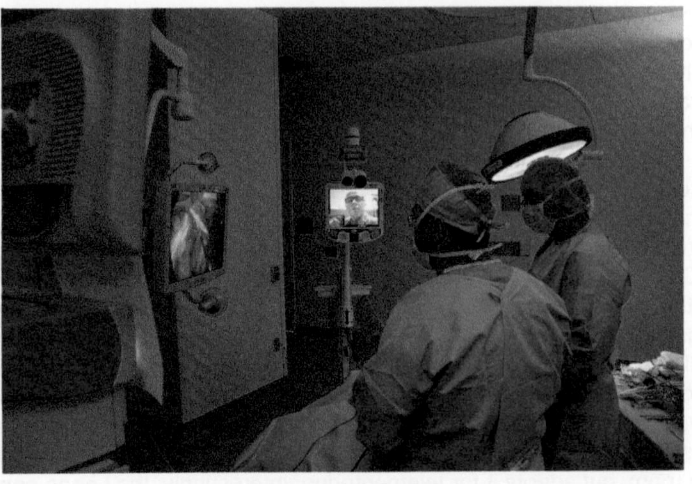

Fig. 7. Telementoring in procedural training laboratory.

Although telementoring is ongoing for the MITIE Lapco program, its early success has resulted in confidence that such a program could be distributed across the United States. Efforts are underway to partner with other ACS AEI institutes to prove that this sophisticated curriculum can be conducted and multiple centers.

## A PROPOSAL TO CREATE A NATIONAL TRAINING INFRASTRUCTURE FOR PRACTICING HEALTH CARE PROFESSIONALS

As described, the Institute of Medicine of the National Academies estimates that if all states in the United States could provide the quality of care provided by the highest-performing states, there would have been 75,000 fewer deaths in 2005 and $210 billion saved. The Institutes vision to address these deficiencies is to create a "learning health care system" that includes a leadership-instilled culture of learning. Organized, ongoing educational efforts focused on helping practicing health care professionals deliver optimal, value-based care is the cornerstone of controlling health care expenditures in the United States. We need as robust of an educational structure to support practicing health care professionals of all specialties as we have for students and postgraduate trainees. If this infrastructure was created, it could embrace the educational home concept for not only practicing surgeons, but all health care professionals. The process for how a national training program could be developed and distributed might proceed as follows.

### *The United States Establishes an Authority on the Management of Health Care Issues Important to the Nation*

This organization would be similar to NICE (National Institute for Health Care Excellence) in the UK, whose mission is to "provide national guidance and advice to improve health and social care" and has the authority to mandate policy. Work by this organization could start by concentrating on the needs of patients who receive care from US-funded programs (eg, Centers for Medicare and Medicaid Services programs) with input from reputable national institutions such as the Centers for Disease Control and Prevention, National Institutes of Health, and the Food and Drug Administration, and medical/surgical professional societies.

### *United States Authority Establishes Guidelines for Managing Diseases of Importance to United States Public Health*

Six of the top 8 health care expenditures in the United States, including heart disease ($107 billion annually), cancer ($82 billion), chronic obstructive pulmonary disease/asthma ($64 billion), joint disease ($62 billion), diabetes ($51 billion), and high blood pressure ($43 billion), would be the initial focus for establishing national, mandated guidelines that decrease variability in the care of these patients and optimize outcomes. If this effort resulted in only a 10% decrease in cost, the result would be more than $40 billion saved annually.

### *Curriculum Developed to Educate United States Health Care Work Force to Implement Guidelines*

Curriculum development can be central or by designated regional training centers. An example of central development would be the Centers for Disease Control and Prevention creating a training program to teach health care professionals the proper management of Ebola-infected patients. An example of developing a training program by a regional training center is the development of a comprehensive curriculum for training surgeons to perform laparoscopic colectomy by MITIE.

### *Curricula Distributed to Approved Training Centers*

These training centers may be located in each state or regionally, depending on the resources available. Centers are chosen based on an accreditation process to ensure they have the appropriate scale and capabilities. Desired features of approved centers include an infrastructure of personnel and technology capable of supporting the training of large numbers of health care professionals across multiple specialties and technology to support this training, both within the center and through telecommunication outside of the center.

### *Approved Training Centers Distribute Curricula into State or Local Training Environments*

Many health care providers may not be able to leave their communities for training, so they must be supported locally. Approved centers must have the capability of distributing training curricula to other centers of smaller scope and scale so that educational solutions can reach into smaller communities. Audiovisual technology can be used for telementoring at a distance.

### *Measurement of Performance*

The effectiveness of the training curricula will be measured through a reporting system that includes approved regional training centers reporting back to the US authority.

### *Government Contributions*

To establish a national training network for practicing health care professionals, the US government will need to dedicate resources and effort to the cause. This includes the following:

1. The United States establishes an authority on the management of health care issues important to the nation.
2. Provide funding to help approved regional training centers to develop and maintain the infrastructure required to provide necessary training.
3. Implement policy changes that enable nationwide training. This system includes eliminating the restriction of telementoring across state lines and consideration

of issuing a "medical education license" that allows practicing health care professionals to participate in hands-on training on real patients under the guidance of experts, just as medical trainees do. Such a license would shelter the professional from unreasonable medicolegal liabilities.

4. Work with telecommunication companies to build a secure, wireless network for broadcast of medical video and images for the purposes of training.

### *Finances*

If one considers only 6 of the top 8 health care expenditures in the United States as described, the results is nearly $410 billion spent annually. Reducing these costs by 10% through a national distributed training network would save $41 billion annually. If only 0.1% is invested in the infrastructure to develop a training network, that would make available $400 million annually. Part of these funds would be used to support the US authority that establishes guidelines on best practices; part to support the training centers for the development, administration, and distribution of curricula; and part to support trainees going through the training.

## SUMMARY

Given the pace of change in surgery today and a growing need to decrease variability in the delivery of health care to optimize quality while minimizing cost, surgeons need an "educational home" to which they can return intermittently through their career to retool. We need as robust of an educational structure to support practicing surgeons as we have for students and postgraduate trainees.

## REFERENCES

1. Hardy KJ. Carl Langenbuch and the Lazarus Hospital: events and circumstances surrounding the first cholecystectomy. Aust N Z J Surg 1993;63(1):56–64.
2. Reynolds W Jr. The first laparoscopic cholecystectomy. JSLS 2001;5(1):89–94.
3. Birkmeyer JD, Finks JF, O'Reilly A, et al. Surgical skill and complication rates after bariatric surgery. N Engl J Med 2013;369:1434–42.
4. Bass BL, Polk HC, Jones RS, et al. Surgical privileging and credentialing: a report of a discussion and study group of the American Surgical Association. J Am Coll Surg 2009;209(3):396–404.

# Advanced Engineering Technology for Measuring Performance

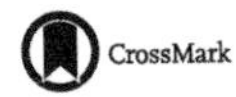

Drew N. Rutherford, MS[a], Anne-Lise D. D'Angelo, MD[a], Katherine E. Law, MS[b], Carla M. Pugh, MD, PhD[a,b,*]

**KEYWORDS**

- Simulation • Technology • Assessment • Sensors • Motion tracking

**KEY POINTS**

- Many technologies can achieve motion tracking of a surgeon's movements, but limitations in the simulation-based and operating room environments constrain their usage.
- Visual attention can reveal the cognitive processes underlying selection of procedural actions.
- Physiologic stress measurement can discern between experience levels of surgeons based on stress response, but it has multiple limitations.
- Evaluation of physical examination skills can be enhanced with the use of sensors to collect data on palpation force, frequency, location, and duration.
- Video-based data collection paired with qualitative analysis tools can be a valuable supplement to traditional observation methods.
- Application of innovative technology-based assessment tools requires a systematic evaluation of validity evidence using the modern construct validity framework.

## INTRODUCTION

Simulation-based clinical skills assessments have become a high priority in helping promote and ensure clinical excellence.[1–5] Trainee competence in the simulated environment can be assessed in numerous ways, including self-assessment measures,[6] observer-generated measures,[7–10] and technology-based performance measures.[2–5] Self-assessment and observer-based scoring are commonly used to assess trainees

[a] Department of Surgery, University of Wisconsin School of Medicine and Public Health, 3236 Clinical Science Center, 600 Highland Avenue, Madison, WI 53792, USA; [b] Department of Industrial and Systems Engineering, University of Wisconsin-Madison, 3215 Mechanical Engineering Building, 1513 University Avenue, Madison, WI 53706, USA
* Corresponding author. Department of Surgery, University of Wisconsin School of Medicine and Public Health, 3236 Clinical Science Center, 600 Highland Avenue, Madison, WI 53792, USA.
*E-mail address:* pugh@surgery.wisc.edu

Surg Clin N Am 95 (2015) 813–826
http://dx.doi.org/10.1016/j.suc.2015.04.005 surgical.theclinics.com
0039-6109/15/$ – see front matter 

but remain subject to bias. In contrast, technology-based measures can objectively quantify clinical and procedural performance and provide patient-centered metrics.[11]

Current technology allows for the collection of a variety of performance measures based on (1) motion,[12] (2) visual attention,[13] (3) physiologic stress,[14] and (4) palpation.[15] In addition, the use of innovative video capture technology and qualitative assessment measures can aid in the evaluation of data gathered from advanced engineering technology. The performance data generated from technology-based assessment tools (**Table 1**) may provide objective and reliable measures not possible with checklists and global rating scales alone. This article provides an overview of advanced engineering technology used to measure performance and the impact on clinical and surgical skills assessment.

## MOTION

A developing field in the assessment of complex surgical skill proficiency is the use of electronic sensors to record movement. Multiple technologies are able to capture the movement of a surgeon's hands and instruments while performing real or simulated procedures. These motion capture technologies record the 3-dimensional (3D) position of a person's body over time, known as kinematics, whereas other sensor technologies focus on recording the forces produced or experienced by a person or object, defined as kinetics.[16]

Various motion measures can be derived from a trace of position over time (**Fig. 1**A). The path length of the hands, straightness of movements, and working volume, defined as the 3D area in which the hands are moving, are obtained from 3D position. Velocity, acceleration (**Fig. 2**B), and motion smoothness profiles can be generated by taking derivatives with respect to time. Time-based measures, such as the number of

**Table 1**
**Examples of data collected from measuring hand movements, visual attention, physiologic responses, and palpation**

| Measurement | Data Outputs (Units) |
|---|---|
| Hand movements<br>Motion tracking | • Path length (m)<br>• Time (s)<br>• Velocity (cm/s)<br>• Acceleration ($cm/s^2$)<br>• Motion smoothness ($cm/s^3$)<br>• 3D position (m)<br>• Working volume ($cm^3$) |
| Visual attention<br>Eye tracking | • Gaze location (m)<br>• Fixation duration (s)<br>• Number of eye movements (#) |
| Physiologic responses<br>Electrodermal activity<br>Thermal imaging | • Temperature (°C)<br>• Thermal emission ($W/m^2$)<br>• Skin conductance (S)<br>• Voltage signal (V)<br>• Heart rate (beats/min)<br>• Respiratory rate (breaths/min) |
| Palpation<br>Force sensors | • Force (N)<br>• Area palpated ($cm^2$)<br>• Pressure ($N/m^2$)<br>• Palpation time (s) |

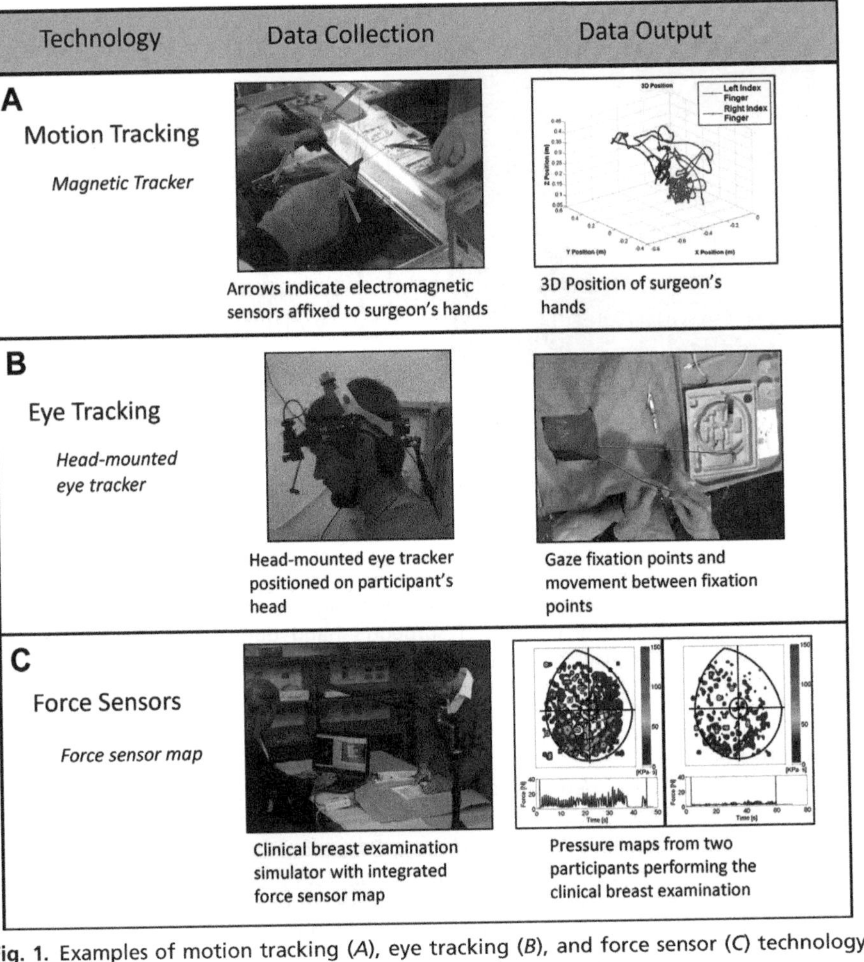


**Fig. 1.** Examples of motion tracking (*A*), eye tracking (*B*), and force sensor (*C*) technology used in research studies and corresponding sample data output.

movements used and time on task, can then be derived from these profiles. Performance in each of these measures is highly procedure specific, but the data provide useful predictors of skill, as they are shown to differ between novices and experts[12,17] as well as with task difficulty.[18]

Motion capture technology spans a variety of methodologies and types of electronic sensors. Those most commonly used in the study of human performance of complex manual skills include (1) optical tracking, (2) accelerometry-based tracking, and (3) magnetic tracking.

### *Optical Tracking*

The most commonly used motion capture technology for optical tracking uses cameras to record infrared light. The light may be reflected or emitted by markers placed on the body or instruments or visible light from the body itself. Three major categories of tracking exist based on the type of light or marker used: passive infrared, active infrared, and markerless visible light. Each technology has a variety of strengths and limitations that make it suitable for different situations.

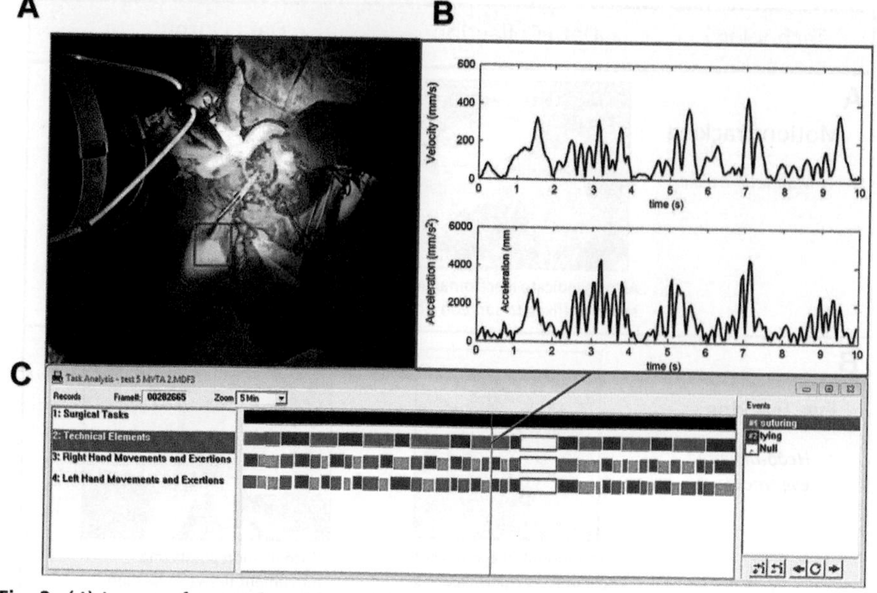


**Fig. 2.** (*A*) Image of operative video with pixel patch tag (*red square*) for motion tracking. (*B*) Acceleration and velocity profiles of surgeon's hand during the highlighted time segment collected with pixel tagging technology. (*C*) Screenshot of Multimedia Video Task Analysis video coding software used for classifying behavior.

### *Passive infrared*

Passive marker systems use multiple infrared cameras placed around a capture volume to track reflective markers (Bonita & T-Series, Vicon Motion Systems Ltd, Oxford, UK; Oqus, Qualisys AB, Gothenburg, Sweden; Raptor series, Motion Analysis Corp, Santa Rosa, CA, USA). People and objects are instrumented with small retroreflective balls that are affixed with tape, hook and loop fasteners, or glue. Each camera is equipped with a bright, near-infrared light that illuminates the capture volume. In each sampling period, the markers reflect the infrared light back to the camera and an image containing all of the markers visible to the camera is obtained. Computer software then calculates the 3D location of each marker by combining and interpolating images from each camera. This technique requires multiple cameras for good accuracy and the capture space to be calibrated before recording live data.

To track limbs and large body segments, preconfigured marker sets must be used with human subjects. Markers are placed on the body, and a set of marker locations are recorded while a subject stands in a neutral orientation. This set is used to infer the identity of markers during actual data collection, as markers that disappear or overlap in a camera view can become confused by the system. Although this system can record dozens of markers, a practical limit to the numbers of markers used exists, because the technology cannot easily distinguish between 2 closely spaced markers.

### *Active infrared*

Active optical systems use markers that are physically connected to power supplies (Visualeyez, Phoenix Technologies, Inc, Burnaby, BC, Canada; Optotrak Certus, Northern Digital, Inc, Waterloo, ON, Canada; Impulse X2, PhaseSpace, San Leandro,

CA, USA). These markers are typically an infrared light emitting diode (IRED) that is connected by wires to a control unit. In this method, the infrared camera system sends a signal independently to each marker and turns it on briefly while the image is captured. The system then moves to the next marker in the cycle and obtains images where only that single marker is visible, thus eliminating possible interference by other markers. The advantage of this technology over passive optical systems is that the identity of markers is never lost. This technology can be highly useful in differentiating individual fingers in the recording of suturing skills where markers operate in close proximity to each other.[18] In addition, the IREDs are much brighter than a reflective marker and can be operated at much higher sampling frequencies and with greater accuracy than a passive system.

**Limitations** Although both the passive and active infrared optical systems can offer excellent accuracy with small markers, their main limitation is the necessity for a direct visual line of sight of the marker to a camera. This requirement can be mitigated by adding more cameras in different locations around the capture space, but such a solution clutters the work area with equipment and cables. In the surgical arena, it is often difficult or impossible to place cameras in locations that can capture the motion of hands in the operative field with reliable line of sight. Placement of markers on hands or tools is also cumbersome and can significantly interfere with the functional operation of instruments. In addition, these systems function poorly in the presence of infrared light sources such as incandescent and halogen light bulbs and sunlight. Although the optical systems provide a high degree of accuracy, the need for direct line of sight, multiple cameras, and calibration makes these optical systems less practical for use in the surgical simulation laboratory or operating room.

### *Markerless tracking*

In recent years, optical tracking using visible light cameras without markers has become a popular alternative to expensive infrared camera systems (OptiTrack, NaturalPoint, Inc, Corvallis, OR, USA; BioStage, Organic Motion, New York, NY, USA). These systems incorporate inexpensive, generic off-the-shelf cameras (eg, webcams, digital cameras, gaming console cameras) and require little setup time or calibration. Software can be configured to track large pixel-based patches (see **Fig. 2**A) of the hands and instruments to obtain position data in 2 dimensions, or in 3D if multiple cameras are used simultaneously. One major drawback when using off-the-shelf cameras, such as the Microsoft (Redmond, WA, USA) Kinect camera for Xbox, is that there are few dedicated software solutions for universal applications. Most researchers require long development time to create their own custom software using machine vision programming platforms such as OpenCV (open-source computer vision) to obtain working simulation and analysis environments.

This method of motion tracking has advantages in that it can be performed post hoc on existing video of a procedure. In addition, markers do not need to be placed on the hands, so this technique avoids a loss of dexterity from foreign objects on the hands and preserves a sterile environment in the operating room. Cameras can be mounted to structures such as overhead lights, but this type of tracking has its own set of limitations. Fixed, mounted cameras can become obstructed by the surgeon's head. Another limitation is that these systems display large amounts of noise and lead to lower spatial resolution and higher variability than passive or active optical systems. They are particularly susceptible to confusion of overlapping body segments and tracking unintended objects in the visual field. Despite the reality that existing operating room video may be suboptimal for tracking, researchers have demonstrated the utility of markerless tracking in open procedures[19] and laparoscopic box trainers.[20]

### *Accelerometry-Based Tracking*

Inertial measurement units use small, lightweight accelerometers to record accelerations applied to the device (Kinesia, Great Lakes NeuroTechnologies, Cleveland, OH, USA; Xsens Technologies, Enschede, The Netherlands). The acceleration signal is integrated twice with respect to time to achieve incremental position data. Because of measurement errors, these devices are highly susceptible to a drift or distortion of the signal over sampling periods lasting longer than a few minutes. This causes large inaccuracies in the position data. One major consideration is that the beginning of each sample must always start with the device in a completely known and stationary neutral position and orientation as the device records only changes in position. An advantage of these inexpensive, lightweight devices is that they are self-contained, requiring no power wires and only elastic bands or adhesive to place on a person; this makes them useful in situations in which portability and limited line of sight are major concerns such as in neurosurgery trainers.[21]

### *Magnetic Tracking*

Magnetic tracking systems offer the best motion capture solution in situations in which high accuracy of position data is necessary and there is not a consistent line of sight between cameras and an individual's hands. Electromagnetic sensors connected by wires to a receiver unit are used in conjunction with a transmitter that generates a pulsed magnetic field in the capture volume (Patriot, Polhemus, Colchester, VT, USA). The sensors record position and orientation (6° of freedom) with very fine spatial resolution. Because the magnetic field can penetrate most materials, the technology functions without direct line of sight. However, the range of the transmitters is typically limited to a few meters. Conductive materials (eg, steel, stainless steel, iron, aluminum, copper, brass) interfere with the shape of the magnetic field and cause distortion in the position data. This limitation can be compensated by mapping any metal in the capture volume, but best practices are to avoid the use of large metal objects and opt for plastic and wood frames for tables or fixtures. The small amount of metal that most surgical tools possess does not largely affect recording. Because these systems operate without the need for direct line of sight, they have become a more popular motion capture method for laparoscopic box trainers and simulation units that lack sufficient views of obstructed tools.[22,23]

Because of the major factors of a limited line of sight to the fingers within surgical procedures and an inability to tolerate data loss, the authors use magnetic tracking technology (trakSTAR, Ascension Technology, Shelburne, VT, USA) for their simulation-based environments. The system provides spatial accuracy with no line-of-sight limitations by using small cylindrical markers (2–3 mm diameter) that provide minimal task interference to users (see **Fig. 1**A). In addition, the short ranges of the magnetic transmitters allow us to capture independent motion from multiple people simultaneously. This multiperson capture is not feasible using traditional optical systems. Magnetic technology provides a single-system solution that is highly practical in various simulation-based scenarios.

## VISUAL ATTENTION

Observing where surgeons place their conscious attention gives one a way to determine the targets of their attentional focus and concentration. The most common way to quantify the objects of visual attention, where the eyes are focused during a task, is through the use of eye tracking technology. Eye tracker devices monitor the orientation of one or both eyes to measure where a person fixes his or her gaze (Eye-Trac, Applied Science Laboratories, Bedford, MA, USA; Tobii Glasses 2, Tobii Technology AB, Stockholm, Sweden). Data from eye tracking systems provide measurements of where a person is placing their central vision; this indicates which objects in their environment are necessary visual cues for them to successfully complete a task.[16] This method can record information only about central vision; it does not properly assess the contribution that peripheral vision can yield during a task.[16] Eye tracking data have been previously used in simulation to assess cognitive processes leading to the selection of surgical procedure actions.[13]

Most hand movements are completed using vision to guide the hands and rapidly account for spatial errors.[24] Movements that present an individual with high demands for accuracy necessitate even greater visual control for error reduction. Using eye trackers to find the gaze of surgeons allows one to infer which objects or steps in a procedure the individual deems more difficult. Their visual attention points out regions where they are struggling and where they gather information for planning upcoming movements.[13]

Eye tracker devices use infrared cameras to record the orientation of the pupil. Similar to how a cat's eye reflects visible light, a human eye reflects near-infrared light striking the retina. Eye trackers shine an infrared light source into an eye and capture an image of the resulting pupil reflection as well as the reflection off of the curved surface of the cornea. The 2 reflections are used to calculate the direction of the eye's gaze with respect to the face. This direction must also be combined with the orientation of the head to obtain the gaze direction of the person's scene, which is typically accomplished by using a motion capture system to record the position and orientation of the frame of the head-mounted eye tracker unit (see **Fig. 1**B). In addition, most head-mounted eye trackers also include a standard video camera pointing forward to record the person's live point of view for later review with the gaze information.

Tracking eye movements can offer useful information for assessing a surgeon's cognitive processes; however, it presents several limitations in the simulation and operating room environment. Individuals are required to wear the eye tracker unit on the head, which typically trails long wires that limit freedom of movement. In addition, the tracker units must be calibrated before a procedure to obtain good accuracy, which is a lengthy process. Any shift in the head gear during a procedure requires a new calibration to be performed. In the operating room, these interruptions can be detrimental; they may pose fewer challenges in less constrained simulation environments.

## PHYSIOLOGIC STRESS

Physiologic stress, also known as physiologic arousal, has been used in multiple fields to understand how the human performs under stress and to determine the level of stress that produces a decrease in performance (Yerkes-Dodson law, 1908). Two main theories on how to measure physiologic stress exist. One approach measures stress through brain activity[25] with the use of functional MRI or electroencephalography.[26] Although measurement of stress via the brain can produce valuable findings, it has not yet reached the point of use in real-time situations, and, therefore, is not addressed further in this article. The alternative perspective measures stress through the body via contact sensors,[27] which can measure pulse, breaths per minute, and perspiration.

### *Electrodermal Activity*

Traditionally, galvanic skin response (GSR) has been the gold standard of tools for measuring electrodermal activity through perspiratory responses in real time. It is typically measured on the finger or palm, where sweat gland activation is the strongest.[28] When the sensor is attached to the skin, electric signals are produced that indicate a change in the electrical properties (conductance) of the skin when the user experiences stress. Few studies have examined GSR in surgical performance as these sensors need to be placed on the hand. However, one study examined the difference between laparoscopic and open surgeries using simulation and used GSR as one indicator of stress experienced by surgeons when performing knot-tying tasks.[29] The study found that stress levels increased in transitioning from open to laparoscopic knot tying, as hypothesized. GSR has been thoroughly studied in different fields. This work helped to develop a well-established understanding of GSR data patterns when subjects are repeatedly aroused.[30] Because the location of GSR sensors could limit surgical dexterity, the authors recommend its use in simulated settings, with alternative methods used in situ.

### *Thermal Imaging*

Thermal imaging has emerged as a method to evaluate stress responses by surgeons in the operating room.[28] Shastri and colleagues[28] found that during stress arousal, additional physiologic signs were indicated on the face, and through monitoring facial imaging the responses are similar to GSR sensing. After multiple experiments,[26] thermal imaging and GSR were used to compare performance between novice and experienced surgeons during laparoscopic tasks; no significant difference between responses was found ($P>.05$).[14]

Thermal imaging of the perinasal area is far easier to use in the operating room because of easier accessibility to the face than to the hands.[14] However, there are multiple contributing thermal factors that can affect the data, such as blood flow, sweat gland activation, and breathing.[28] In addition, the raw facial signals need to be transformed to make meaning of the data through techniques such as wavelets analysis[28] or signal extraction.[26]

Although each method of physiologic stress measurement has its limitations, both approaches are grounded in well-understood theory. Because of the evolving nature of surgical technique, surgeons will continue to experience increasing stress to maintain optimal performance, making techniques such as GSR and thermal imaging relevant today.

## PALPATION

Surgery has long been a profession that relies on the ability to gain knowledge through the use of touch to examine the human body, termed palpation. However, teaching proper physical examination techniques can be challenging. Experts may have difficulty verbalizing the process of gaining information through touch and assessing how the trainee is actually using palpation to gather information. The study of physical examination techniques in the simulation-based environment may help us to teach and objectively evaluate hands-on performance.[15] The theoretic basis for this line of research comes out of work by cognitive psychologists Roberta Klatzky and Susan Lederman. These researchers have produced a large body of work on the exploration, recognition, and perception of objects.[31–33]

The use of palpation to examine the human body includes the use of pressure. Pressure (force/area) can be measured with the use of multiple types of force sensors, including sensors that detect force based on properties such as electrical resistance or capacitance. The authors' laboratory uses sensors called force-sensing resistors (FSRs) that detect force application by changes in electrical resistance. Integration of these sensors into a simulator allows for the measurement of palpation force while a participant performs a physical examination. This technology gives us the ability to quantify characteristics of physical examination skills with measurements of palpation force, frequency, time, area, and pressure.

Integration of sensor technology into physical examination simulators was first pioneered in the clinical pelvic examination (CPE)[34–37] and later expanded to the digital rectal examination (DRE),[38] clinical breast examination (CBE) (see **Fig. 1**C),[5,39–41] and endotracheal intubation with direct laryngoscopy.[11] Incorporation of sensor technology into physical examination simulators provides quantification of trainees' palpation. This measurement is especially beneficial when the physical examination occurs in an enclosed space not visible to the instructor (CPE, DRE, endotracheal intubation) or requires specific levels of pressure (CBE).

Prior work with sensor-based simulation-based research on the performance of the DRE,[38,42,43] CPE,[34–37] and CBE[5,39–41] has revealed that differences in palpation technique can relate to accuracy and proficiency. For example, integration of sensors into the anorectal canal of a DRE simulator demonstrated that practicing clinicians and trainees had specific, quantifiable differences in palpation technique.[38] Practicing clinicians performed their examination with increased palpation pressure and frequency compared with trainees. In addition, clinicians palpated a greater number of anatomic locations across a wider area than the trainees. These findings were consistent with observations that students are more focused on pronating and supinating their fingers than purposeful abduction/adduction and flexion/extension of the examining finger.[38] This body of research demonstrates how force sensors can be integrated into simulators and used to assess examination and procedural techniques. These data can serve an important role in both education as well as competency-based examinations.

The wide range of available product dimensions allows for the integration of these products into multiple anatomic surfaces. Sensors can be purchased as individual units (Interlink Electronics, Camarillo, CA, USA) or as integrated force sensing maps (TEKSCAN, Boston, MA, USA; XSENSOR, Calgary, AB, Canada; Pressure Profile Systems, Los Angeles, CA, USA). The smaller individual units can be replaced easily and are inexpensive, at less than $10.00 for an individual FSR (Interlink Electronics, Camarillo, CA, USA). The sensors are paper thin, which allows them to be more easily integrated into simulators in embedded locations or affixed to superficial features. However, the sensors tend to be made out of a stiff material that can sometimes be detected with palpation when placed in a superficial location. The authors' laboratory has been investigating the use of a conductive cloth that is able to detect force, allowing for seamless integration into simulator surfaces.[44]

Overall, force sensors provide an objective means to capture how people use touch to perform physical examinations or procedures. The information gathered by the physician during palpation is important to the practice of medicine; however, little research exists on how practicing clinicians perform examinations and also on how trainees learn to use their sense of touch. By instrumenting the simulators with sensors, one can gain insight regarding patient-centered examination factors, including the amount and type of palpation pressure used in specific anatomic locations.[15] In addition, changes in palpation characteristics relative to clinical anatomy and pathology can be assessed.[40] The use of force sensors in the simulation-based environment may help us develop better physical examination assessment tools that are more accurate and reliable than those based on observation alone.

## VIDEO-BASED OBSERVATION AND ANALYSIS

As technology has advanced, so have the tools used to conduct observational research. Video and audio-based recording methods can aid in both understanding and improving performance on a smaller scale, such as individual performance,[45] as well as on a larger system scale, like teamwork.[46] The ability to review the same moment multiple times allows for a richer understanding of human interaction and context than with real-time observation alone.[47] Although it is impossible to process completely everything that is happening, video recording can provide a more objective perspective than the subjective view of the researcher in observation.[48]

Video recorders developed for use during high-action sports and the introduction of mass-market wearable technologies have slowly gained use in the surgical domain. Recorders such as the GoPro (San Mateo, CA, USA) and Google Glass (Mountain View, CA, USA) can record for long periods; based on where the camera is located in the operating room, it can provide an environmental view or an individual's perspective during surgery.

In conjunction with video and audio recording, video analysis software such as Transana (Madison, WI, USA) (**Fig. 3**) and Multimedia Video Task Analysis (MVTA) (Madison, WI, USA) (see **Fig. 2**C) allows for tagging and annotating large numbers of videos to obtain data-rich moments and classify behaviors. After coding the media files, the data can be extracted into usable files such as Microsoft Excel for further analysis.

Integrating audio and video recording into data collection presents some challenges. Additional cost and time are necessary to install and implement new equipment. In addition, gaining clinician trust is fundamental to this approach and can be a significant roadblock if not obtained. Clinicians require time to show buy-in for consistently using recording equipment and complying with its constraints.[47,49] In addition, the time involved postrecording in data analysis can be excessive and requires interrater reliability assessments to ensure validity.

## TECHNOLOGY-BASED ASSESSMENTS

The growing need for competency-based assessments in surgical education requires the development of performance measures that are innovative with robust validity evidence.[50] In 2013, Cook and colleagues[50] systematically reviewed the literature for the type of validity evidence evaluated in technology-enhanced simulation-based assessments in medicine. Only 64% of the studies reviewed actually included methods for interpreting the evidence of validity. The framework for evaluating validity evidence has moved away from making claims of formal validation of instruments and considering discrete sources of validity (face, content, criterion, and concurrent). Rather, modern frameworks describe a more unitary view of validity, fitting all these forms of validity under construct validity as detailed in Downing's[51] comprehensive review of the topic. This work demonstrates the need for continuous assessment of validity evidence with different user groups in different venues. The goal is to have a series of experiments that clarify for which users the assessment is best suited.

To provide appropriate sources of validity evidence, the choice of technology and performance metric used depends on the goals of the assessment and venue. Technology-based assessments allow for a variety of measures that can be combined to further assess validity. In the authors' laboratory, they use mixed methods and combine multiple techniques for measuring performance. Video recording allows for in depth performance analysis that can support the findings from technology-based metrics. This combined approach enables us to evaluate better the data outputs and provides a means for assessing validity evidence.

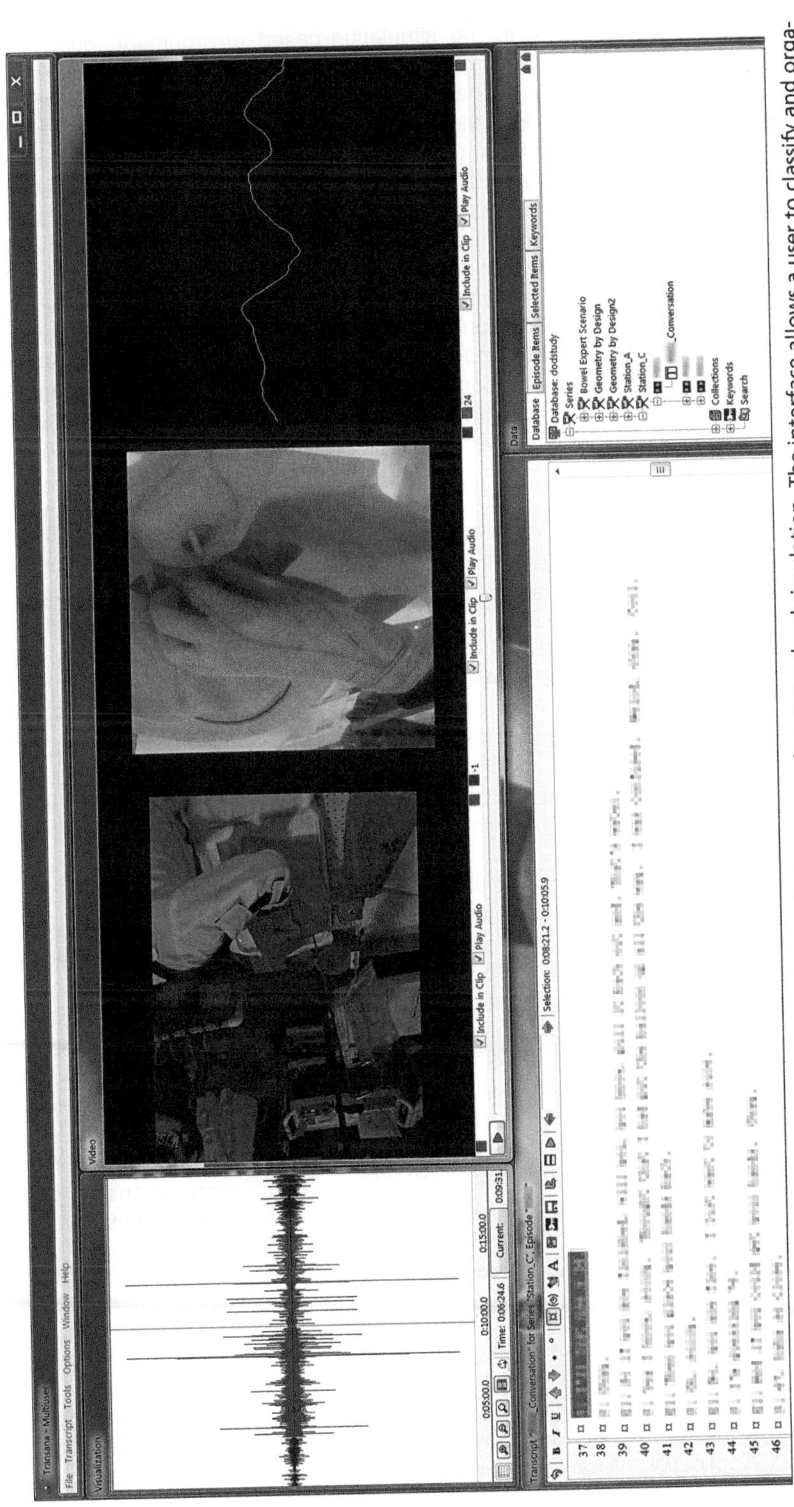


**Fig. 3.** Transana software package[53] used for transcribing verbal responses in a procedural simulation. The interface allows a user to classify and organize behaviors observed and to export media clips of highlighted times of interest. (*From* Woods D, Fassnacht C. Transana v2.61a. Madison (WI): The Board of Regents of the University of Wisconsin System; 2012. Available at: http://www.transana.org; with permission.)

When assessing performance in the simulation-based environment, numerous opportunities exist to conduct controlled experiments with multiple technology-based systems. However, research has also focused on the translation of these technology-based assessments into the operating room.[52] There are several challenges to bringing the technologies discussed earlier into the operating room, including reduced surgeon dexterity, the need for sterilization, concern for patient safety, and the cost of added equipment and time in the operating room. It is thought that the simulation-based environment can serve as an appropriate venue for evaluating clinical and procedural skills in a safer, more cost-efficient manner.

The inclusion of advanced engineering technology in clinical and procedural skills assessment may provide innovative tools for objectively assessing hands-on clinical skills that go beyond the traditional competency assessments based on self-report logbooks, amount of time spent training, or pen and paper tests. Future work should focus on using mixed methods (observation and technology-based metrics) for developing a process for evaluating clinical competency that demonstrates validity evidence.

## REFERENCES

1. The American Board of Surgery. Training Requirements – General Surgery Certification. 2014. Available at: http://www.absurgery.org/default.jsp?certgsqe_training. Accessed November 25, 2014.
2. Datta V, Chang A, Mackay S, et al. The relationship between motion analysis and surgical technical assessments. Am J Surg 2002;184(1):70–3.
3. Dosis A, Aggarwal R, Bello F, et al. Synchronized video and motion analysis for the assessment of procedures in the operating theater. Arch Surg 2005;140(3):293–9.
4. Chmarra M, Bakker N, Grimbergen C, et al. TrEndo, a device for tracking minimally invasive surgical instruments in training setups. Sens Actuators A Phys 2006;126(2):328–34.
5. Salud LH, Ononye CI, Kwan C, et al. Clinical breast examination simulation: getting to real. Stud Health Technol Inform 2012;173:424–9.
6. Eva K, Regehr G. Self-assessment in the health professions: a reformulation and research agenda. Acad Med 2005;80(10):S46–54.
7. Martin JA, Regehr G, Reznick R, et al. Objective structured assessment of technical skill (OSATS) for surgical residents. Br J Surg 1997;84(2):273–8.
8. Fried G, Feldman L. Objective assessment of technical performance. World J Surg 2008;32(2):156–60.
9. Regehr G, MacRae H, Reznick R, et al. Comparing the psychometric properties of checklists and global rating scales for assessing performance on an OSCE-format examination. Acad Med 1998;73(9):993–7.
10. Epstein R. Assessment in medical education. N Engl J Med 2007;356(4):387–96.
11. Issa N, Salud L, Kwan C, et al. Validity and reliability of a sensor-enabled intubation trainer: a focus on patient-centered data. J Surg Res 2012;177(1):27–32.
12. Chmarra M, Klein S, de Winter J, et al. Objective classification of residents based on their psychomotor laparoscopic skills. Surg Endosc 2010;24(5):1031–9.
13. James A, Vieira D, Lo B, et al. Eye-gaze driven surgical workflow segmentation. Med Image Comput Comput Assist Interv 2007;4792:110–7.
14. Pavlidis I, Tsiamyrtzis P, Shastri D, et al. Fast by nature-how stress patterns define human experience and performance in dexterous tasks. Sci Rep 2012;2:305.
15. Pugh C. Application of national testing standards to simulation-based assessments of clinical palpation skills. Mil Med 2013;178(10):55–63.

16. Magill R. Motor learning and control: concepts and applications. 9th edition. New York: McGraw-Hill; 2011.
17. Oropesa I, Chmarra M, Sanchez-Gonzalez P, et al. Relevance of motion-related assessment metrics in laparoscopic surgery. Surg Innov 2013;20(3): 299–312.
18. D'Angelo A, Rutherford D, Ray R, et al. Idle time: an underdeveloped performance metric for assessing surgical skill. Am J Surg 2015;209(4):645–51.
19. Glarner C, Hu Y, Chen C, et al. Quantifying technical skills during open operations using video-based motion analysis. Surgery 2014;156(3):729–34.
20. Oropesa I, Sanchez-Gonzalez P, Chmarra M, et al. EVA: laparoscopic instrument tracking based on endoscopic video analysis for psychomotor skills assessment. Surg Endosc 2013;27(3):1029–39.
21. Zecca M, Sessa S, Lin Z, et al. Development of the ultra-miniaturized inertial measurement unit WB3 for objective skill analysis and assessment in neurosurgery: preliminary results. Med Image Comput Comput Assist Interv 2009;12: 443–50.
22. Hofstad E, Vapenstad C, Chmarra M, et al. A study of psychomotor skills in minimally invasive surgery: what differentiates expert and nonexpert performance. Surg Endosc 2013;27(3):854–63.
23. Mackay S, Datta V, Mandalia M, et al. Electromagnetic motion analysis in the assessment of surgical skill: relationship between time and movement. ANZ J Surg 2002;72(9):632–4.
24. Keele S, Posner M. Processing of visual feedback in rapid movements. J Exp Psychol 1968;77(1):155.
25. McEwen BS. Physiology and neurobiology of stress and adaptation: central role of the brain. Physiol Rev 2007;87(3):873–904.
26. Shastri D, Papadakis M, Tsiamyrtzis P, et al. Perinasal imaging of physiological stress and its affective potential. IEEE Trans Affect Comput 2012;3(3):366–78.
27. Cohen S, Kessler R, Gordon L. Measuring stress: a guide for health and social scientists. New York: Oxford University Press; 1997.
28. Shastri D, Merla A, Tsiamyrtzis P, et al. Imaging facial signs of neurophysiological responses. IEEE Trans Biomed Eng 2009;56(2):477–84.
29. Berguer R, Smith WD, Chung YH. Performing laparoscopic surgery is significantly more stressful for the surgeon than open surgery. Surg Endosc 2001; 15(10):1204–7.
30. Montagu JD, Coles EM. Mechanism and measurement of the galvanic skin response. Psychol Bull 1966;65(5):261–79.
31. Lederman S, Klatzky R. Hand movements: a window into haptic object recognition. Cogn Psychol 1987;19(3):342–68.
32. Lederman S, Klatzky R. Haptic classification of common objects: Knowledge-driven exploration. Cogn Psychol 1990;22(4):421–59.
33. Klatzky R, Lederman S. The haptic identification of everyday life objects. In: Hatwell Y, Streri A, Gentaz E, editors. Touching for knowing: cognitive psychology of haptic manual perception. Amsterdam: John Benjamins Publishing Co; 2003. p. 105.
34. Pugh CM, Youngblood P. Development and validation of assessment measures for a newly developed physical examination simulator. J Am Med Inform Assoc 2002;9(5):448–60.
35. Pugh CM, Rosen J. Qualitative and quantitative analysis of pressure sensor data acquired by the E-Pelvis simulator during simulated pelvic examinations. Stud Health Technol Inform 2002;85:376–9.

36. Mackel T, Rosen J, Pugh C. Data mining of the E-Pelvis simulator database: a quest for a generalized algorithm for objectively assessing medical skill. Stud Health Technol Inform 2006;119:355–60.
37. Mackel T, Rosen J, Pugh C. Markov model assessment of subjects' clinical skill using the E-Pelvis physical simulator. IEEE Trans Biomed Eng 2007;54(12): 2133–41.
38. Balkissoon R, Blossfield K, Salud L, et al. Lost in translation: unfolding medical students' misconceptions of how to perform a clinical digital rectal examination. Am J Surg 2009;197(4):525–32.
39. Laufer S, Cohen ER, Maag AL, et al. Multimodality approach to classifying hand utilization for the clinical breast examination. Stud Health Technol Inform 2014; 196:238–44.
40. Pugh CM, Domont ZB, Salud LH, et al. A simulation-based assessment of clinical breast examination technique: do patient and clinician factors affect clinician approach? Am J Surg 2008;195(6):874–80.
41. Laufer S, Rasske K, Stopfer L, et al. Undetectable force sensors for characterizing the clinical breast exam. Engineering in Medicine and Biology Society (EMBC), 2014 36th Annual International Conference of the IEEE. 2014. Chicago, August 26-30, 2014.
42. Wang N, Gerling G, Childress R, et al. Quantifying palpation techniques in relation to performance in a clinical prostate exam. IEEE Trans Inf Technol Biomed 2010;14(4):1088–97.
43. Wang N, Gerling G, Krupski T, et al. Using a prostate exam simulator to decipher palpation techniques that facilitate the detection of abnormalities near clinical limits. Simul Healthc 2010;5(3):152–60.
44. Salud LH, Pugh CM. Use of sensor technology to explore the science of touch. Stud Health Technol Inform 2011;163:542–8.
45. D'Angelo A, Law K, Cohen E, et al. Use of error analysis to assess resident performance. Surgery, in press.
46. Catchpole K, Giddings A, Wilkinson M, et al. Improving patient safety by identifying latent failures in successful operations. Surgery 2007;142(1):102–10.
47. Mackenzie C, Xiao Y. Video techniques and data compared with observation in emergency trauma care. Qual Saf Health Care 2003;12:II51–7.
48. Mays N, Pope C. Qualitative research: observational methods in health care settings. BMJ 1995;311(6998):182–4.
49. Law K, Hildebrand E, Oliveira-Gomes J, et al. A comprehensive methodology for examining the impact of surgical team briefings and debriefings on teamwork. Proc Hum Factors Ergon Soc Annu Meet 2014;58:703–7.
50. Cook DA, Brydges R, Zendejas B, et al. Technology-enhanced simulation to assess health professionals: a systematic review of validity evidence, research methods, and reporting quality. Acad Med 2013;88(6):872–83.
51. Downing S. Validity: on the meaningful interpretation of assessment data. Med Educ 2003;37(9):830–7.
52. Stefanidis D, Sevdalis N, Paige J, et al. Simulation in surgery: what's needed next? Ann Surg 2015;261(5):846–53.
53. Woods D, Fassnacht C. Transana v2.61a. Madison (WI): The Board of Regents of the University of Wisconsin System; 2012. Available at: http://www.transana.org.

# Moving the Needle

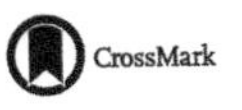

## Simulation's Impact on Patient Outcomes

Tiffany Cox, MD[a], Neal Seymour, MD[b], Dimitrios Stefanidis, MD, PhD[c,*]

**KEYWORDS**

- Simulation • Surgery • Kirkpatrick level • Virtual reality • Transfer of skills
- Operating room • Patient outcomes

**KEY POINTS**

- Acquisition of surgical skill on simulators has led to improved trainee performance in the clinical environment and the operating room.
- Patient benefits as a result of simulation training have been demonstrated for central line placement, obstetric emergencies, cataract surgery, laparoscopic inguinal hernia repair, crisis resource management, and team training.
- Limitations of the existing literature include a paucity of available studies, mainly single-institutional studies and studies retrospective in nature with inadequate controls that introduce bias into their results.
- Further high-quality research is necessary to solidify the evidence in support of the value of simulation training in improving patient outcomes.

## INTRODUCTION

Simulation training is a mainstream educational method experienced by medical care workers in numerous job types and areas of specialization. It has become an important part of the surgical training experience, and residents have been mandated to have access to simulation centers during training by the Residency Review Committee[1] to complete certifications such as the Fundamentals of Laparoscopic Surgery[2] and Fundamentals of Endoscopic Surgery.[3] These surgical training curricula, which have validated evidence-based simulation components, are now required for American Board of Surgery certification eligibility. The development of a comprehensive simulation-based skills curriculum for surgical residents[4] by the American College of Surgeons (ACS) and Association of Program Directors in urgery, as well as the advent

[a] Department of Surgery, Carolinas Medical Center, 1025 Morehead Medical Drive, Suite 300, Charlotte, NC 28204, USA; [b] Department of Surgery, Baystate Medical Center, 759 Chestnut Street, Springfield, MA 01199, USA; [c] Department of Surgery, Carolinas Simulation Center, Carolinas Medical Center, Carolinas Healthcare System, 1025 Morehead Medical Drive, Suite 300, Charlotte, NC 28204, USA
* Corresponding author.
*E-mail address:* dimitrios.stefanidis@carolinashealthcare.org

Surg Clin N Am 95 (2015) 827–838
http://dx.doi.org/10.1016/j.suc.2015.03.005
surgical.theclinics.com
0039-6109/15/$ – see front matter 

of the ACS Consortium of Accredited Education Institutes, signal a dramatically increased role of simulation in the training and certification of surgeons.

However, simulation training requires significant material and personnel resources and can be costly.[5–7] Coupled with increasing financial pressures on surgical departments and resident work hour limitations, wide implementation of simulation training is challenging.[8] To facilitate broader acceptance and implementation, evidence of effectiveness of the highest level is needed.[7] Such evidence would ideally demonstrate that simulation-based training improves patient outcomes and achieves health care system benefits. This review identifies existing studies providing such high-quality evidence.

## METHODS

The authors conducted a literature search (**Fig. 1**) using MEDLINE to identify studies that evaluated the impact of simulation training on patient outcomes. Methods considered included laboratory-based training models or low-fidelity simulation and technology-based methods such as virtual reality or high-fidelity simulation. Two independent investigators reviewed the retrieved abstracts of the literature search and further studied the full papers of those relevant to the topic. The references cited in these articles were further searched to identify any additional relevant articles. The Kirkpatrick model[9] of training evaluation adapted to medical education[10] was used to assign each reviewed paper to the specific level of educational outcome it examined. The 4 Kirkpatrick levels as they pertain to simulation are as follows:

- Level 1, Reaction: Did the learner perceive value in using a simulator or participating in simulation training?
- Level 2, Learning: Did the learner's knowledge, skill, or attitude improve as a result of simulation training?
- Level 3, Behavioral Change: Did the knowledge, skills, and attitudes acquired during simulator training transfer to the clinical environment (ie, bedside, operating room)?
- Level 4, Results: Did the simulation training program lead to improved patient outcomes?

For the purposes of this article, only level 4 studies were included, the most impactful and important means to demonstrate the value of simulation training.

## RESULTS

### *Available Evidence of Effectiveness*

To date, 12 papers[11–22] reporting Kirkpatrick level 4 outcomes and 3 systematic reviews[23–25] have been published. Perhaps the best-known studies are from Barsuk and colleagues,[19] who assessed the impact of simulator-based mastery learning of central line placement by internal medicine residents on patient outcomes. The investigators assessed central line–associated blood stream infections (CLABSIs) during a 32-month period in the medical intensive care unit (ICU) before and after their intervention. They demonstrated an 85% reduction in CLABSIs after the trained residents rotated through the ICU (0.50 infections per 1000 catheter days) compared with the same unit before the intervention (3.20 infections per 1000 catheter days, $P \leq .001$) and with another ICU in the same hospital throughout the study period (5.03 infections per 1000 catheter days, $P \leq .001$).[19] The same researchers also reported in a later study that their intervention resulted in significant medical care cost savings, mainly as a result of decreased complications, which led to a 7:1 return on investment, further

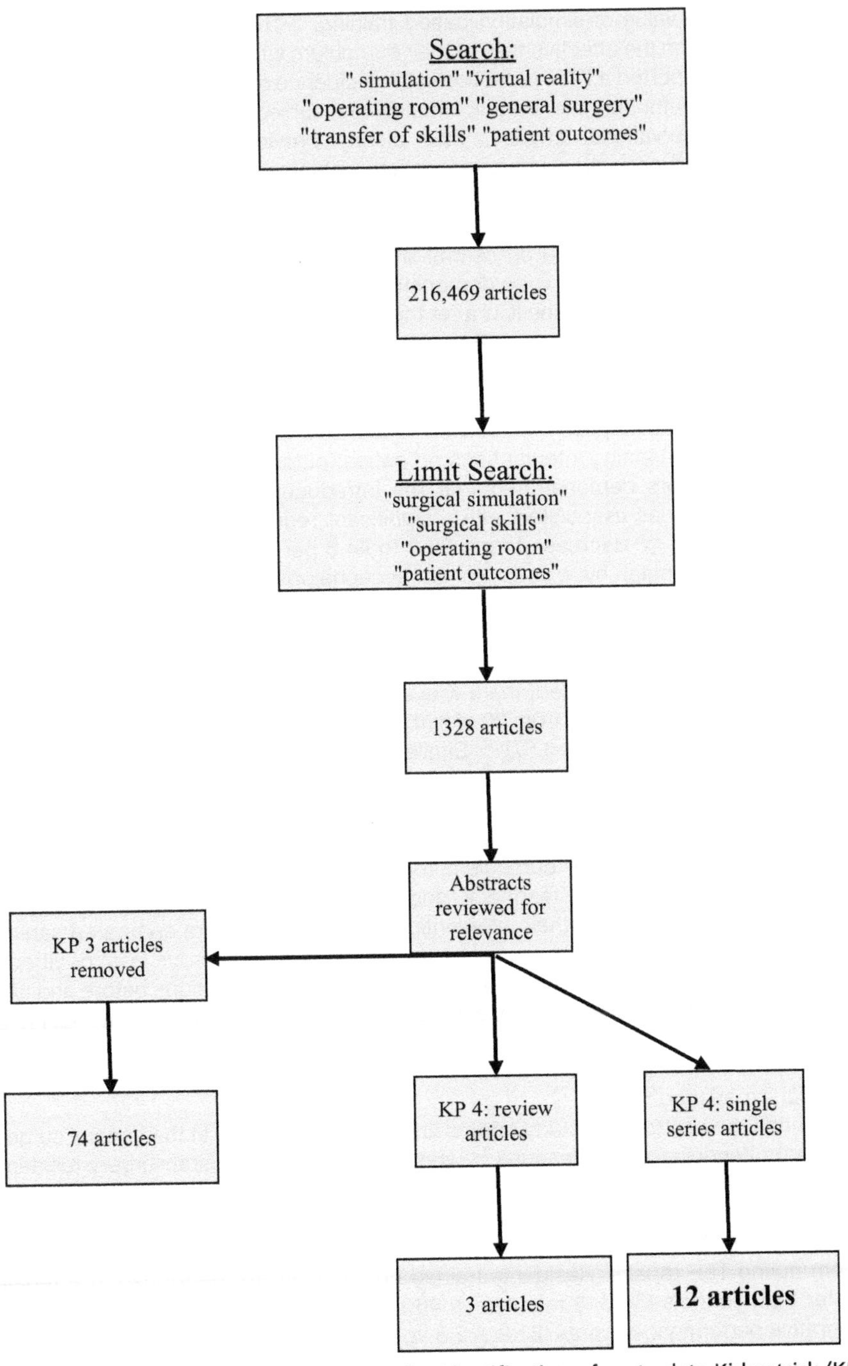


**Fig. 1.** Literature search through MEDLINE for identification of up-to-date Kirkpatrick (KP) level 4 articles.

highlighting the value of simulation-based training.[26] The researchers published an updated report on the effectiveness of their curriculum when disseminated to other institutions and reported a 74% reduction in the incidence of CLABSIs as a result of their intervention.[11] Although the Barsuk studies are subject to limitations and biases related to observational studies, they clearly provide a strong link between simulation-based education–improved patient outcomes and return on investment. This same type of patient outcome analysis was replicated by another study; Khouli and colleagues[14] randomized residents to a simulator and video trained group and to a video-only trained group on central line insertion and followed CLABSIs in the ICU after their intervention. They demonstrated that there was a 70% reduction in the incidence of CLABSIs in the ICU after the intervention compared with before, confirming a similar reduction noted by Barsuk and colleagues, and that simulation-based training in sterile techniques during central venous catheter was superior to traditional training or video training alone.

Draycott and colleagues[22] published 2 studies demonstrating the impact of simulation-based training interventions on patient outcomes in the United Kingdom. These investigators demonstrated that the introduction of obstetric emergencies training courses was associated with a significant reduction in low 5-minute Apgar scores (scores of $\leq$6 decreased from 86.6 to 44.6 per 10,000 births; $P<.001$) and a decrease in neonatal hypoxic-ischemic encephalopathy from 27.3 to 13.6 per 10,000 births ($P = .032$). They later demonstrated that the introduction of shoulder dystocia training for all maternity staff was associated with improved management and neonatal outcomes of births complicated by shoulder dystocia.[21]

After training was introduced, there was a significant reduction in neonatal injury at birth after shoulder dystocia, from 30 of 324 (9.3%) to 6 of 262 (2.3%) (relative risk 0.25 [confidence interval (CI) 0.11–0.57]).[21] Similar to the Barsuk studies, these reports suggest a strong link between the simulation-based training intervention and patient outcomes but are subject to methodological design bias.

In the ophthalmologic surgical spectrum, Rogers and colleagues[20] implemented an intense, structured surgical curriculum for ophthalmology residents that included simulator training, formative feedback, and deliberate practice of capsulorhexis. To assess the effectiveness of their intervention, these investigators compared sentinel events, defined as a posterior capsule tear (with or without vitreous loss) or vitreous loss (from any cause), during resident performed cataract operations before and after curriculum implementation. The researchers demonstrated a statistically significant reduction in the sentinel event rate, from 7.17% before the curriculum introduction to 3.77% after the simulation-based curriculum ($P = .001$) even after adjusting for surgical experience.[20]

Perhaps the best-quality study addressing patient outcomes in the general surgery field is by Zendejas and colleagues,[17] who randomized 50 general surgery residents (postgraduate year 1–5) to a mastery learning group who trained to proficiency on a laparoscopic totally extraperitoneal (TEP) hernia repair simulator and a traditionally trained group. The performance of both groups was then compared in the operating room during TEP repairs. Residents trained on the simulator performed TEP repairs faster than controls (34 $\pm$ 8 minutes vs 48 $\pm$ 14 minutes; $P<.001$), achieved higher operative performance scores (21.9 $\pm$ 2.8 vs 18.3 $\pm$ 3.8 on Global Operative Assessment of Laparoscopic Skill assessment; $P = .001$), and caused fewer intraoperative (peritoneal tear, procedure conversion; adjusted odds ratio [OR], 0.15; CI, 0.04–0.59) and postoperative complications (urinary retention, seroma; adjusted OR, 0.17; CI, 0.4–0.74).[17] Furthermore, the need for overnight stay of patients was less likely in the simulator-trained group (OR, 0.23; CI, 0.05–1.0). This study provided high-quality evidence on the effectiveness of simulator-based training on improving patient outcomes, even though the complications recorded were minor in nature.

In respect to team dynamics, multiple studies have evaluated the effect of simulation-based team training on patient outcomes. Andreatta and colleagues[13] conducted a study using simulation-based pediatric mock codes and identified improved survival rates for pediatric patients with cardiopulmonary arrest (CPA). From 2005 to 2009, mock codes were called in the same format as a real code on at least a monthly basis. Video recordings assisted in postprocess debrief training. Survival rates for CPA went from 33% in 2005 to 56% in 2008 after simulation mock code training; specifically, pulseless survival rate improved from 15% to 56%.[13] Phipps and colleagues[12] applied crew resource management (CRM) training using simulation in a Labor and Delivery unit. This study was prospective and carried out for 30 months, with evaluation of patient outcomes before and after training; outcomes of 8 quarters pretraining were compared with outcomes of 6 quarters posttraining. The training consisted of 4-hour didactics with 4 hours of simulation and debriefing within 1 week. They demonstrated a decrease in the Adverse Outcomes Index (AOI) score from 0.052 (range, 0.048–0.055) during a period of 8 quarters in the baseline pre-CRM AOI compared with an AOI score of 0.043 (range, 0.040–0.047) for the 6 quarters of posttraining scores.[12] The 2 quarters during training were excluded. The large number of staff involved having this shared learning experience to create a common vocabulary and frame of reference was attributed to improving patient outcomes in this manner. An additional study in the obstetric literature was published by Riley and colleagues,[15] evaluating randomized assignment of training programs to 3 separate hospitals; no intervention, team strategies and tools to enhance performance and patient safety (TeamSTEPPS), and a full intervention group consisting of TeamSTEPPS with adjunct simulation training exercises. The in situ simulation training component consisted of a 30- to 45-minute scenario from triage, to labor and the operating room, followed by recovery unit, and concluded with a debriefing session. Perinatal outcomes were measured by the Weighted Adverse Outcomes Score (WAOS), demonstrating a statistically significant decrease in the full intervention group from a WAOS score of 1.15 to 0.72, representing a 37.4% decrease in adverse event rates.[15] This study demonstrated the value of simulation training in further improving nontechnical skills and patient outcomes compared with commonly used curricula.

Two studies were identified on team training in Trauma Critical Care. The first was by Capella and colleagues[18] who conducted a study to investigate if formal team training would improve team behaviors in the trauma resuscitation bay and ultimately improve clinical outcomes. A pretraining and posttraining comparison was performed, with the training component based on TeamSTEPPS with supplemented simulation-based curriculum graded by the Trauma Team Performance Observation Tool. The training involved a 2-hour didactic session and additional 2 hours of simulation sessions, which were scenario based and video recorded for debriefing; some participants required additional scenario-based simulation training compared with the average to attain similar levels of confidence and similar accomplishment of the scenario objectives. All aspects of team performance, including leadership, monitoring, mutual support, and communication, were improved after TeamSTEPPS and simulation training compared with pretraining for live resuscitations. With respect to patient outcomes, in-hospital mortality was reduced from 13.1% pretraining to 8.5% posttraining, but because of the small sample size, this finding was not statistically significant ($P = .12$).[18]

Further investigation into trauma team training was evaluated by Steinemann and colleagues[16] in a prospective study using human patient simulator-based training in conjunction with didactics. A total of 141 live resuscitations pretraining were compared with 103 live resuscitations posttraining from 2009 to 2010; no difference between patient demographics or Injury Severity Score were identified between the 2 populations.[16] Mortality was observed in 4 patients posttraining compared with 8 patients pretraining, and average ICU days (0.3 vs 19) and hospital days (3.4 vs 5.1) were reduced, but these differences were not statistically significant[16]; however, immediate improvement in acute care in the trauma bay with reduction in resuscitation time was noted (26 vs 32 minutes, $P<.05$).

## SUMMARY

The use of medical simulation training is supported by a growing body of evidence suggesting the effectiveness in achieving educational outcomes of various types. Specifically in surgery, these outcomes include transfer of surgical skill to bedside procedures,[27–39] endoscopy,[40–62] and in the operating room.[63–98] This body of work also suggests, however, that the allotment of time alone for simulation training is not sufficient. Good educational outcomes, from technical skills to specific learner performance-related behaviors, require a protected and proctored experience within a curriculum with proficiency-based goals. To investigate the effects of simulation training on patient outcomes, study design and measurement methods that capture the data relevant to the training paradigm are more complex and difficult. The number of studies that have specifically examined patient outcomes (Kirkpatrick model level 4 investigations) is lesser than those studies that have examined outcomes at lower levels of the Kirkpatrick evaluation framework. However, the evidence for effectiveness of simulation training on patient outcomes tends to be strong for the selected simulation interventions used in the studies identified. Among the most compelling data are those showing that catheter-related bloodstream infections can be reduced by training in a simulation platform before actual patient procedures. This training additionally demonstrated ability to reduce the immediate complications of the procedure and even costs that would have been incurred by the added care of such complications that were avoided. Data of this type demand the attention of educational leaders and should prompt extensive use of the suggested training methods if the benefits are substantial.

In surgical education, simulation training has been shown to result in shorter procedure duration, reduction in the occurrence of highly specified errors observed during live patient procedures, and, most significantly, improvement in the rates of long-term patient outcomes. Achievement of measurable patient outcome benefits is associated not only with simulation of selected procedures or procedural components but also with simulation aimed at development of nontechnical skills critical to teamwork. Arguably, these are the most important outcomes to optimize given current perceptions that poor performance in nontechnical skills areas is a major contributor to errors and adverse patient outcomes.[99–101] The complexity of studying the impact of simulation training on outcomes of this type is considerable. Yet, as the review suggests, this objective is feasible, amenable to measurement, and has demonstrated direct patient benefit.

## FUTURE DIRECTIONS

The current and potential future uses for simulation for surgical training are vast. Although proof of improved patient outcomes with simulation-based education is not a necessity for development and deployment of new simulators or training protocols (and may not even be possible in some situations), the value of such proof is inestimable to justify necessary effort and expenditure on such training. Although substantial progress has been made, most notably outside of the surgical field, this has been modest at best. A more complete understanding of the impact of simulation training on patient outcomes requires ongoing work. If accomplished with carefully designed, high-quality studies, expanded simulation-based preparation of surgeons and other surgical providers for their clinical responsibilities would be inevitable.

The resources to investigate the impact of simulation training on nontechnical, and to some extent technical, skills should be facilitated by increased reliance of health care institutions on quality measurement processes to meet requirements for reporting and reimbursement. Database collection systems such as the National Surgical Quality Improvement Program could be adapted and used to yield information relevant to the expected outcomes of surgical simulation rather than building such tools de novo. Informing such databases with objective performance data collection obtained from simulation training would allow one to directly link the impact of education interventions on patient outcomes and identify in parallel training needs of health care providers.

## REFERENCES

1. ACGME. Program Requirements for Graduate Medical Education in General Surgery. April 16, 2015. Available at: http://www.acgme.org/acgmeweb/portals/0/pfassets/programrequirements/440_general_surgery_07012014.pdf.
2. Fried GM, Feldman LS, Vassiliou MC, et al. Proving the value of simulation in laparoscopic surgery. Ann Surg 2004;240(3):518–25 [discussion: 525–8].
3. Society of American Gastrointestinal and Endoscopic Surgeons. Surgical Fundamentals. April 16, 2015. Available at: http://www.fundamentals-didactics.com.
4. American College of Surgeons. ACS/APDS Surgery Resident Skills Curriculum. April 16, 2015 Available at: https://www.facs.org/education/program/apds-resident/.
5. Orzech N, Palter VN, Reznick RK, et al. A comparison of 2 ex vivo training curricula for advanced laparoscopic skills: a randomized controlled trial. Ann Surg 2012;255(5):833–9.
6. Scott DJ, Ritter EM, Tesfay ST, et al. Certification pass rate of 100% for fundamentals of laparoscopic surgery skills after proficiency-based training. Surg Endosc 2008;22(8):1887–93.
7. Stefanidis D, Sevdalis N, Paige J, et al. Simulation in surgery: what's needed next? Ann Surg 2015;261(5):846–53.
8. Korndorffer JR Jr, Arora S, Sevdalis N, et al. The American College of Surgeons/Association of Program Directors in Surgery National Skills Curriculum: adoption rate, challenges and strategies for effective implementation into surgical residency programs. Surgery 2013;154(1):13–20.
9. Kirkpatrick DL, Kirkpatrick JD. Evaluating training programs: the four levels. 3rd edition. San Francisco (CA): Berrett-Koehler; 2006.
10. Bewley WL, O'Neil HF. Evaluation of medical simulations. Mil Med 2013;178(10 Suppl):64–75.
11. Barsuk JH, Cohen ER, Potts S, et al. Dissemination of a simulation-based mastery learning intervention reduces central line-associated bloodstream infections. BMJ Qual Saf 2014;23(9):749–56.
12. Phipps MG, Lindquist DG, McConaughey E, et al. Outcomes from a labor and delivery team training program with simulation component. Am J Obstet Gynecol 2012;206(1):3–9.

13. Andreatta P, Saxton E, Thompson M, et al. Simulation-based mock codes significantly correlate with improved pediatric patient cardiopulmonary arrest survival rates. Pediatr Crit Care Med 2011;12(1):33–8.
14. Khouli H, Jahnes K, Shapiro J, et al. Performance of medical residents in sterile techniques during central vein catheterization: randomized trial of efficacy of simulation-based training. Chest 2011;139(1):80–7.
15. Riley W, Davis S, Miller K, et al. Didactic and simulation nontechnical skills team training to improve perinatal patient outcomes in a community hospital. Jt Comm J Qual Patient Saf 2011;37(8):357–64.
16. Steinemann S, Berg B, Skinner A, et al. In situ, multidisciplinary, simulation-based teamwork training improves early trauma care. J Surg Educ 2011;68(6):472–7.
17. Zendejas B, Cook DA, Bingener J, et al. Simulation-based mastery learning improves patient outcomes in laparoscopic inguinal hernia repair: a randomized controlled trial. Ann Surg 2011;254(3):502–9 [discussion: 509–11].
18. Capella J, Smith S, Philp A, et al. Teamwork training improves the clinical care of trauma patients. J Surg Educ 2010;67(6):439–43.
19. Barsuk JH, Cohen ER, Feinglass J, et al. Use of simulation-based education to reduce catheter-related bloodstream infections. Arch Intern Med 2009;169(15):1420–3.
20. Rogers GM, Oetting TA, Lee AG, et al. Impact of a structured surgical curriculum on ophthalmic resident cataract surgery complication rates. J Cataract Refract Surg 2009;35(11):1956–60.
21. Draycott TJ, Crofts JF, Ash JP, et al. Improving neonatal outcome through practical shoulder dystocia training. Obstet Gynecol 2008;112(1):14–20.
22. Draycott T, Sibanda T, Owen L, et al. Does training in obstetric emergencies improve neonatal outcome? BJOG 2006;113(2):177–82.
23. Boet S, Bould MD, Fung L, et al. Transfer of learning and patient outcome in simulated crisis resource management: a systematic review. Can J Anaesth 2014;61(6):571–82.
24. Zendejas B, Brydges R, Hamstra SJ, et al. State of the evidence on simulation-based training for laparoscopic surgery: a systematic review. Ann Surg 2013;257(4):586–93.
25. McGaghie WC, Draycott TJ, Dunn WF, et al. Evaluating the impact of simulation on translational patient outcomes. Simul Healthc 2011;6(Suppl):S42–7.
26. Cohen ER, Feinglass J, Barsuk JH, et al. Cost savings from reduced catheter-related bloodstream infection after simulation-based education for residents in a medical intensive care unit. Simul Healthc 2010;5(2):98–102.
27. Ahya SN, Barsuk JH, Cohen ER, et al. Clinical performance and skill retention after simulation-based education for nephrology fellows. Semin Dial 2012;25(4):470–3.
28. Bagai A, O'Brien S, Al Lawati H, et al. Mentored simulation training improves procedural skills in cardiac catheterization: a randomized, controlled pilot study. Circ Cardiovasc Interv 2012;5(5):672–9.
29. Hseino H, Nugent E, Lee MJ, et al. Skills transfer after proficiency-based simulation training in superficial femoral artery angioplasty. Simul Healthc 2012;7(5):274–81.
30. Andreatta P, Chen Y, Marsh M, et al. Simulation-based training improves applied clinical placement of ultrasound-guided PICCs. Support Care Cancer 2011;19(4):539–43.
31. Jiang G, Chen H, Wang S, et al. Learning curves and long-term outcome of simulation-based thoracentesis training for medical students. BMC Med Educ 2011;11:39.

32. Evans LV, Dodge KL, Shah TD, et al. Simulation training in central venous catheter insertion: improved performance in clinical practice. Acad Med 2010;85(9):1462–9.
33. Smith CC, Huang GC, Newman LR, et al. Simulation training and its effect on long-term resident performance in central venous catheterization. Simul Healthc 2010;5(3):146–51.
34. Barsuk JH, McGaghie WC, Cohen ER, et al. Simulation-based mastery learning reduces complications during central venous catheter insertion in a medical intensive care unit. Crit Care Med 2009;37(10):2697–701.
35. Barsuk JH, McGaghie WC, Cohen ER, et al. Use of simulation-based mastery learning to improve the quality of central venous catheter placement in a medical intensive care unit. J Hosp Med 2009;4(7):397–403.
36. Britt RC, Novosel TJ, Britt LD, et al. The impact of central line simulation before the ICU experience. Am J Surg 2009;197(4):533–6.
37. Duncan DR, Morgenthaler TI, Ryu JH, et al. Reducing iatrogenic risk in thoracentesis: establishing best practice via experiential training in a zero-risk environment. Chest 2009;135(5):1315–20.
38. Sotto JA, Ayuste EC, Bowyer MW, et al. Exporting simulation technology to the Philippines: a comparative study of traditional versus simulation methods for teaching intravenous cannulation. Stud Health Technol Inform 2009;142:346–51.
39. Chaer RA, Derubertis BG, Lin SC, et al. Simulation improves resident performance in catheter-based intervention: results of a randomized, controlled study. Ann Surg 2006;244(3):343–52.
40. Gomez PP, Willis RE, Sickle KV. Evaluation of two flexible colonoscopy simulators and transfer of skills into clinical practice. J Surg Educ 2014;72:220–7.
41. Deutschmann MW, Yunker WK, Cho JJ, et al. Use of a low-fidelity simulator to improve trans-nasal fibre-optic flexible laryngoscopy in the clinical setting: a randomized, single-blinded, prospective study. J Otolaryngol Head Neck Surg 2013;42(1):35.
42. Ende A, Zopf Y, Konturek P, et al. Strategies for training in diagnostic upper endoscopy: a prospective, randomized trial. Gastrointest Endosc 2012;75(2):254–60.
43. Fried MP, Kaye RJ, Gibber MJ, et al. Criterion-based (proficiency) training to improve surgical performance. Arch Otolaryngol Head Neck Surg 2012;138(11):1024–9.
44. Ferlitsch A, Schoefl R, Puespoek A, et al. Effect of virtual endoscopy simulator training on performance of upper gastrointestinal endoscopy in patients: a randomized controlled trial. Endoscopy 2010;42(12):1049–56.
45. Fried MP, Sadoughi B, Gibber MJ, et al. From virtual reality to the operating room: the endoscopic sinus surgery simulator experiment. Otolaryngol Head Neck Surg 2010;142(2):202–7.
46. Haycock A, Koch AD, Familiari P, et al. Training and transfer of colonoscopy skills: a multinational, randomized, blinded, controlled trial of simulator versus bedside training. Gastrointest Endosc 2010;71(2):298–307.
47. Schout BM, Ananias HJ, Bemelmans BL, et al. Transfer of cysto-urethroscopy skills from a virtual-reality simulator to the operating room: a randomized controlled trial. BJU Int 2010;106(2):226–31 [discussion: 231].
48. Chandra DB, Savoldelli GL, Joo HS, et al. Fiberoptic oral intubation: the effect of model fidelity on training for transfer to patient care. Anesthesiology 2008;109(6):1007–13.
49. Shirai Y, Yoshida T, Shiraishi R, et al. Prospective randomized study on the use of a computer-based endoscopic simulator for training in esophagogastroduodenoscopy. J Gastroenterol Hepatol 2008;23(7 Pt 1):1046–50.

50. Yi SY, Ryu KH, Na YJ, et al. Improvement of colonoscopy skills through simulation-based training. Stud Health Technol Inform 2008;132:565–7.
51. Park J, MacRae H, Musselman LJ, et al. Randomized controlled trial of virtual reality simulator training: transfer to live patients. Am J Surg 2007;194(2):205–11.
52. Sedlack RE. Validation of computer simulation training for esophagogastroduodenoscopy: Pilot study. J Gastroenterol Hepatol 2007;22(8):1214–9.
53. Cohen J, Cohen SA, Vora KC, et al. Multicenter, randomized, controlled trial of virtual-reality simulator training in acquisition of competency in colonoscopy. Gastrointest Endosc 2006;64(3):361–8.
54. Hochberger J, Matthes K, Maiss J, et al. Training with the compact EASIE biologic endoscopy simulator significantly improves hemostatic technical skill of gastroenterology fellows: a randomized controlled comparison with clinical endoscopy training alone. Gastrointest Endosc 2005;61(2):204–15.
55. Knoll T, Trojan L, Haecker A, et al. Validation of computer-based training in ureterorenoscopy. BJU Int 2005;95(9):1276–9.
56. Blum MG, Powers TW, Sundaresan S. Bronchoscopy simulator effectively prepares junior residents to competently perform basic clinical bronchoscopy. Ann Thorac Surg 2004;78(1):287–91 [discussion: 287–91].
57. Sedlack RE, Kolars JC. Computer simulator training enhances the competency of gastroenterology fellows at colonoscopy: results of a pilot study. Am J Gastroenterol 2004;99(1):33–7.
58. Sedlack RE, Kolars JC, Alexander JA. Computer simulation training enhances patient comfort during endoscopy. Clin Gastroenterol Hepatol 2004;2(4):348–52.
59. Gerson LB, Van Dam J. A prospective randomized trial comparing a virtual reality simulator to bedside teaching for training in sigmoidoscopy. Endoscopy 2003;35(7):569–75.
60. Rowe R, Cohen RA. An evaluation of a virtual reality airway simulator. Anesth Analg 2002;95(1):62–6 Table of contents.
61. Ost D, DeRosiers A, Britt EJ, et al. Assessment of a bronchoscopy simulator. Am J Respir Crit Care Med 2001;164(12):2248–55.
62. Tuggy ML. Virtual reality flexible sigmoidoscopy simulator training: impact on resident performance. J Am Board Fam Med 1998;11(6):426–33.
63. Bansal VK, Raveendran R, Misra MC, et al. A prospective randomized controlled blinded study to evaluate the effect of short-term focused training program in laparoscopy on operating room performance of surgery residents (CTRI/2012/11/003113). J Surg Educ 2014;71(1):52–60.
64. Cannon WD, Garrett WE Jr, Hunter RE, et al. Improving residency training in arthroscopic knee surgery with use of a virtual-reality simulator: a randomized blinded study. J Bone Joint Surg Am 2014;96(21):1798–806.
65. Kurashima Y, Feldman LS, Kaneva PA, et al. Simulation-based training improves the operative performance of totally extraperitoneal (TEP) laparoscopic inguinal hernia repair: a prospective randomized controlled trial. Surg Endosc 2014;28(3):783–8.
66. Palter VN, Grantcharov TP. Individualized deliberate practice on a virtual reality simulator improves technical performance of surgical novices in the operating room: a randomized controlled trial. Ann Surg 2014;259(3):443–8.
67. Gala R, Orejuela F, Gerten K, et al. Effect of validated skills simulation on operating room performance in obstetrics and gynecology residents: a randomized controlled trial. Obstet Gynecol 2013;121(3):578–84.

68. McCannel CA, Reed DC, Goldman DR. Ophthalmic surgery simulator training improves resident performance of capsulorhexis in the operating room. Ophthalmology 2013;120(12):2456–61.
69. Palter VN, Orzech N, Reznick RK, et al. Validation of a structured training and assessment curriculum for technical skill acquisition in minimally invasive surgery: a randomized controlled trial. Ann Surg 2013;257(2):224–30.
70. Pokroy R, Du E, Alzaga A, et al. Impact of simulator training on resident cataract surgery. Graefes Arch Clin Exp Ophthalmol 2013;251(3):777–81.
71. van Det MJ, Meijerink WJ, Hoff C, et al. Effective and efficient learning in the operating theater with intraoperative video-enhanced surgical procedure training. Surg Endosc 2013;27(8):2947–54.
72. Franzeck FM, Rosenthal R, Muller MK, et al. Prospective randomized controlled trial of simulator-based versus traditional in-surgery laparoscopic camera navigation training. Surg Endosc 2012;26(1):235–41.
73. Pollard TC, Khan T, Price AJ, et al. Simulated hip arthroscopy skills: learning curves with the lateral and supine patient positions: a randomized trial. J Bone Joint Surg Am 2012;94(10):e68.
74. Belyea DA, Brown SE, Rajjoub LZ. Influence of surgery simulator training on ophthalmology resident phacoemulsification performance. J Cataract Refract Surg 2011;37(10):1756–61.
75. Beyer L, Troyer JD, Mancini J, et al. Impact of laparoscopy simulator training on the technical skills of future surgeons in the operating room: a prospective study. Am J Surg 2011;202(3):265–72.
76. Palter VN, Grantcharov T, Harvey A, et al. Ex vivo technical skills training transfers to the operating room and enhances cognitive learning: a randomized controlled trial. Ann Surg 2011;253(5):886–9.
77. Calatayud D, Arora S, Aggarwal R, et al. Warm-up in a virtual reality environment improves performance in the operating room. Ann Surg 2010;251(6):1181–5.
78. Gauger PG, Hauge LS, Andreatta PB, et al. Laparoscopic simulation training with proficiency targets improves practice and performance of novice surgeons. Am J Surg 2010;199(1):72–80.
79. Kallstrom R, Hjertberg H, Svanvik J. Impact of virtual reality-simulated training on urology residents' performance of transurethral resection of the prostate. J Endourol 2010;24(9):1521–8.
80. Sroka G, Feldman LS, Vassiliou MC, et al. Fundamentals of laparoscopic surgery simulator training to proficiency improves laparoscopic performance in the operating room-a randomized controlled trial. Am J Surg 2010;199(1):115–20.
81. Tongprasert F, Wanapirak C, Sirichotiyakul S, et al. Training in cordocentesis: the first 50 case experience with and without a cordocentesis training model. Prenat Diagn 2010;30(5):467–70.
82. Wohaibi EM, Bush RW, Earle DB, et al. Surgical resident performance on a virtual reality simulator correlates with operating room performance. J Surg Res 2010;160(1):67–72.
83. Kundhal PS, Grantcharov TP. Psychomotor performance measured in a virtual environment correlates with technical skills in the operating room. Surg Endosc 2009;23(3):645–9.
84. Larsen CR, Soerensen JL, Grantcharov TP, et al. Effect of virtual reality training on laparoscopic surgery: randomised controlled trial. BMJ 2009;338:b1802.
85. Siassakos D, Hasafa Z, Sibanda T, et al. Retrospective cohort study of diagnosis-delivery interval with umbilical cord prolapse: the effect of team training. BJOG 2009;116(8):1089–96.

86. Howells NR, Gill HS, Carr AJ, et al. Transferring simulated arthroscopic skills to the operating theatre: a randomised blinded study. J Bone Joint Surg Br 2008;90(4):494–9.
87. Van Sickle KR, Ritter EM, Baghai M, et al. Prospective, randomized, double-blind trial of curriculum-based training for intracorporeal suturing and knot tying. J Am Coll Surg 2008;207(4):560–8.
88. Ahlberg G, Enochsson L, Gallagher AG, et al. Proficiency-based virtual reality training significantly reduces the error rate for residents during their first 10 laparoscopic cholecystectomies. Am J Surg 2007;193(6):797–804.
89. Banks EH, Chudnoff S, Karmin I, et al. Does a surgical simulator improve resident operative performance of laparoscopic tubal ligation? Am J Obstet Gynecol 2007;197(5):541.e1–5.
90. Aggarwal R, Tully A, Grantcharov T, et al. Virtual reality simulation training can improve technical skills during laparoscopic salpingectomy for ectopic pregnancy. BJOG 2006;113(12):1382–7.
91. Schijven MP, Jakimowicz JJ, Broeders IA, et al. The Eindhoven laparoscopic cholecystectomy training course–improving operating room performance using virtual reality training: results from the first E.A.E.S. accredited virtual reality trainings curriculum. Surg Endosc 2005;19(9):1220–6.
92. Grantcharov TP, Kristiansen VB, Bendix J, et al. Randomized clinical trial of virtual reality simulation for laparoscopic skills training. Br J Surg 2004;91(2):146–50.
93. McClusky DA 3rd, Gallagher AG, Ritter EM, et al. Virtual reality training improves junior residents' operating room performance: results of a prospective, randomized, double-blinded study of the complete laparoscopic cholecystectomy. J Am Coll Surg 2004;199(3):73.
94. Lin E, Szomstein S, Addasi T, et al. Model for teaching laparoscopic colectomy to surgical residents. Am J Surg 2003;186(1):45–8.
95. Hamilton EC, Scott DJ, Fleming JB, et al. Comparison of video trainer and virtual reality training systems on acquisition of laparoscopic skills. Surg Endosc 2002;16(3):406–11.
96. Seymour NE, Gallagher AG, Roman SA, et al. Virtual reality training improves operating room performance: results of a randomized, double-blinded study. Ann Surg 2002;236(4):458–63 [discussion: 463–4].
97. Hamilton EC, Scott DJ, Kapoor A, et al. Improving operative performance using a laparoscopic hernia simulator. Am J Surg 2001;182(6):725–8.
98. Reznick R, Regehr G, MacRae H, et al. Testing technical skill via an innovative "bench station" examination. Am J Surg 1997;173(3):226–30.
99. Hu YY, Arriaga AF, Roth EM, et al. Protecting patients from an unsafe system: the etiology and recovery of intraoperative deviations in care. Ann Surg 2012;256(2):203–10.
100. Catchpole K, Mishra A, Handa A, et al. Teamwork and error in the operating room: analysis of skills and roles. Ann Surg 2008;247(4):699–706.
101. Rothschild JM, Landrigan CP, Cronin JW, et al. The critical care safety study: the incidence and nature of adverse events and serious medical errors in intensive care. Crit Care Med 2005;33(8):1694–700.

# Conducting Elite Performance Training

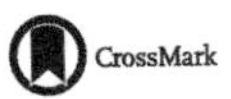

Elliott Silverman, PA-C, MSHS[a,b,*], Scott A. Tucker, MA[b], Solveig Imsdahl, BA[b], Justin A. Charles, BS[b], Mallory A. Stellato, BS[c], Mercy D. Wagner, MD[a], Kimberly M. Brown, MD[d]

**KEYWORDS**

- Simulation • Performance • Coaching • Conducting • Leadership • Music • Sports • Training • Surgical education • Medical leadership development

**KEY POINTS**

- In elite-level music and sports, the skills and strategies of the performance coach affect the achievement of mastery performance.
- Simulation-based training in surgery functions as a rehearsal or practice, during which the desired performance is practiced and refined until proficiency is achieved.
- Specific, reproducible techniques are used to coach elite-level athletes and musicians, and these techniques have direct applications in simulation-based training of surgeons and surgical teams.
- Constants are strategies used in every simulation and include coaching team (CT), warm-up, bilateral active engagement (BAE), and momentum arc.
- Planned variables are strategies that are used on an as-needed basis.

## INTRODUCTION

Within undergraduate, graduate, and postgraduate surgical practice, a need exists to acquire and maintain proficiency of core skills before when they are clinically applied. In the context of higher-than-acceptable adverse event rates in health care,[1,2] work hour restrictions for residents, evermore complex and technologically advanced surgical procedures, and an increased sense among chief residents of not being fully prepared to enter independent practice,[3] a clear need to improve training methods that

[a] Department of Surgery, Walter Reed National Military Medical Center, Uniformed Services University, 4301 Jones Bridge Road, Bethesda, MD 20814, USA; [b] The Choral Arts Society of Washington, DC, 5225 Wisconsin Ave, Washington, DC 20015, USA; [c] Cornell University, Ithaca, NY 14850, USA; [d] Department of Surgery, University of Texas Medical Branch, 301 University Boulevard, Galveston, TX 77554-0737, USA
* Corresponding author. Department of Surgery, Walter Reed National Military Medical Center, Uniformed Services University, 4301 Jones Bridge Road, Bethesda, MD 20814.
*E-mail address:* elliott@conductingperformance.org

Surg Clin N Am 95 (2015) 839–854
http://dx.doi.org/10.1016/j.suc.2015.04.011
0039-6109/15/$ – see front matter Published by Elsevier Inc.
surgical.theclinics.com

translate to iterative skill and confidence building for the learners is evident. Faculty development with respect to the skill of coaching is needed to accomplish this goal. Coaching to elite performance is a skill in and of itself. This article provides surgical educators with a step-by-step coaching model, consisting of techniques and strategies from the rehearsals of an elite musical ensemble and athletic sports training performance, which have been identified and deconstructed for use in medical education. This method is named the Conducting Elite Performance Training in Medicine (CEPTiM) model.

Medical simulation is similar to penicillin. It can be lifesaving but if applied incorrectly, it is ineffective. It is not an all-encompassing solution, and a critical need exists to create new versions of it in surgical training to adapt to rapidly emerging problems and resistant pathogens that contribute to global morbidity and mortality. Innovative and efficient training models are needed to address the challenges of increasingly complex surgical procedures. When applied as a complete framework, the techniques and strategies that comprise the CEPTiM model operate synergistically to allow for increasingly iterative training sessions that lead to elite performance in simulated and nonsimulated events.

The traditional training paradigm is that the more experience one has, the better the person's performance will be. It has been demonstrated, however, that, more so than experience, deliberate practice (DP) is crucial to expert performance and avoidance of arrested development in a particular task or skill.[4] DP entails setting a well-defined goal, being motivated to improve, and having adequate opportunities for practice and refinement of performance through structured feedback. This process has been documented to be effective for skill acquisition in medical and surgical training.[5]

Engaging in DP alone, however, is not sufficient for an individual to reach maximal performance. The CEPTiM model has been created for surgical educators to integrate and apply a defined coaching construct to medical education that includes an emphasis on team-based and procedural skills. These techniques and strategies can be integrated and applied separately, yet have a multiplying effect when used in tandem, maximizing each other's efficiency and effectiveness.

The model described in this article is derived from a collaboration among experts in health care, music, and sports training. Scott Tucker serves as the Conductor and Artistic Director of the Choral Arts Society of Washington D.C. Solveig Imsdahl is a 2-time member of the US National Rowing Team. Elliott Silverman has spent 7 years as a surgical education coach, served a year as the Visiting Fellow in the Cornell University Department of Music, trained for 2 years with Scott Tucker, and collaborated with Solveig Imsdahl to identify and distill the elements from elite music and sports that could form a standardized model for direct application to surgical coaching.

## CONDUCTING ELITE PERFORMANCE TRAINING IN MEDICINE MODEL OVERVIEW

The CEPTiM model has the ability to improve medical education by providing a reproducible, standard lexicon and an iterative surgical coaching model to attain proficiency of core skills before when they are needed.

The techniques and strategies are classified as either constants or planned variables. A constant technique or strategy is defined as one that is fundamental to and occurs at each and every simulation or training session. Planned variable techniques and strategies are used by coaches in moments when they have planned to highlight critical steps or when the trainees unexpectedly need correction or refinement. The component strategies that comprise the CEPTiM model are summarized in **Table 1**.

## CONDUCTING ELITE PERFORMANCE TRAINING IN MEDICINE—CONSTANTS

CEPTiM contains 4 constant training strategies as delineated in the following.

### *Warm-up*

Every training session begins with a 5- to 10-minute warm-up that serves 2 main purposes. The first is an active opportunity for coached refinement of fundamentals that is strategically designed to set conditions for the group of individuals to become a team. One of the most important elements of a successful team is alignment toward a common goal, with each member feeling vital and important to achieving this goal.[6] By developing this mind-set at the start of each training session, the team functions at the highest level throughout training and eventual performance. The most important part of a coach's job is to guide the team. To make this guidance effective, however, a few fundamental steps are required. First, a common vision must be communicated to and comprehended by the team. Second, this vision needs to be broken down into smaller, more digestible fragments, giving each member a specific and achievable goal. Third, the coach must act as a constant and confident supporter of the team's ability, regardless of the obstacles they encounter. This support fosters team confidence, which serves as a foundation for the mindfulness necessary to gain the most out of training. The coach's guidance can provide a sense of security so that the individual team members can focus on the present moment, without distraction about nonperformance-related past or future events. The coach can offer positive, specific, and realistic encouragement along the way by reminding the team about the progress they have made, pointing out where they currently stand, and informing them what they need to do to achieve their goal.

### *Examples*

#### *Music*

The choral warm-up is done in 2 stages. First, the singers concentrate on their own physical technique; this involves stretching, awareness of posture and breathing, and attention to maximizing the resonance of the voice for both beauty and power. Next, the singers are directed to extend their attention beyond their own sound to that of those around them and the whole choir. This attention hones the intonation, vowel production, balance, and rhythmic coordination needed for a chorus to perform at its best. All of this is guided by the conductor, who feeds information to the choral singers and aids them in the goal of perfect choral unity. During the course of the warm-up, group focus intensifies, and by the end of the warm up, the entire ensemble is ready to tackle the challenges of the specific music to be rehearsed.

#### *Sports*

It is essential for an athlete to warm up in training or competition because it prepares the athlete both physically and mentally. A mental warm-up could include, for example, listening to music to create focus and block out other distractions, visualizing success, or simply changing into uniform to set the mood. A physical warm-up is important for increasing body temperature, blood flow, and heart rate for better circulation, which ultimately accelerates the athlete's progress, because the muscles are able to contract and relax faster. Teams often have specific routines that they perform as a group to create immediate unity and shared focus from the beginning, such as group runs or sport-specific exercises (eg, high-kicks, lunges, squats, push-ups) that are performed in sync. This routine helps create a sense of alignment toward the team's goal, making each athlete feel important from the start.

**Table 1**
**Component Strategies and Techniques of the CEPTiM Model**

| | Strategy | Technique | Description | Application in Surgical Training |
|---|---|---|---|---|
| CEPTiM model | Constant | Warm-up | Starting a training session with performance of basic or fundamental skills to prepare the trainees mentally and physically for the planned activity and to create team alignment toward a common goal | Residents start a laparoscopic skills workshop with basic laparoscopic surgical tasks on a box trainer; trauma team starts workshop by performing a resuscitation on a simulated patient with straightforward injuries |
| | | Coaching team | Conducting simulation-based training with a team of 2 or more coordinated instructors who work together to maintain unbroken communication with the trainees | Head faculty instructor facilitates debrief of team training scenario while assistant cues up the appropriate video clip to illustrate teaching point |
| | | Bilateral active engagement | Maintaining active focus and mindfulness to the training and performance, such that learners are maximally prepared for any planned or unplanned event in the training and therefore learn to maintain mindfulness in actual performance | Planning a simulation-based training workshop to anticipate equipment/ supply/audiovisual needs and ensure that all are present so instructor does not have to turn attention from trainees to attend to other issues |
| | | Momentum arc | Creating a training experience in which learners are given goals that are challenging yet achievable within the allotted time; learners are motivated by progressive success and awareness of performance improvement throughout the training | Designing a simulation-based training workshop that teaches a skill that is appropriately matched to the level of learner, such as an ultrasound-guided central line insertion for a fourth year medical student, and breaking down the procedure into discrete tasks, such as cannulating the vein under ultrasound guidance, that can then be performed together as the full procedure, once each subtask is mastered |

| | | | |
|---|---|---|---|
| Planned variables | Clear performance excellence parameters | Providing a description of mastery performance and outlining steps needed to achieve mastery | Watching a video of a laparoscopic Nissen fundoplication with trainees and discussing what elements of the performance constitute the masterful execution of the operation |
| | Immediate feedback corrective coaching with immediate practice opportunity | Stopping the training to point out performance deviation from expectation and to provide feedback on how to achieve expected performance | Stopping a trauma resuscitation team training scenario to point out incorrect cervical spine immobilization during intubation, giving a demonstration and instructions on how to do it properly, allowing the team to practice, then restarting the scenario |
| | Intraprocedural guidance | Providing corrective coaching during the skill training or performance without stopping the learner's actions | Talking a trainee through a live-animal or cadaveric surgical procedure, giving feedback on how to adjust dissection plane or angle of needle driver to improve performance while the trainee continues to operate |
| | Midtraining refinement brief | Pausing the training to reorient learners to the underlying concepts or overall goal | Stopping a team training scenario to reestablish role clarity when the leader engages in a task rather than appropriately delegating |
| | Refinement of balance | Combining performances of well-trained individuals or teams to create a larger high-performing team | Conducting a simulation involving the transfer of a patient from the trauma bay to the operating room or from the operating room to the intensive care unit |

### *Surgery*

Many hospitals have mandated team huddles at the start of the day that, when well performed, can most certainly function as a team warm-up. It is an effective way to communicate goals and strategies for the day's operations. In addition, the team can share knowledge of each member's role, critical clinical steps, and what is needed to maximize the ability to perform them. Huddles typically proceed by individual members introducing themselves and their role for the day. The team leader, often the staff surgeon, should facilitate this interchange and encourage and define the active roles of the members. The team leader outlines the specific expected challenges to be managed, the needs of individual members to maximize their chance of success, and irregularities to be rapidly identified to all, which is no different than a brief before team training or mock codes. These indoctrinated rituals (instincts) can become truly robust if used to transform a group of individuals into a team.

## *Coaching Team*

The CT comprises coaches (eg, head coach and assistant coach) who train together to most effectively and efficiently lead each iterative rehearsal. The goals of each individual rehearsal (ie, simulation) are distilled from the needed elements required to peak at performance. When a CT is present, the head coach can efficiently and instantaneously communicate with the other members of the CT so that a break does not occur in focused communication with the trainees. This sustained focus is of special importance for continuous monitoring and instantaneous corrective actions of the learners' performance. Moreover, it allows for a more unified front as perceived by the learners. Communication skills have been shown to be a main differentiating factor between successful and unsuccessful coaches.[7]

The CT also provides a second layer of identification and correction compared with a single coach. However, it is the rehearsed teamwork and effortless communication between coaches that makes this technique so effective. Because alignment does not happen on its own, the group of coaches must become a CT for maximal efficiency.[8] Teams not only are more efficient at communicating but also have been demonstrated to make fewer mistakes in high-risk and high-intensity work environments, compared with individuals. This fact is of greater relevance when performance requires multiple skills, judgments, and experiences.[9]

## *Examples*

### *Music*

The choral conductor generally works in tandem with a skilled accompanist at the piano. Teamwork between the conductor and the accompanist greatly enhances the effectiveness of the rehearsal. As the conductor gives verbal feedback, the accompanist is poised to demonstrate or underline the points made by the conductor, and this requires a common understanding of the goals of the rehearsal as well as a shared skill set in identifying and correcting the problems encountered. In addition, in a large ensemble, there are often section leaders (appointed sopranos, altos, tenors, and basses) who communicate the conductor's information to their respective sections between rehearsals and who bring questions from the ensemble to the conductor.

### *Sports*

Team boats in rowing have a coxswain sitting at the end of the boat, who is in charge of steering, giving commands, and making sure the crew is synchronized. In addition to the in-boat coach, there is also a coach riding alongside the crew in a launch giving additional advice. As a rehearsed team, the coxswain and coach are able to give more thorough feedback, because the coach has a broader, more distant perspective, whereas the coxswain is moving with the crew, feeling the rhythm, set, and speed of the boat as they make changes. Communication between the coxswain and coach make for quicker and more efficient development of the crew.

### *Surgery*

In running simulations, it is often necessary to have facilitators to assist the primary training faculty coach to allow for the necessary engagement among all the learners and to keep the simulation moving forward according to the momentum arc strategy (see later section). A surgical CT is neither a faculty member attempting to teach a simulation skill by himself or herself to a large group of learners nor a faculty member working alongside simulation technicians who are generally familiar with the simulation center and equipment. A surgical CT comprises a head coach (lead faculty member) and 1 or more assistant coaches (fellow advanced practice clinician, nurse, or simulation technician). This team has deliberately rehearsed the simulation, including the starting point and endpoint goals, critical steps, and equipment needed for each step and restep. They have anticipated unexpected moments when the head coach will need to use the CEPTiM model method to immediately cease incorrect performance and redirect to demonstrate correct performance, as described later in this article. The head coach is set up for success for this crucial role via the CT constant. The assistant coaches facilitate the progression of the training session by continuously anticipating the needs of both the head coach and the learners so that there is no break in engagement between the learners and head coach. For example, a break in engagement might be a participant or coach momentarily leaving the group to get the correct piece of equipment or alter the state of a mannequin. The CT provides the constant framework to eliminate these interruptions.

### *Bilateral Active Engagement*

BAE occurs when the team (CT and learners) is actively engaged throughout the simulation and ready to anticipate the next unknown training direction. It functions best when it is established during the warm-up period and then proceeds without interruption through the rest of the training session. BAE is a critical skill that allows the CT to instantaneously choose the most effective CEPTiM corrective action tool when needed. BAE increases motivation and continued active engagement of the learners during the often multihour rehearsal/simulation/practice. Engagement can be defined as the simultaneous occurrence of high concentration, enjoyment, and motivation in achieving higher levels of performance. All 3 of these aspects lead to flow, the feeling of buoyancy or effortlessness plus high mental output, and, as a result, more effective learning.[10]

BAE encourages a harmonious learning environment, so intelligence, capabilities, and motivation momentum can be amplified. When each coach and trainee allows the others to contribute at their highest capacity, it leads to a multiplying effect on the team as a whole, resulting in elite performance as a team, rather than a group of individuals.[11]

To be adequately prepared for future real-life scenarios, learners must constantly be engaged, even when they are not immediately involved in the training. Each individual must be aware of the current situation and not mentally check out, so they can match the appropriate style and intensity of performance when they are needed again, even on short notice. The CT sets the conditions for success for BAE via the head coach's ability to focus without interruption on the training element at the given moment.

Traditional leadership/medical training often involves instructors who lead by knowing and doing everything with little input from those who are learning. Although it is undoubtedly important that the learners are actively engaged with their CT to best learn,[4,7] it is not enough for learners to be unilaterally engaged with their coaches. The coaches need to be equally actively tuned in to the cognitive, physiologic, and emotional status of the team they are coaching.

Learners must constantly be engaged to be adequately prepared for the next step of the procedure, for identification of irregularities, and for constructive response to potential unknown scenarios. Each person must be constantly aware of the situation and not cognitively lose focus.

### *Examples*

#### *Music*

The best example of team members not losing focus is in Beethoven's Ninth Symphony, the Ode to Joy. In the middle of the final movement (the only movement where the chorus sings) there is a tenor solo, followed by an extended orchestral interlude. This interlude quiets down into what seems like a holding pattern, 18 measures of soft offbeats in the French Horn and false starts in the strings. The music becomes so soft that it sounds like it might disappear altogether. Then, without warning, the Chorus erupts into a full-throated exposition of the main theme, forte and at the top of their range: "Freude schoener Goetterfunken, Tochter aus Elysium!..." Each chorus member must have the tempo, dynamic, and spirit of the phrase fully placed at the front of their mind to enter here with accuracy. One can always tell if a chorus is well prepared at moments like this.

#### *Sports*

If a basketball player is on the bench and the coach says "get in there," the player cannot be fumbling to warm up as he or she is on the way to the court. The player must be mentally present at all times to be ready to perform at a level that matches, or even improves on, the dynamics of the rest of the team. The other team members may have been active for a while. If another member joins in, it has to be as if the member has been playing for the entire time with them.

#### *Surgery*

Imagine a trocar lacerating a major vessel and causing a massive hemorrhage during a routine laparoscopic surgery. There is no time for warm up. When a patient has a sudden code or life-threatening event on the operating table, each member of the surgical team must be alert and performing at 100% capacity from time zero. This kind of performance does not just happen. Team members need to be attentive and engaged with a sense of personal responsibility to the patient that is fostered by the team leader and their interactions. Continually challenging the team, engaging the individuals in critical steps in the case, and fostering this sense of patient ownership are just a few ways to keep the members actively engaged. Team training with simulation scenarios can replicate these high-stakes, critical, rare events and condition members to remain alert and engaged and empower them to help when the timing from the bench to action is critical.

### *Momentum Arc*

The momentum arc describes how the CT should map out the overall scope of each training session to foster a sense of momentum so that the learners feel like they are presented with problems that they either overcome or come close to overcoming over the course of the session. This way, they are energized by their progress rather than exhausted by the end of a training session. The learners should feel a sense of energy that flows right through the end of the training session so when they return for further training, they anticipate the same arc.

It is important to strike a balance between a sense of accomplishment and maintenance of real, high standards through honest feedback. Incessant stopping and correcting can rapidly lead to defeat, while letting too many teachable moments pass results in missed opportunities for learning and can lead to the incorporation of poor performance habits. The art of creating a Momentum Arc is in ensuring that standards do not drop, but at the same time, the learners are not defeated in their attempts to uphold the standards. The continuity from one simulation to another allows for sustained iterative motivation for peak performance through the entirety of the training continuum. By maintaining BAE, the CT can best assess this balance for each aspect of the simulation and monitor the momentum arc for the duration of the training.

### Examples

#### Music

The best rehearsals are ones in which there is a genuine sense of progress toward that common goal and interruptions by the conductor decrease during the course of the rehearsal. Long passages of music where problems have been solved and musical goals reached are satisfying to the singers, and this motivates them to work just as hard or even harder at the next rehearsal. Conversely, if a conductor constantly stops to correct the ensemble, the performers become demoralized and their performance level will drop as they seek approval from the conductor rather than achievement of the shared vision.

#### Sports

Coaches break down lifetime goals into smaller, more achievable goals, so that the athlete is able to approach the ultimate goal 1 step at a time; this helps create the sustained momentum required, because the athlete feels energized by each accomplished benchmark, rather than being overwhelmed by the entire process.

#### Surgery

Taking residents through complex procedures can be exhausting for both the resident and the faculty. Maintaining engagement, energy, and active learning throughout the experience is crucial, which then sets the grounds to perform a successful team task. It is now the coaches' job to maintain this energy through the balance of the procedure. Trainees should be guided with precise, directed feedback to help maintain the previously set standards that are appropriate for their skill level. Expecting first-year residents to perform a bowel anastomosis at the level of a chief resident, although flattering, likely leaves them feeling defeated. Inversely, only praising a chief resident on their trocar placement during a routine cholecystectomy might induce apathy and fail to progress their skills past their current level. Maintaining the momentum arc requires an active, engaged coach who is aware and willing to continuously adjust his or her strategy to meet the needs of the team and leave them with a true sense of accomplishment and excitement that they then expect for the next iterative simulation.

## CONDUCTING ELITE PERFORMANCE TRAINING IN MEDICINE—PLANNED VARIABLES

The constants take place in every training session, whereas planned variables are used only when necessary. Key techniques are highlighted in the following.

## CLEAR PERFORMANCE EXCELLENCE PARAMETERS

Setting clear performance excellence parameters (CPEP) provides the boundaries of performance excellence that outline what elite status is and exactly what the trainees need to do to reach it. Goal setting alone is an important aspect of successful coaching, but CPEP has more components.[7] CPEP involves clear, bilateral goal setting; demonstration of proper technique; and requirement of excellence before continuing. Often, the CT has a vision of success, but the learners may not yet subscribe to that same vision. It is the CT's job to guide the learners' performance toward their vision, as well as to incorporate their vision of elite team performance to maximize their own performance as a CT. This strategy is akin to the shared mental model in TeamSTEPPS (Team Strategies and Tools to Enhance Performance and Patient Safety) lexicon. This way, all members of the team are oriented to collectively move toward the exact same visualized outcome.

The process begins in the head coach's mind. The coach thinks about the image of what the desired outcome looks like, sounds like, and feels like. The learners usually start with an image that is different from the head coach's. Therefore, part of the process is changing what the learners present with to what the head coach is imagining. The CT informs the learners what that end-product performance image is so everybody is moving in the same direction toward the same exact vision. CPEP is not only correcting the learners and having them demonstrate to all that the excellence parameters can be reached in practicum, but also feeding them the vision of what it should be so they incorporate it in themselves.

Having a shared understanding is a crucial tenet of teamwork that allows for identification of errors and their resulting correction.[7] The CT should not move on with instruction until learners demonstrate that they can perform within the parameters established by the head coach. This requirement confirms that the learners understand the excellence parameters and are able to achieve at the required level before moving through the rest of the training. At this step, the learners assimilate the shared vision of the goal and begin to understand what it looks like, what it sounds like, and what it feels like. CPEP is not a single checkpoint done only once at the beginning of training but rather an active demonstration of parameters throughout the skill acquisition sessions. The CT should frequently ensure that everyone shares the same vision of operating inside the CPEP and make the proper adjustments if deviations occur, as demonstrated in further planned variable techniques in the CEPTiM model.

### *Examples*

#### *Music*

The best conductors achieve momentum by instilling in their ensemble a common vision of the end goal. This common vision is sometimes expressed through imagery and sometimes through technical explanation. When everyone in the room has a clear vision of what the end result should be, there is a natural drive that occurs. For example, each singer in a chorus needs to consider how his or her sound output integrates with the sound of the rest of the group. A soloist may be able to sing different syllables quickly, but as an ensemble, this simply would not work. The words are like ingredients, and each singer must focus on singing the vowels and consonants in a uniform and beautiful way so that they blend seamlessly together when sung simultaneously by many different voices. The words emerge from the broken down components when they are given this level of attention. A skilled conductor knows instinctively when to interrupt the flow of the music and when to trust the performers to self-correct.

***Sports***

Having athletes visualize success is an effective strategy to helping them succeed. A coach explains how the team is going to achieve their goal, painting the picture by giving specific details (eg, cheering fans, weather conditions, game development) to create that shared vision of success throughout the team. For example, a basketball coach may have the team cut down the nets at the beginning of the year to simulate winning the championship. The best coaches are able to show their team that there is a difference between what you think you are capable of and what you are actually capable of, ever pushing through—thereby raising the bar anew on—the limits you set for yourself; this is a sign of progress. A team that has experienced performing beyond their imagined limits knows how to remain focused throughout the iterative continuum of training. They may also become more goal oriented in unexpected, emergency (low-frequency high-stakes) situations, because their early training has instilled focus and adherence to high performance standards at the limits of their comfort zones.

***Surgery***

Despite memorizing the surgical atlas and knowing the steps of the operation, a surgical resident may still struggle through the operation or even fail to live up to the faculty's expectations. This failure can be largely due to not knowing these expectations or failing to have a shared vision. A quick brief before a specific operation can really bring the operating team together as a unit and verbalize these expectations to include critical points in the procedure, skills the resident is expected to perform, skills with which they might need assistance or extra guidance, and possible troubleshooting strategies. If the faculty surgeon envisions the mesh placed in a certain way with a certain tack using a particular strategy, this can be communicated to the resident as part of their goals and expectations. The team then spends the time during the procedure meeting or working to meet these goals, performing as a team and focusing on the patient, instead of backtracking to communicate these goals or being frustrated with each other.

## IMMEDIATE FEEDBACK CORRECTIVE COACHING WITH IMMEDIATE PRACTICE OPPORTUNITY WITH OR WITHOUT REFINEMENT

Immediate feedback corrective coaching (IFCC) is when the CT stops the training at the first sign of deviation from the CPEP to offer immediate identification and begin immediate corrective coaching to reenter the CPEP. The immediate practice opportunity (IPO) always follows the IFCC; they are coupled as IFCC + IPO and describe a crucial component of DP.[4] This combination provides an opportunity for learners to demonstrate to the instructor, and to each other, their strengthened ability to adjust their understanding and actions to be able to perform within the CPEP again. The training session does not move on to other areas until the trigger for the IFCC + IPO is resolved. It may take several IFCC + IPO attempts in rapid-cycle form before the group has demonstrated the corrected action and is prepared to move on. It is a key responsibility of the CT to not create a sand castle that can be washed away with a wave. The immediacy of both the feedback and opportunity for practice is essential to guarantee that the foundation of performance excellence has been strengthened rather than temporarily patched. Stopping and correcting as soon as the problem is recognized not only increases the number of times it is performed correctly but also minimizes the number of times it is performed incorrectly. This technique allows conditioning (opportunity to instill instincts) for only the correct response and the skill of immediately identifying internal irregularities for correction.

In certain cases, deviation from CPEP can provide an opportunity to further refine the parameters for even finer performance standards. In order for a team to progress iteratively, clearly defined rules, expectations, and a standard lexicon of communication need to exist. Coaches can accelerate the process of getting the team on the same page by repeatedly using clear, comprehensible terms. A common language (of terms, expressions, and signals) enables the team to exchange information efficiently and clearly. By reinforcing the boundaries while staying open to feedback, the coach creates a virtual CPEP box around the team that includes the rules needed to elicit elite performance. If a coach is not required to identify individuals who break rules, the team more often stays inside the box. It is not meant to be a box of restrictions, but rather a box of security, allowing the team to develop mutual trust and proceed iteratively within a common structure and direction. Teams with consistent coaches are able to perform to their highest ability and grow faster than teams who are unaware of the boundaries of their work environment.

In an analysis of 252 laparoscopic common bile duct injuries, 97% of the time the injury was not recognized. This type of injury results in part from a visual perception illusion that IFCC + IPO in a simulated setting might help in decreasing morbidity.[12,13] Telementoring and teleproctoring opportunities and formalized fellowships by the Society of American Gastrointestinal and Endoscopic Surgeons are leading the way in the continuum of training and guided practice in the clinical setting for nonnovice performers.

## *Examples*

### *Music*

It is the conductor's job to hold the ensemble to the highest standard. The conductor keeps the fundamentals in good form (eg, proper vocal tone, sensitivity to the ensemble), reminds the chorus of common pitfalls (eg, descending patterns often flat, soft passages unintentionally slow, certain syncopations tend to drag, other common rhythms rush), and monitors the specific musical passages for accurate notes, rhythms, articulations, and dynamics. Instant decisions are made during the course of the rehearsal about what to correct and in what order of priority. If a specific mistake that falls in the category of a fundamental, or a common pitfall, is being made, that mistake is high priority and used as a teachable moment. All corrections are done within the context of the ultimate goal and musical vision that has been established for that rehearsal.

### *Sports*

Especially in sports that involve choreographed routines (such as gymnastics or dancing) it would be time consuming and less productive for a coach to wait until the athlete has completed the entire routine before providing feedback. Therefore, stopping the athlete immediately provides the opportunity to correct specific skills and refine technique. Immediate feedback also ensures that the athlete is more likely to know what the coach is referring to, as opposed to recalling a particular action later.

### *Surgery*

Surgical residents are continually learning and refining new technical skills. Guided practice with immediate feedback and refinement toward defined objectives is the basis of DP. This strategy has been proved to improve skill mastery. Laparoscopic skills training is the perfect time to have one-on-one coaching with the residents that can then be translated and continued into the operating room. Dangerous maneuvers, such as handling a sharp off screen, can be corrected and exterminated immediately, and inefficient moves can be brought to the residents' attention and refined through continued practice. As their skills increase, the bar can be raised to promote continued refinement, skill acquisition, and engagement by the learners.

### *Intraprocedural Guidance*

Intraprocedural guidance (IPG) is the act of guiding learners through a procedure without stopping them. Although major deviations from CPEP require IFCC + IPO, at times it is appropriate to adjust external goal-focused performance without stopping action. This adjustment enables the coach to continuously finely guide learners while they are performing the skill, rather than stopping and restarting the whole procedure. IPG can also be done using nonverbal communication, which more realistically portrays true performance conditions. In medicine, midprocedural guidance coupled with postprocedural feedback can increase motivation and reduce anxiety and perceived workload compared with only postprocedural feedback.[14]

### *Examples*

#### *Music*

In rehearsal, sometimes the singers quickly raise their hand if they have made a mistake. This action acknowledges that they are aware and will self-correct, and it is then not necessary to interrupt the flow of the music for an individual's error.

#### *Sports*

The stroke in rowing is a fluid and continuous motion comprising the catch, drive, finish, and recovery. A coach often provides feedback on individual parts without interrupting the continuous flow of the stroke, as rowers make fine adjustments to their technique. This method gives rowers a more natural practice environment, allowing them to perceive how distinct corrections affect the entire stroke as well.

#### *Surgery*

IPG is a core component to the traditional style of medical education. Walking an intern through a bedside procedure, such as central line insertion, or the staff first assisting a resident during a cholecystectomy are common examples of this technique. Barring unsafe maneuvers, the learner can continue through the procedure uninterrupted, following clear commands and directions.

### *Midtraining Refinement Brief*

In the midst of training, the learners may hyperfocus on minute details of the simulation, blurring the big picture. The midtraining refinement brief (MTRB) is a pause in training to remind the learners of major underlying concepts to apply to specific situations and the process as a whole. During an MTRB, the CT should aim to provide a greater understanding of the context, allowing the learners to refocus during training roadblocks. For example, during suturing training, the CT would stop practice if a learner is breaking sterile and safe technique and then reinforce to the team the importance of patient and fellow clinician safety during suturing. Mindfulness toward the group's vision, objectives, and standards, as well as the roles of the learners and CT, amplifies the capacity of the team to perform at an elite level.[11]

### *Examples*

#### *Music*

When focused on a particular phrase of a piece of music, choir members may lose sight of the mood of the piece. For example, they may be singing a soft hymn too loud and with too much intensity, or they might have a frown on their face while singing happy lyrics. Another common error is singing with the music folders angled parallel to their face so that the sound at the level of the audience is muted and muffled. By taking the time to tell the choir about the context of the piece and its overall vision, the CT can ensure more aligned performance moving forward.

#### *Sports*

It is a common occurrence that athletes get caught up in the details of the current training, resulting in unnecessary anxiety or stress. The coach's responsibility in this situation is to remind the athletes of the overall goal (for instance, winning a race or qualifying for the Olympics), with the intention of redirecting the athletes' energy and recreating momentum and focus.

#### *Surgery*

Running a mock trauma code can be the controlled, and sometimes uncontrolled, chaos. Team members can become anxious or focused on a specific task or feature of the patient and lose sight of the resuscitation goals. Just like in a real code, the facilitator can give a quick brief on what has happened, what the priorities are, the goals of resuscitation, and if any goals have changed since the start. If this particular patient calls for expedited transfer to the operating room, the team may need to be refocused toward this goal, which can decrease the stress and feeling of being overwhelmed.

## *Refinement of Balance*

Refinement of balance (RoB) is the art of combining several elite teams together to function as 1 large elite team. "Teamwork is not an automatic consequence of placing people together."[8] It is more than several individuals performing separately as a group. Interprofessional teams often train separately before meeting for simultaneous care of a patient (surgery team, anesthesia team, perioperative nursing team). A uniformity of goal-centered care and cooperation to achieve elite performance must be present. Balance is a key element for cooperation, especially between interdisciplinary teams. As the profession of medicine evolves, a need for additional training to promote such interprofessionalism exists.[9] RoB tends to have much greater emphasis toward the end of a training cycle and closer to performance. At this point, each separate group has reached elite team performance within themselves. That the different sections are proficient in their roles separately, however, does not necessarily mean they are proficient at working together. RoB is about overcoming this disconnect and creating synergy between all groups. By being engaged, but as outside observers, the CT is in the ideal position to give such feedback from an outside vantage point.

### *Examples*

#### *Music*

For a symphony performance, the choir, orchestra, band, and soloists must be able to reach the same balance in volume and harmony with each other as they did separately. Sometimes, one of the members of the CT sits in the audience and uses simple nonverbal cues (thumbs up, thumb to the side, thumbs down) to alert the conductor how and where the balance is lacking. For example, are the primary elements of the piece being clearly heard where the audience is sitting, or is one or more sections performing too loudly to hear the soloists? Then the conductor can give appropriate feedback, such as telling the choir to sing louder, to refine the balance between the 4 groups.

#### *Sports*

When rowers compete, they often face numerous crews in the water that they have never raced with before. In this scenario, the coxswains in each boat become responsible for coordinating a harmonized performance as the 60-foot-long boats race side by side, only a few feet apart from each other. It is critical that each boat's trajectory is on course to win and to never collide. The rowers rely on the coxswains to lead several individual team boats down the race course, functioning as one greater unit. Although coxswains have experience training next to other boats, they need to be able to make fine adjustments and find the right balance whenever they line up next to other elite teams, because the rowers (faced in the opposite direction) are not in a position to evaluate themselves.

### *Surgery*

Taking an entire operating room team through a mock code is a perfect opportunity to work on RoB. The training consists of several high-functioning, efficient teams that must come together synergistically to efficiently manage a life-threatening event. If the surgical team is taking too much of the room nurse's attention, then the anesthesia team might not be able to communicate the need for blood products. The facilitator can help guide communication and make sure all the teams are truly working as one cohesive unit with one goal.

## SUMMARY

The CEPTiM model can be approached in 2 ways. The first is as a tool belt from which to pull strategies and apply to coaching and teaching methods as needed. Although this model is useful, the true utility is as an all-inclusive framework to prime, initiate, sustain, and refine educational or coaching activities. The elements of the model interact synergistically, intertwining, overlapping, and building on each other to yield the highest educational results. The authors have proposed this model as a single, complete method for surgical CTs to practice during simulation and real-time training in clinical environments.

The application of adult learning theory and DP[4] to medical education is evident and imperative. By enhancing educators' skills and creating elite-level coaches, learners can be trained into elite performing teams, secondarily teaching them to also be elite coaches and promoting lifelong learning through a self-perpetuating cycle.

## REFERENCES


1. Kohn LT, Corrigan J, Donaldson MS. To err is human: building a safer health system. Washington, DC: National Academy Press; 2000.
2. Institute of Medicine, Committee on Quality Health Care in America. Crossing the quality chasm: a new health system for the 21st century. Washington, DC: Committee on Quality of Health Care in America; National Academies Press; 2001.
3. Pugh CM, DaRosa DA, Bell RH. Residents' self-report learning needs for intraoperative knowledge: are we missing the bar? Am J Surg 2010;199(4):562–5.
4. Ericsson KA. Deliberate practice and acquisition of expert performance: a general overview. Acad Emerg Med 2008;15(11):988–94.
5. Palter VN, Grantcharov TP. Individualized deliberate practice on a virtual reality simulator improves technical performance of surgical novices in the operating room. Ann Surg 2014;259(3):443–8.
6. Katzenbach JR, Smith DK. The discipline of teams. Harv Bus Rev 1993;71:111–20.
7. Greenberg CC, Ghousseini HN, Quamme SRP, et al. Surgical coaching for individual performance improvement. Ann Surg 2014;261:32–4.

8. Salas E, Sims DE, Klein C, et al. Can teamwork enhance patient safety? Forum Risk Manage Found Harv Med Inst 2003;23:5–9.
9. Lerner S, Magrane D, Friedman E. Teaching teamwork in medical education. Mt Sinai J Med 2009;76(4):318–29.
10. Shernoff DJ, Csikszentmihalyi M. Flow in schools. In: Furlong MJ, Gilman R, Huebner ES, editors. Handbook of positive psychology in schools. London: Routledge; 2014. chap 11. p. 75–108.
11. Wiseman L, Bradwejn J, Westbroek EM. A new leadership curriculum. Acad Med 2014;89(3):376–9.
12. Way LW, Stewart L, Gantert W, et al. Causes and prevention of laparoscopic bile duct injuries. Ann Surg 2003;237(4):460–9.
13. Lipshy KA. Crisis management leadership in the operating room. San Diego: Creative Team Publishing; 2013.
14. O'Connor A, Schwaitzberg SD, Cao CGL. How much feedback is necessary for learning to suture? Surg Endosc 2008;22(7):1614–9.

# Emotional Intelligence and Simulation

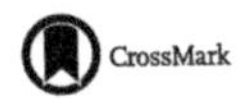

Sophia K. McKinley, MD, EdM[a], Roy Phitayakorn, MD, MHPE (MEd)[b,*]

**KEYWORDS**

- Emotional intelligence • Simulation • Graduate medical education
- ACGME core competencies

**KEY POINTS**

- Emotional intelligence (EI) is how an individual manages his or her own emotions and the emotions of others; this concept is well established in the business literature but is still a nascent field of research in medical education.
- Simulation has many characteristics that make it well suited to deliver EI development interventions because of its safe, standardized environment.
- Effective simulations to develop EI in surgery will likely require preparatory work, occur during protected education time, and provide participants with immediate feedback or assessment.

## EMOTIONAL INTELLIGENCE: BACKGROUND

### *Definition and Conceptual Models*

A commonly cited definition of EI is the "ability to monitor one's own and others' emotions, to discriminate among them, and to use this information to guide one's thinking and actions."[1] More succinctly, EI describes how an individual manages his or her own emotions and the emotions of others. Salovey and Mayer[2] introduced their theory of EI in 1990, and the topic has since gained both academic and popular interest, most notably through the writings of Harvard Business School Professor Dan Goleman[3–6] who wrote in his 1998 essay "What Makes a Leader?" that "emotional intelligence is the *sine qua non* of leadership."

Although the idea of EI was introduced more than 20 years ago, there continues to be academic debate regarding the nature of EI. Several researchers embrace the conceptualization of EI as an ability, either as a social intelligence or a type of cognitive skill.[1,4,7–9] Others have promoted a trait conceptualization of EI in which an individual's

[a] Department of Surgery, Massachusetts General Hospital, Harvard Medical School, 55 Fruit Street, GRB-425, Boston, MA 02114, USA; [b] Department of Surgery, Massachusetts General Hospital, Harvard Medical School, 55 Fruit Street, Boston, MA 02114, USA
* Corresponding author.
*E-mail address:* rphitayakorn@mgh.harvard.edu

Surg Clin N Am 95 (2015) 855–867
http://dx.doi.org/10.1016/j.suc.2015.03.003 surgical.theclinics.com
0039-6109/15/$ – see front matter 

EI reflects disposition and personal characteristics.[10,11] The particular stance toward EI influences the approach to EI measurement and assessment.[12,13] Within an ability construction of EI, self-report is inadequate to capture how an individual performs with regard to managing his emotions and the emotions of others. Furthermore, an ability model of EI presents the challenge of determining objective standards against which ability should be measured. For the trait model of EI, pure self-report can be an effective way to determine an individual's tendencies and characteristics but may not adequately reflect how the individual performs in reality.[10,11,14] For example, people who have low trait assertiveness may, through self-awareness and practice, succeed in negotiations, even though it may be more effortful for them compared with a colleague who has high trait assertiveness. Both the trait and ability frameworks of EI reject the hypothesis that EI is fixed and immutable. Rather, proponents of both models assert that EI can be taught, learned, and developed and that it responds to life experiences and the conscious self-development efforts of an individual.[5,14,15]

### *Emotional Intelligence in the Workplace*

Much of the increasing interest in EI is driven by research that demonstrates a positive relationship between EI and work performance characteristics, primarily in the corporate setting. In a study of executives in a multinational food and beverage company, McClelland[16] found that those hired based on emotional competencies had a 6% 2-year turnover rate compared with the 50% turnover rate experienced by those hired through traditional methods. Furthermore, executives with strong EI exceeded annual earning goals by 20%, whereas their colleagues with lower EI underperformed relative to targets. There were similar findings in the European and Asian divisions, suggesting that the importance of EI is not limited to particular cultural contexts. Other researchers demonstrated that the emotional competency of stress management was positively correlated with job performance in retail store managers as measured by net profits, sales per square foot, sales per employee, and sales per dollar inventory investment.[17] Goleman[5] claims that EI is twice as important as technical skill and traditional intelligence quotient as an ingredient to excellent job performance across all employment levels and business sectors. He asserts that the importance of EI increases with position, with up to 90% of the difference in performance of senior leaders attributed to differences in EI factors.

A meta-analysis of 57 published research articles that included more than 12,000 individuals also supports the claim that EI is a valid predictor of job performance.[18] EI may also influence group functioning, with high-EI teams demonstrating a high level of performance throughout a task, in contrast to low-EI teams, which start out at lower levels of performance and eventually catch up to the performance level of the high-EI teams.[19] In short, the business community has embraced EI and the view that by placing a high value on the skill of emotion management, a company can improve performance and consequently profits, optimize employee hiring and retention, and create a more satisfying customer experience.[20,21]

## EMOTIONAL INTELLIGENCE IN SURGERY

### *Rationale for Increased Interest in Physician Emotional Intelligence*

Perceiving and managing emotions is fundamental to medicine as physicians must navigate their own emotions as well as the emotions of patients and other team members, often in high-tension and charged situations, to succeed as effective practitioners. The Accreditation Council for Graduate Medical Education (ACGME) has defined 6 core competencies—Patient Care, Professionalism, Systems-based

Practice, Interpersonal and Communication Skills, Medical Knowledge, and Practice-based Learning and Improvement—that trainees are expected to attain by the conclusion of residency.[22] Intuitively, EI is applicable to interpersonal skills and communication. However, if one considers all of the scenarios in medicine that require careful management of emotion, it becomes apparent that EI may underpin other ACGME competencies as well. A literature review of EI in health care settings demonstrated the broad relevance of EI to medicine, including domains related to the competencies of Interpersonal Skills and Communication, Patient Care, Professionalism, Medical Knowledge and Practice-based Learning and Improvement.[12] As such, there has been an increasing call for incorporating the development of EI into medical training.[12,13,23–26]

### *Emotional Intelligence in Surgery: Studies to Date*

Despite the interest in EI and its potential role in multiple ACGME core competencies, only a handful of studies have attempted to characterize the EI profiles of resident physicians, and even fewer have focused on surgery. Jensen and colleagues[27] described the EI of 74 surgical residents at a university program using the Bar-On Emotional Quotient Inventory (EQ-i), a self-report tool rooted in the ability conceptualization of EI in which 133 items cluster to 5 composite scores and 15 content subscores.[28] Although there was a wide range of individual scores, mean group scores were higher than the national average overall and for each of the 5 composite and 15 content scales. Residents scored highest in stress tolerance and lowest in social responsibility, a component of the composite interpersonal score. EI did not correlate with age or training level. This descriptive study did not comment on gender differences within the resident group nor did it attempt to establish the predictive validity of EI on resident performance.

The authors' multi-institutional education research group studied the trait EI of 139 resident physicians across multiple specialties, including 85 general surgery residents.[29] The authors used the Trait Emotional Intelligence Questionnaire (TEIQue, **Table 1**), a 153-item self-assessment of trait EI, which clusters to 15 independent facets and 4 composite factors, and found that there were fewer gender differences among the general surgery residents than across all the specialties combined, a finding that suggested that individuals with similar trait EI characteristics self-select into surgery and/or that the process of surgical training leads the development of a particular EI profile. This study also demonstrated that different specialties exhibited different profiles of relative high and low trait EI development areas, a finding that was interpreted to demonstrate a need for specialty-specific, targeted EI development interventions.[30] One conclusion from this study was that baseline trait EI assessment could be used to identify the areas in which different groups of residents would benefit most from additional, intentional growth.

Lin and colleagues[31] also used the TEIQue and examined the EI of medical student applicants to a general surgery residency program. These investigators examined whether EI was correlated with traditional measures of applicant quality, such as United States Medical Licensing Examination (USMLE) scores, clerkship grades, number of publications, honors society status, faculty evaluation of the interview, and faculty evaluation of applicant EI using the TEIQue 360° Short Form (360° SF). A total of 53 applicants participated in the study. Applicants scored statistically significantly higher in overall EI when compared with the general population, and there was no difference between men and women applicants. Age was the only demographic predictor of EI, with EI increasing modestly with age. There was no correlation between EI scores and any academic parameter except USMLE score, for which there

**Table 1**
**Sample items from the Trait Emotional Questionnaire, a psychometrically validated EI tool**

| | Disagree Completely | | | | | | | Agree Completely |
|---|---|---|---|---|---|---|---|---|
| 1 | I am usually able to control other people | 1 | 2 | 3 | 4 | 5 | 6 | 7 |
| 2 | Generally, I do not take notice of other people's emotions | 1 | 2 | 3 | 4 | 5 | 6 | 7 |
| 3 | When I receive wonderful news, I find it difficult to calm down quickly | 1 | 2 | 3 | 4 | 5 | 6 | 7 |
| 4 | I tend to see difficulties in every opportunity rather than opportunities in every difficulty | 1 | 2 | 3 | 4 | 5 | 6 | 7 |
| 5 | On the whole, I have a gloomy perspective on most things | 1 | 2 | 3 | 4 | 5 | 6 | 7 |
| 6 | I do not have a lot of happy memories | 1 | 2 | 3 | 4 | 5 | 6 | 7 |
| 7 | Understanding the needs and desires of others is not a problem for me | 1 | 2 | 3 | 4 | 5 | 6 | 7 |
| 8 | I generally believe that things will work out fine in my life | 1 | 2 | 3 | 4 | 5 | 6 | 7 |
| 9 | I often find it difficult to recognize what emotion I am feeling | 1 | 2 | 3 | 4 | 5 | 6 | 7 |
| 10 | I am not socially skilled | 1 | 2 | 3 | 4 | 5 | 6 | 7 |

*From* Petrides KV. Technical manual for the Trait Emotional Intelligence Questionnaire (TEIQue). 1st edition. 5th printing ed. London: London Psychometric Laboratory; 2012; with permission.

was a slight negative correlation. There was no correlation between applicant TEIQue score and faculty 360° SF. Furthermore, TEIQue scores did not correlate with faculty evaluation of the applicant's interview. Despite the lack of correlation between measured EI and traditional admission parameters, there was a modest correlation between EI and rank status, with unranked candidates scoring significantly lower in EI than ranked candidates. Given the mixed findings, the authors concluded that it was too early to include EI as a parameter for selecting general surgery residents.

In another study of medical students, Arora and colleagues[32] investigated the relationship between the stress experienced by subjects before, during, and after a surgical task and trait EI. They assessed the trait EI of medical students and then measured the heart rate as well as reported stress levels of medical students who completed a task using the Minimally Invasive Surgical Trainer–Virtual Reality, a validated virtual reality simulator. Medical students who had high trait EI reported higher levels of stress and also had higher heart rates during the simulated surgical task, which may suggest that high trait EI may not necessarily always be beneficial. These same students, however, also demonstrate more rapid recovery to before-task stress levels than lower–trait EI peers. Overall, this study demonstrated that simulation can effectively draw out individual differences in responses to simulated scenarios and that there may be an interaction between EI and simulation, which can be exploited or used for educational purposes. One avenue of future investigation is to use collected data on an individual's trait EI or stress response to tailor future simulated experiences such that the individual develops more effective stress-coping strategies.

Weng and colleagues[33] have demonstrated a positive relationship between physician EI and patient satisfaction for attending level surgeons in Taiwan. In a study of 50 surgeons and 549 patients, there was a statistically significant positive correlation between surgeon EI and the presurgical patient-doctor relationship. This research used the Wong and Law Emotional Intelligence Scale, a 16-item tool based on an ability conceptualization of EI. In one study, the investigators computed physician EI based on both self-rating and nursing director ratings.[34] Data regarding the patient-doctor relationship was collected both from physicians and nursing directors using the 9-item Patient-Doctor Relationship Questionnaire-9.[35] Postoperatively, however, physician EI did not have a significant correlation with the patient-doctor relationship.

### *Emotional Intelligence in Surgery: Unanswered Questions*

To summarize, studies of EI in surgery have focused on describing the EI levels of surgical residents or surgical applicants. As such, there are multiple unanswered questions with regard to EI and surgery. The first is whether EI is predictive of a surgical trainee's performance. To the authors' knowledge, no study has examined whether a surgical resident's EI corresponds to his or her clinical performance by any measure. In one multi-institutional study, researchers recruited residents from anesthesiology residencies at 5 academic institutions to determine if a correlation existed between resident EI and clinical performance as measured by faculty evaluation of the 6 ACGME core competencies.[36] Only 86 of 339 invited residents completed the study, but researchers concluded that several of the EI scores and subscores were statistically significantly correlated with all 6 of the ACGME core competencies with a modest effect size. These scores were measured using the EQ-i instrument and included total EI score, intrapersonal composite score, self-regard, self-actualization, and stress tolerance. There were no statistically significant gender differences in EQ-i total score, composite scale, or content score aside from empathy, although the investigators did not indicate which gender scored higher. Again, descriptive statistics of the residents as a group were not published, but these findings suggest that given a large enough number of participating resident physicians, EI may have predictive validity for resident physician performance.

A second unexplored question about EI and surgery is whether targeted EI development leads to improved clinical performance. There are at least 2 approaches to the selection and design of an EI development program. One could first assess the baseline EI characteristics of surgical residents and then specifically address areas of low development. This strategy embraces the view that well-rounded development would aid clinical performance by arming residents with the skills and confidence in EI strategies they are less comfortable with or inclined to use, in essence increasing the number of tools at their disposal when encountering the diversity of emotionally demanding hospital scenarios. Another approach to selecting EI targets for development is to determine which areas of EI most correlate with strong clinical performance and then design educational programming intended to augment these particular areas regardless of a group's baseline EI profile. This method reflects the view that well roundedness in itself may not be essential to superior performance; rather, specific traits are more essential than others in enabling clinical effectiveness. It remains to be seen whether EI development does indeed lead to gains in clinical performance and whether there is an optimal strategy in choosing EI targets.

A third frontier in EI research is the role that simulation would have in EI development, if any. The remainder of this article is devoted to outlining the benefits that simulation may bring to EI development, exploring the variety of forms in which simulation might support the development of EI, and reviewing the evidence that simulation may be an effective way to augment EI development with the ultimate goal of improved clinical performance.

## EMOTIONAL INTELLIGENCE AND SIMULATION

### *Benefits of Incorporating Simulation into Emotional Intelligence Development*

Simulation has the potential to facilitate several goals of EI development. One of the key first steps of EI development is increased self-knowledge. Simulation rooms may be equipped with video capture and replay technology, which would allow trainees to watch themselves after the simulated experience is over and gain clearer understanding of their own performance. Self-knowledge is also augmented through simulation because of the way in which simulations frequently end with reflective debriefing sessions in which participants are asked to describe their subjective experience of the simulation. These types of replay and reflection opportunities are not typical of clinical work and are one of the distinguishing features of simulation that lends it an advantage in enlightening simulation participants to their own patterns of thought and behavior. One could imagine individuals believing themselves to be good listeners and then on review of a simulation session, realize that they interrupted a simulated patient multiple times.

Simulation is also ideal for EI development because it provides an arena in which patients can come to no harm. This feature of simulation can be used to maximally support participants as they test out emotional management strategies in which they are not well developed or do not feel comfortable using. It is precisely the low-stakes environment of simulation that makes it the ideal training ground for participants as they practice the EI strategies with which they are least comfortable. For example, baseline EI assessment may demonstrate that a surgical resident has a low level of development in assertiveness. Simulation may provide the kind of low stakes, safe context in which that resident could practice assertiveness before engaging in assertiveness strategies on the wards with real patients.

Finally, the structured nature of simulation could benefit EI development because it allows for standardization of scenarios that demand engaging in emotional management. One benefit of standardization is that it can provide the opportunity for controlled repetition and practice of situations with which participants struggle. Standardization also makes possible the fair comparison of individuals. Creating standardized emotional experiences may allow for discrimination between individuals to identify strengths and areas for future improvement, and it also enables accurate measurement of EI development gains by creating the possibility of repeated testing of an individual within an emotionally charged experience after that individual has undergone some other type of EI development intervention.

### *Current Uses of Simulation in Medicine Relevant to Emotional Intelligence*

Simulation is already being used across a broad range of specialties and training levels to target interpersonal skills, communication, professionalism, and team functioning, all domains that EI is thought to underpin.[37–44] For example, in one study of 55 interns from multiple specialties, researchers used simulation via standardized patient actors to improve performance of the residents in disclosing medical error, a task that requires sensitivity to one's own and others emotions.[42] The investigators incorporated a debriefing session after the medical disclosure scenario in which simulation participants reviewed a video recording of their simulation exercise either alone or with a faculty member. In the following month, the interns completed an online tutorial aimed at increasing their knowledge of medical error disclosure guidelines before returning for a second simulation session. Both self-rating and external reviewer ratings of the interns' interpersonal skills and communication and professionalism in medical disclosure encounter improved significantly by the second session. This combined use of simulation with a didactic curriculum demonstrates the potential of simulation to provide feedback and an opportunity for reflection as well as the benefit of repetition.

Within emergency medicine, simulation has been used to assess resident professionalism in a variety of ethically challenging scenarios such as withdrawing care, engaging in an end-of-life conversation with a terminally ill patient, or refusing an attending physician's request to allow a medical student to practice intubation on a recently deceased patient.[39] Residents in this study benefited from the fact that simulation can provide standardized scenarios to residents in a safe and supportive way; no patients are actually harmed as the consequence of the ethical decision making, and they have the opportunity to practice refusing an unethical request from an attending physician without fear of retribution.

Different researchers have aimed to use simulation to assess and develop nontechnical skills in surgery as well. Kneebone and colleagues[45] have designed a carotid endarterectomy simulator that, in addition to addressing a surgeon's technical ability to complete the procedure, assesses an individual's ability to gain informed consent, maintain appropriate patient communication, and manage stress during an operation that is sometimes done on a conscious patient.[46,47] Part of the design of this simulator was to incorporate a real standardized patient as a means to activate a rich and complex emotional response to the simulation scenario, thus making it more similar to real clinical encounters when compared with mannequin-based simulation.

### *Simulation and Emotional Intelligence in Business*

Although the authors are unaware of any surgical simulation that is specifically targeted to developing EI, several products exist in the business world that are designed to spur the growth of an individual's skills and comfort in managing the emotions of oneself and others. Citing the relationship between increased work achievement and EI, multiple companies have marketed simulation-based EI training as a path toward greater career success. In 2009, the Harvard Business Review published a computer-based simulation entitled Leading Teams with Emotional Intelligence.[48] The simulation is described as "an interactive case" that will "hone your leadership skills in a safe environment" and enable you to "apply the tools immediately to your current job." The listed price is $225, and unfortunately few details of the simulation are readily available without purchase of the product.

Simulearn Inc (Norwalk, CT, USA), has also published a computer-based simulation product entitled "vLeader," which has been marketed as a program that increases EI as a means to increase personal effectives and leadership ability.[49] vLeader learners participate in a gamelike program in which they virtually attend meetings simulated by actors (**Fig. 1**). Simulearn advertises the benefits of simulated learning as being a safe environment for practicing, experimenting, and exploring different strategies of solving interpersonal dilemmas. vLeader simulates situations that are emotionally demanding. They cite a handful of research studies in which use of vLeader was associated with positive outcomes such as an increase in the 360° ratings of managers or in the measured EI scores of college students participating in a business course.[50,51]

Blueline Simulations takes a slightly different approach to simulation and EI by offering to build custom simulated environments for companies to use in employee training.[52] Blueline states that it will recreate a corporation's business in a simulated gaming environment so that employees can practice interaction with clients, use a company's software, or manipulate complex or dangerous equipment in a safe, engaging environment. Although not specifically geared toward the development of EI, Blueline does emphasize that its simulations lead to more effective interactions

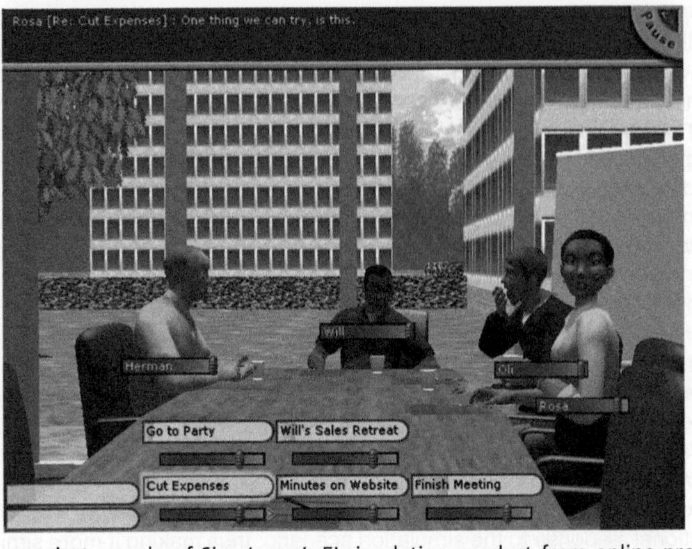


**Fig. 1.** Screen shot sample of SimuLearn's EI simulation product from online promotional video. (*From* SimuLearn Inc. Available at: http://www.simulearn.net/; with permission.)

with customers and teamwork skills, both of which require identification and management of one's own and other's emotions.

At least 2 companies have created games aimed at increasing EI. Planet Jockey has published a computer game in which players must act as chief executive officer in response to scenarios provided by executives at Fortune 500 companies.[53] Players are provided with mentorship throughout the different levels, which is specifically targeted toward EI and leadership development. The If You Can Company published a game entitled *If You Can* that is marketed as a game that develops the EI of children as the foundation to academic and life achievement.[54] Players navigate a planet in which there is a long-standing conflict between cats and dogs, and they must make emotionally wise decisions to reunify the 2 warring populations. Given the prominence that EI has had in academic and lay news, it would be not be surprising if more private entities developed EI development games and simulations aimed toward different markets ranging from elementary school to the corporate level. The existence of such products demonstrates a belief that such simulations are feasible and effective, or that in the least, there exists a demand for tools that use simulation to cultivate EI.

### *Designing Effective Simulation for Emotional Intelligence Development*

Given the limited number of hours available for training, it is crucial to design simulation for EI development that is as effective and efficient as possible. Several published studies provide guidance on characteristics of educational interventions that are either effective or ineffective. Perhaps the most critical aspect of future EI simulations is that they be mandatory activities for residents that occur during protected educational time. In one study of family medicine residents, investigators designed an EI intervention that consisted of one-on-one EI coaching by a certified individual.[26] No resident completed the intervention arm of the study, and the investigators attributed this to the fact that these coaching sessions did not occur during protected time and that the residents had too many competing clinical and academic responsibilities to prioritize participating in the intervention regardless of how useful it might have been. In another study on voluntary participation in simulation by surgical residents, Chang and colleagues[55] found that, even though surgical residents found simulators to be helpful, the frequency with which the residents practiced technical skills on the simulator was low. For example, 0% of postgraduate year (PGY) 4 and PGY5 residents returned to the simulator after an introductory session. These investigators also concluded that to be effective, an educational intervention for busy residents must be mandatory.

Several studies have demonstrated the performance gains that can be made when simulation is mandatory and afforded protected time for residents. In one study by Seymour,[56] a structured simulation curriculum was associated with an increase in resident technical skills in laparoscopic surgery. Within the realm of nontechnical skills, protected simulation to learn how to break bad news has been shown to be well liked and well received by resident physicians across multiple specialties including surgery, emergency medicine, and pediatrics.[43,57,58] Furthermore, these studies demonstrated that performance of residents breaking bad news as rated by a faculty reviewed improved after participating in the simulation curriculum.

The other critical lesson from the studies on breaking bad news, which is highly relevant to designing simulation for developing EI, is that simulation is only 1 piece of the overall intervention. Before simulation, the residents or medical students who participated in the simulation were required to prepare for the simulation session by completing readings, watching videos, or attending more traditional didactic sessions. This preparatory work was then followed by the simulations that provided an opportunity for the trainees to enact the lessons they learned from their previous work. Feedback was provided to the trainees so that they would have the opportunity to improve on future sessions, which highlights the importance of spaced or intermittent sessions. By creating a more longitudinal design with repeated observations, the trainees are afforded the opportunity to demonstrate improvement and consequently the effectiveness of prior intervention sessions. Multiple sessions also provide the space for formative as well as summative feedback and assessment.

To summarize, the authors believe that effective simulation interventions aimed at EI will demonstrate the following characteristics:

- Occur during protected educational time without competing academic or clinical responsibility
- Require preparatory work before the simulation session
- Provide postsimulation feedback/assessment and allow postsimulation review of behavior and performance to allow for self-reflection with opportunities for deliberate practice
- Be longitudinal in nature to allow for tracking of progression

## FUTURE RESEARCH

The use of simulation for EI development or assessment is rich with opportunities for research and investigation. One fundamental area of research is the development of appropriate EI simulation cases. This process may require a presimulation needs assessment, as well as iterative creation of standardized, simulated cases that present emotionally demanding scenarios to simulation participants. Residents, patients, nurses, program directors, and attending surgeons could all be polled to identify the types of situations that are most commonly faced or most commonly strain EI. Then, standardized case scenarios based on these needs assessments could be drafted, piloted, and revised.

Another area of research is evaluating the effectiveness of simulation to discriminate between individuals with different EI profiles. Standardized performance metrics could be designed that allow easy identification of an individual's EI strengths and areas for potential improvement. These metrics would also facilitate comparisons between the trait and ability models of EI. Individuals could see how they self-report their EI traits and also see how they actually use those EI skills during a high-fidelity simulation. Creating effective EI assessment during simulation also enables faculty to measure the effectiveness of EI development throughout a longitudinal curriculum.

A third area of research is whether simulation itself can be used to deliver EI development. Essentially, do participants in simulation undergo EI gains? One could envision comparing simulation versus other modes of EI interventions, such as classroom learning, webinars, or self-study. The authors predict that given the realism of simulation and the consequent effectiveness of simulation to provoke an emotional reaction in participants, simulation will outperform other methods of EI development interventions.

The ultimate goal in using simulation for EI development is to achieve measurable gains in clinical performance and patient care. Faculty assessment of resident physicians or patient satisfaction scores may be used to determine whether resident participation in EI-targeted simulation improves resident performance. Patient satisfaction surveys of faculty or 360° evaluations may also serve to demonstrate whether faculty-level surgeons benefit from simulation-based EI training.

## SUMMARY

To summarize, EI is an established concept in the business literature with evidence that it is an important factor in determining career achievement. At present, there is increasing interest in the role that EI has in medical training, although it is still an unexplored area. This article summarizes the EI literature most relevant to surgical training and outlines the reasons that simulation would offer many benefits to the development of EI. Several companies have already begun to develop simulations for development of EI within a business context. Although there are many unanswered questions, it is anticipated that future research will demonstrate the effectiveness of using simulation to develop EI within surgery.

## REFERENCES


1. Mayer J, Salovey P. What is emotional intelligence?. In: Salovey P, Sluyter DJ, editors. Emotional development and emotional intelligence: educational implications. New York: Basic Books; 1997. p. 3–31.
2. Salovey P, Mayer J. Emotional intelligence. Imagination, cognition, and personality. 9;1990;185–211.
3. Goleman D. Emotional intelligence. New York: Bantam Books; 1995. p. 352, xiv.
4. Goleman D. Working with emotional intelligence. New York: Bantam Books; 1998. p. 383, xi.
5. Goleman D. What makes a leader? Harv Bus Rev 1998;76(6):93–102.
6. Goleman D. The focused leader. (cover story). Harv Bus Rev 2013;91(12):50–60.
7. Bar-On R, Parker JD. The handbook of emotional intelligence: theory, development, assessment, and application at home, school, and in the workplace. 1st edition. San Francisco (CA): Jossey-Bass; 2000. p. 528, xv.
8. Mayer JD, Salovey P, Caruso DR, et al. Measuring emotional intelligence with the MSCEIT V2.0. Emotion 2003;3(1):97–105.
9. Roberts RD, Zeidner M, Matthews G. Does emotional intelligence meet traditional standards for an intelligence? Some new data and conclusions. Emotion 2001; 1(3):196–231.

10. Petrides KV, Furnham A. Trait emotional intelligence: psychometric investigation with reference to established trait taxonomies. Eur J Pers 2001;15(6):425–48.
11. Petrides KV, Pita R, Kokkinaki F. The location of trait emotional intelligence in personality factor space. Br J Psychol 2007;98(2):273–89.
12. Arora S, Ashrafian H, Davis R, et al. Emotional intelligence in medicine: a systematic review through the context of the ACGME competencies. Med Educ 2010; 44(8):749–64.
13. Lewis NJ, Rees CE, Hudson JN, et al. Emotional intelligence medical education: measuring the unmeasurable? Adv Health Sci Educ Theory Pract 2005;10(4): 339–55.
14. Petrides KV. Technical manual for the Trait Emotional Intelligence Questionnaire (TEIQue). 1st edition. London: London Psychometric Laboratory; 2012. 5th printing ed.
15. Salovey P, Sluyter DJ. Emotional development and emotional intelligence: educational implications. 1st edition. New York: BasicBooks; 1997. p. 288, xvi.
16. McClelland DC. Identifying competencies with behavioral-event interviews. Psychol Sci 1998;9(5):331–9.
17. Lusch RF, Serpkenci RR. Personal differences, job tension, job outcomes, and store performance - a study of retail store managers. J Mark 1990;54(1):85–101.
18. Van Rooy DL, Viswesvaran C. Emotional intelligence: a meta-analytic investigation of predictive validity and nomological net. J Vocat Behav 2004;65(1):71–95.
19. Jordan PJ, Ashkanasy NM, Härtel CEJ, et al. Workgroup emotional intelligence: scale development and relationship to team process effectiveness and goal focus. Hum Resource Manag Rev 2002;12(2):195–214.
20. Freedman J. The business case for emotional intelligence. [White Paper]. 2010. Available at: http://www.6seconds.org/2010/10/06/the-business-case-for-emotional-intelligence-2010/. Accessed October 1, 2010.
21. Cherniss C. The business case for emotional intelligence. 1999. Available at: http://www.eiconsortium.org/pdf/business_case_for_ei.pdf. Accessed December 29, 2013.
22. Stewart M. Core competencies. 2001. Available at: https://www.acgme.org/acWebsite/RRC_280/280_coreComp.asp. Accessed September 26, 2012.
23. Grewal D, Davidson HA. Emotional intelligence and graduate medical education. JAMA 2008;300(10):1200–2.
24. Pilkington A, Hart J, Bundy C. Training obstetricians and gynaecologists to be emotionally intelligent. J Obstet Gynaecol 2012;32(1):10–3.
25. Taylor C, Farver C, Stoller JK. Perspective: can emotional intelligence training serve as an alternative approach to teaching professionalism to residents? Acad Med 2011;86(12):1551–4.
26. Webb AR, Young RA, Baumer JG. Emotional intelligence and the ACGME competencies. J Grad Med Educ 2010;2(4):508–12.
27. Jensen AR, Wright AS, Lance AR, et al. The emotional intelligence of surgical residents: a descriptive study. Am J Surg 2008;195(1):5–10.
28. Bar-On R. The Bar-On Emotional Quotient Inventory (EQ-i): rationale, description and psychometric properties. In: Geher G, editor. Measuring emotional intelligence: common ground and controversy. New York: Nova Science Publishers; 2004. p. 277, xiv.
29. McKinley SK, Petrusa ER, Fiedeldey-Van Dijk C, et al. Are there gender differences in the emotional intelligence of resident physicians? J Surg Educ 2014; 71(6):e33–40.
30. McKinley SK, Petrusa ER, Fiedeldey-Van Dijk C, et al. A multi-institutional study of the emotional intelligence of resident physicians. Am J Surg 2015;209(1):26–33.

31. Lin DT, Kannappan A, Lau JN. The assessment of emotional intelligence among candidates interviewing for general surgery residency. J Surg Educ 2013;70(4):514–21.
32. Arora S, Russ S, Petrides KV, et al. Emotional intelligence and stress in medical students performing surgical tasks. Acad Med 2011;86(10):1311–7.
33. Weng HC, Steed JF, Yu SW, et al. The effect of surgeon empathy and emotional intelligence on patient satisfaction. Adv Health Sci Educ Theory Pract 2011;16(5):591–600.
34. Weng HC, Chen HC, Chen HJ, et al. Doctors' emotional intelligence and the patient-doctor relationship. Med Educ 2008;42(7):703–11.
35. Van der Feltz-Cornelis CM, Van Oppen P, Van Marwijk HW, et al. A patient-doctor relationship questionnaire (PDRQ-9) in primary care: development and psychometric evaluation. Gen Hosp Psychiatry 2004;26(2):115–20.
36. Talarico JF, Varon AJ, Banks SE, et al. Emotional intelligence and the relationship to resident performance: a multi-institutional study. J Clin Anesth 2013;25(3):181–7.
37. Abdelshehid CS, Quach S, Nelson C, et al. High-fidelity simulation-based team training in urology: evaluation of technical and nontechnical skills of urology residents during laparoscopic partial nephrectomy. J Surg Educ 2013;70(5):588–95.
38. Bearman M, O'Brien R, Anthony A, et al. Learning surgical communication, leadership and teamwork through simulation. J Surg Educ 2012;69(2):201–7.
39. Gisondi MA, Smith-Coggins R, Harter PM, et al. Assessment of resident professionalism using high-fidelity simulation of ethical dilemmas. Acad Emerg Med 2004;11(9):931–7.
40. Harnof S, Hadani M, Ziv A, et al. Simulation-based interpersonal communication skills training for neurosurgical residents. Isr Med Assoc J 2013;15(9):489–92.
41. Peterson EB, Porter MB, Calhoun AW. A simulation-based curriculum to address relational crises in medicine. J Grad Med Educ 2012;4(3):351–6.
42. Sukalich S, Elliott JO, Ruffner G. Teaching medical error disclosure to residents using patient-centered simulation training. Acad Med 2014;89(1):136–43.
43. Tobler K, Grant E, Marczinski C. Evaluation of the impact of a simulation-enhanced breaking bad news workshop in pediatrics. Simul Healthc 2014;9(4):213–9.
44. Tofil NM, Morris JL, Peterson DT, et al. Interprofessional simulation training improves knowledge and teamwork in nursing and medical students during internal medicine clerkship. J Hosp Med 2014;9(3):189–92.
45. Kneebone R, Nestel D, Wetzel C, et al. The human face of simulation: patient-focused simulation training. Acad Med 2006;81(10):919–24.
46. Black SA, Nestel D, Tierney T, et al. Gaining consent for carotid surgery: a simulation-based study of vascular surgeons. Eur J Vasc Endovasc Surg 2009;37(2):134–9.
47. Black SA, Nestel DF, Kneebone RL, et al. Assessment of surgical competence at carotid endarterectomy under local anaesthesia in a simulated operating theatre. Br J Surg 2010;97(4):511–6.
48. Leading teams with emotional intelligence. 2014. Available at: http://www.harvardbusiness.org/sites/default/files/16303_CL_LTEI_Sheet_Oct10.pdf. Accessed November 16, 2014.
49. SimuLearn Inc. Available at: http://www.simulearn.net/. Accessed April 27, 2015.
50. Aldrich C. Learning by doing: a comprehensive guide to simulations, computer games, and pedagogy in e-learning and other educational experiences. San Francisco (CA): Pfeiffer; 2005. p. 353, xli.

51. Sidor SM. The impact of computer based simulation training on leadership development, in Department of Educational Research, Technology, and Leadership. Orlando (FL): University of Central Florida; 2007. p. 142.
52. Blue Line Simulations, L. Available at: http://www.bluelinesimulations.com/. Accessed November 16, 2014.
53. Jocket P. Available at: http://planetjockey.com/. Accessed November 16, 2014.
54. Company, I.Y.C. 2014. Available at: http://www.ifyoucan.org/. Accessed November 16, 2014.
55. Chang L, Petros J, Hess DT, et al. Integrating simulation into a surgical residency program: is voluntary participation effective? Surg Endosc 2007;21(3):418–21.
56. Seymour NE. Integrating simulation into a busy residency program. Minim Invasive Ther Allied Technol 2005;14(4):280–6.
57. Bowyer MW, Hanson JL, Pimentel EA, et al. Teaching breaking bad news using mixed reality simulation. J Surg Res 2010;159(1):462–7.
58. Park I, Gupta A, Mandani K, et al. Breaking bad news education for emergency medicine residents: a novel training module using simulation with the SPIKES protocol. J Emerg Trauma Shock 2010;3(4):385–8.

# Advances in Teaching and Assessing Nontechnical Skills

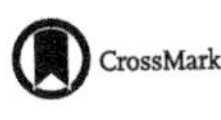


Louise Hull, PhD[a,*], Nick Sevdalis, PhD[b]

**KEYWORDS**

- Nontechnical skills • Teamwork • Training • Education • Assessment

**KEY POINTS**

- The importance of surgeons' nontechnical skills is gaining widespread recognition as a critical element of high-quality and safe surgical care.
- The fundamental nontechnical skills that have been identified to contribute to safety and efficiency in the operating room (OR) include:
  - Communication, teamwork, leadership (social skills).
  - Decision making, situational awareness (cognitive skills).
  - Managing stress and coping with fatigue (personal resource skills).
- Surgeons' nontechnical and teamwork skills are typically trained in an informal and unstructured manner (the so-called hidden curriculum). This informal and unstructured approach is neither optimal nor adequate.
- The need to provide formal and structured training in nontechnical aspects of surgical performance has never been so widely accepted by the surgical community, and consequently initiatives to train these skills have gained increasing prominence in the surgical literature over the past 10 years.
- Despite clear progress in the training and assessment of nontechnical skills, more work is needed to integrate these skills into undergraduate and postgraduate surgical education and training as well as into the continuing professional development of surgeons throughout their careers.

---

Funding: L. Hull is affiliated with the Imperial Patient Safety Translational Research Center; N. Sevdalis research was funded by the National Institute for Health Research (NIHR) Collaboration for Leadership in Applied Health Research and Care South London at King's College Hospital NHS Foundation Trust. The views expressed are those of the authors and not necessarily those of the NHS, the NIHR or the Department of Health.
Conflicts of interest: L. Hull and N. Sevdalis provide team skills training and advice on a consultancy basis in the United Kingdom and internationally.
[a] Department of Surgery and Cancer, Patient Safety Translational Research Center, St Mary's Hospital, Imperial College London, Wright Fleming Building, Norfolk Place, London W2 1PG, UK; [b] Health Service & Population Research Department, Institute of Psychiatry, Psychology & Neuroscience, King's College London, PO29 David Goldberg Centre, De Crespigny Park, Denmark Hill, London SE5 8AF, UK
* Corresponding author.
*E-mail address:* l.hull@imperial.ac.uk

Surg Clin N Am 95 (2015) 869–884
http://dx.doi.org/10.1016/j.suc.2015.04.003 surgical.theclinics.com
0039-6109/15/$ – see front matter 

## INTRODUCTION

This article reviews the knowledge base on training and assessing surgeons, and entire operating room (OR) teams, in nontechnical aspects of their performance. Drawing predominantly on the surgical literature, it first defines nontechnical skills in the context of the OR and reviews some of the key assessment instruments that have been developed to capture these skills. It then reviews key developments that have taken place in the past decade on formal skills training, including recently developed guidelines regarding how best to train faculty to evaluate and train nontechnical and team skills in the OR context. In addition, recommendations to further advance nontechnical skill and team-based training and assessment in surgery are presented.

## NONTECHNICAL SKILLS IN THE OPERATING ROOM AND PERIOPERATIVE CARE: WHAT ARE THEY AND HOW CAN THEY BE EVALUATED?

Nontechnical skills have emerged as key components of high performance in the OR in the past 10 to 15 years.[1] Major publications in the United States, United Kingdom, and internationally have identified that, in addition to the technical performance of surgeons, additional skills are required to ensure safety and efficiency in the OR and the wider perioperative care pathway. The realization that technical ability alone does not equate with superior surgical performance and/or better patient outcomes arose following analyses of incidents that revealed that key problems in perioperative care related to communication and team factors rather than simply deficiencies and failures in surgeons' technical performance.[2,3] Additional factors were thus identified as important determinants of surgical outcomes. This systemic perspective on what determines surgical outcomes explicitly articulated the need to focus on nontechnical aspects of performance in the OR as key components of surgical safety and outcomes.

Nontechnical skills have been defined as "the cognitive, social and personal resource skills that complement technical skills and contribute to safe and efficient task performance."[4] This broad definition applies not only to ORs but across health care settings and also across industries (eg, aviation) in which expert performance and ongoing mitigation of risk are required. Key nontechnical skills applicable to the OR that are within this definition include the following:

- Communication, teamwork, leadership: these are social skills (ie, they refer to how surgeons behave and interact as members of the OR team).
- Decision making, situational awareness: these are cognitive skills (ie, they refer to how surgeons think, both in routine situations and also when crises arise).
- Managing stress and coping with fatigue: these are personal resource skills (ie, they refer to how surgeons manage themselves as health care professionals under the time pressure and stressful conditions that are often the reality of surgical care).

More specifically within the OR and with a surgical focus, several instruments have been developed to capture a range of nontechnical elements of surgeons' performances. A systematic review of the literature, published in 2011, identified 11 articles detailing 4 tools developed to capture the quality of surgeons' nontechnical and teamwork skills.[5] The assessment tools identified in the review are presented in **Box 1**. Key nontechnical skill assessment tools developed since the publication of Ref.[5] are also included (in italics) to provide an up-to-date picture.

Review of the instruments summarized in **Box 1** reveals significant overlap in the nontechnical skills identified and captured across assessment instruments, which is an important positive factor in the development of clinicians' understanding of what

**Box 1**
**Nontechnical skills assessment tools in surgery, including date of development/publication and skills included**

- OTAS, 2006: communication, coordination, cooperation/backup behavior, leadership, team monitoring/situation awareness[6]
- Revised NOTECHS (Nontechnical Skills), 2008: communication/interaction, situation awareness/vigilance, cooperation/team skills, leadership/managerial skills, decision making[7]
- Nontechnical Skills for Surgeons (NOTSS), 2006: communication/teamwork, leadership, situation awareness, decision making[8]
- Oxford NOTECHS, 2008 and *Oxford NOTECHS II, 2014*: teamwork/cooperation, leadership/management skills, problem solving/decision making, situation awareness[9,10]
- *Trauma NOTECHS (T-NOTECHS), 2012*: leadership, cooperation/resource management, communication/interaction, assessment/decision making, situation awareness/coping with stress[11]
- *Surgeons' Leadership Inventory (SLI), 2013*: maintaining standards, managing resources, making decisions, directing, training, supporting others, communicating, coping with pressure[12]
- *NOTECHS for Ward-based Care (W-NOTECHS), 2014*: communication/interaction, situation awareness/vigilance, cooperation/team skills, leadership/managerial skills, decision making[13]
- *Teamwork Skills Assessment for Ward Care: (T-SAW-C), 2014*: communication, cooperation/backup behavior, coordination, leadership, team monitoring/situational awareness, decision making[14]

Italics denote tools developed since the publication of Ref.[5]
*Data from* Refs.[6–14]

these skills are in the OR and how to train them. The overlap suggests that different academic surgical teams working across different health care systems have arrived at largely similar systems for evaluating nontechnical skills; the overlap cross-validates these instruments and shows that the skills listed in **Box 1** can to some degree be generalized.

The tools summarized in **Box 1** also reveal a trend in the surgical nontechnical skills literature: although early instruments had a clear OR focus, more recently developed instruments take nontechnical elements of performance outside the OR and apply them to more specialized care settings in which surgeons care for critically ill patients (eg, trauma care) and also across other parts of the surgical care pathway, such as the surgical ward. This development is important because it shows the quest for a more holistic approach to surgical performance and safety. It is not enough to have good communication and leadership in the OR; the same should apply in ward-based patient care.

In terms of how they can be used, the assessment instruments discussed earlier typically provide specific definitions and examples of behaviors that contribute to superior or substandard performance in the OR or other care settings. For example, OTAS (Observational Teamwork Assessment for Surgery) consists of more than 100 exemplar behaviors that contribute to effective team function and patient safety in the OR. These are used to train surgeons in nontechnical aspects of performance via articulation of what constitutes effective and ineffective OR behaviors (**Box 2**).

Identification of these exemplar behaviors and skills has proved to be important in guiding the development of training programs to teach nontechnical and teamwork

**Box 2**
**What makes effective surgical communication across the surgical pathway (ie, preoperatively, intraoperatively, and postoperatively)? Examples from the OTAS instrument**

Surgeon's preoperative communications:

- Communicates changes to operation or case list
- Talks to team and encourages communication from subteams (anesthesiologist, OR nurses, technicians)
- Verbal confirmation of procedure and intraoperative requirements

Surgeon's intraoperative communications:

- Asks team whether all members are prepared to begin the operation
- Requests and instructions to team communicated clearly and effectively
- Provides information to whole team on progress
- Informs team of technical difficulties/changes of plan

Surgeon's postoperative communications:

- Discusses requirements for next case
- Debriefs team members

skills, including the production of simulated video clips for skill identification and the design of simulation-based skills training scenarios for hands-on skills application.

## THE PARADOX OF NONTECHNICAL SKILLS: CLINICIANS KNOW WHAT THEY ARE BUT ASSESSING THE QUALITY OF NONTECHNICAL PERFORMANCE IS DIFFICULT

One of the barriers in the delivery of nontechnical skills training is that evaluating these skills is difficult. This fact is a paradox; surgeons are able to identify what is wrong with team leadership or communication when they are asked to analyze or review an incident in the OR. The problem here is that terms from everyday language are being used to describe specific behaviors and skills in the OR. The tools that are reviewed earlier (see **Box 1**) offer an important first step in recognizing what these skills are and how they can be defined to achieve a certain degree of consistency between different users, training programs, hospitals, and even countries or cultures. The next step that is required is to develop faculty who are able to use these tools to assess and train residents and also their peers.

**Fig. 1** presents a simple summary of what needs to be in place when a skills assessment is initiated. There is a need for trained faculty assessors who understand how to

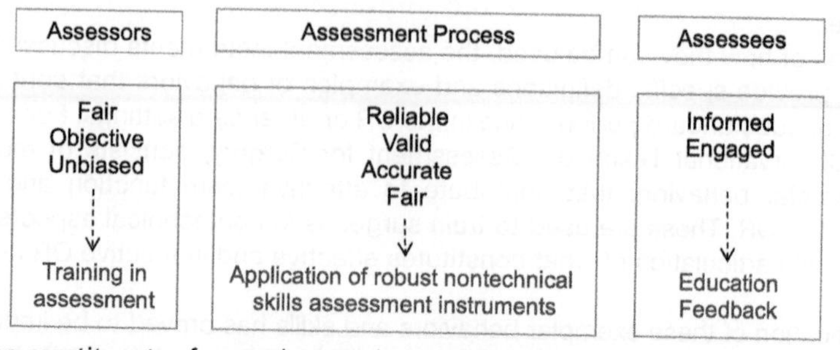


**Fig. 1.** The constituents of a good nontechnical skills assessment.

conduct a nontechnical skills assessment and what its implications are for those who are being assessed. In contrast, those being assessed need to be informed and engaged; these conditions are necessary requirements if the assessment aspires to have an educational impact and to be taken seriously. Practically, the delivery of the assessment should be done via instruments that have undergone some validation, and hence we recommend careful consideration of the tools listed in **Box 1** as a first step, because there are now several tools that can be used with minor, if any, modifications to suit a surgical skills evaluation and training program.

What are the challenges that nontechnical assessments pose to faculty? Assessing someone's skill is a multistage process, which can be described in simple terms as follows:

Observation: the skill in question is observed by the faculty evaluator. For example, in the context of simulation-based leadership training, a fourth-year resident is being observed in the management of a progressively deteriorating patient as the lead surgeon in the OR.

Recording: evaluators either use audiovisual recording equipment or their working memory to create a record of the performance that has just taken place. In our example, the resident is being recorded on a hand-held camera, or the evaluator takes notes during the simulation. Audiovisual recordings allow performances to be reviewed in more detail at a later date and address the issue of the evaluator forgetting what took place, but they are not always feasible, especially outside the simulated environment.

Interpretation: the evaluator has to make an interpretation of what is seen. In our example, the evaluator needs to identify potential reasons why some behaviors were present and others absent while the resident managed the deteriorating patient, interacted with the OR team, and judged their appropriateness.

Evaluation: the evaluator may be asked to produce a numerical rating or to use a checklist to evaluate the level of skill observed.

Feedback/debriefing: if the skill is observed in a training or simulation-based context, the final step of the assessment, and arguably the most important, would be for the evaluator to review and debrief the performance with the participant. In this example, the evaluator would review how the resident managed the deteriorating patient (eg, how the deterioration was discussed with the anesthesiologist and what the decision making was like) and how the OR team was handled, with or without camera footage from the simulation.

Evaluating skills such as leadership, communication, and others that reveal themselves through team interactions in the OR is mentally complex and hence prone to biases. Some of the biases to consider include the following:

- Halo and horns effects: a single aspect of nontechnical performance is overemphasized and inflates (halo) or reduces (horns) the evaluations of other nontechnical skills. This type of bias is important because it is unlikely that a trainee would have done everything right or wrong, but excessive focus on a single element of performance may color the evaluation accordingly.
- Primacy and recency biases: these affect long procedures or tasks. Evaluators tend to recall better the first (primacy) and last (recency) parts of the procedure they are training or assessing; as a result their evaluations neglect the parts of the procedure that took place in the middle. Audiovisual recordings may address these biases, but they come with their own feasibility limitations.
- Nonblinded evaluations: when the faculty and the trainees are known to each other the observed performance may become colored by this knowledge (eg,

"He is not normally like this, he is having a bad day," for a resident performing poorly on a simulation-based exercise. This inference may be true, but it may also obscure true gaps in performance).

- Hawthorne effect: the psychological response of people knowing they are being evaluated is often to assume their best performance, although they may do things differently in everyday life. This behavior produces inflated performances that may not reflect reality.
- Rating biases: these biases relate to how a numerical scale or checklist is used. Leniency bias is present when the evaluator has the tendency to score everyone high on the scale; severity bias is present when the evaluator has the tendency to score everyone low on the scale; central tendency bias is present when the evaluator has the tendency to score everyone on the middle of the scale. All of these biases are addressed with good-quality scales and faculty training.

## FACULTY DEVELOPMENT: A CORNERSTONE FOR MEANINGFUL NONTECHNICAL SKILLS TRAINING AND EVALUATION

As discussed earlier, evaluating someone's nontechnical skills at a surgical task or procedure is a skill in itself, and thus, like all other skills, it requires training and it has a learning curve. We have recently found that it is possible to train surgical and nonclinical evaluators (eg, psychologists) to evaluate nontechnical skills within the OR setting; all evaluators had a learning curve.[15]

Surgery, and health care more broadly, is not the first industry to recognize that training and assessment of nontechnical skills is required to optimize safety and efficiency. Commercial aviation has long accepted the need and importance of training pilot instructors to evaluate crew performance. They therefore developed a structured approach to training their instructor faculty; not every senior pilot automatically qualifies for this task. The brief review *A Gold Standards Approach to Training Instructors to Evaluate Crew Performance*[16] offers a comprehensive overview of the approach this industry has taken; it comes with competitive selection of instructors among senior airline pilots, structured training in how to observe and rate performance, clear explanation of what constitutes good/poor skills, and practice in rating video-recorded performances.

To address the existing gap in developing surgical and educationalist faculty to deliver nontechnical skills training and assessment, our group recently developed a set of consensus-based guidelines derived from experts (who included many of the tool developers listed in **Box 1**).[17] The experts recommended proficiency-based training delivered over 2 full days from interdisciplinary clinical and psychological/human factors faculty with a specified curriculum to cover the theory and practice of nontechnical skills evaluation, hands-on practice sessions in assessing and debriefing nontechnical skills, and understanding of limitations and consequences for the individual of nontechnical skills evaluation. These guidelines sound ambitious but reflect the ultimate aim of such faculty development programs, which is to allow faculty to recognize their own prejudices, make them explicit, and keep them under check when delivering training and assessing skill levels. Based on these guidelines, we have developed a feasible training and development program for faculty, which is reviewed later.

## OBSERVATIONAL TEAMWORK ASSESSMENT FOR SURGERY FACULTY DEVELOPMENT WORKSHOP

Over the past few years, we have developed and refined a training program to train faculty to assess OR nontechnical and teamwork skills using the OTAS tool. The course is delivered as a 1-day or half-day session, depending on requirements and feasibility. The primary objectives of this course are to facilitate the assessment and debriefing of nontechnical and team skills in surgery. Details of the course structure and content are presented in **Fig. 2** and **Table 1**.

## OTHER FACULTY DEVELOPMENT PROGRAMS: NONTECHNICAL SKILL FOR SURGEONS MASTERCLASS

Since 2006, the Royal College of Surgeons of Edinburgh has developed the NOTSS (Nontechnical Skill for Surgeons) Masterclass to train faculty to observe, rate, and provide feedback on nontechnical skills for attending surgeons. This 1-day course, targeted specifically at attending surgeons and higher surgical residents, explores in depth the key nontechnical skills that have been identified to underpin safer surgery. The course consists of didactic sessions (with short talks) and practice in observing and assessing nontechnical skills using the NOTSS instrument. The learning objectives of this course are to equip delegates with an understanding of the theories and research relating to adverse events in surgery and other high-risk industries; and to enhance their ability to apply the NOTSS system to observe, rate, and provide feedback on nontechnical aspects of performance in the OR.

## INSTRUCTIONAL STRATEGIES FOR TRAINING IN NONTECHNICAL AND TEAMWORK SKILLS: INFORMATION, DEMONSTRATION, AND PRACTICE-BASED EDUCATION AND TRAINING

The quest to ensure that the next generation of surgeons and OR teams is equipped with the nontechnical skills to optimize the safety and quality of surgical care has received much attention and has resulted in the development of multiple training interventions targeted at improving nontechnical and teamwork skills.

The 3 most common training strategies used to deliver training are information based (eg, lecture), demonstration based (eg, trainees observe the required skills on recorded video clips), and practice based (eg, role play, simulation). These training strategies have been used independently of each other, but most often in combination; for instance, within a training curriculum that covers both basic lectures (information-based training) and also hands-on simulation-based training (practice-based training). These approaches are reviewed later.

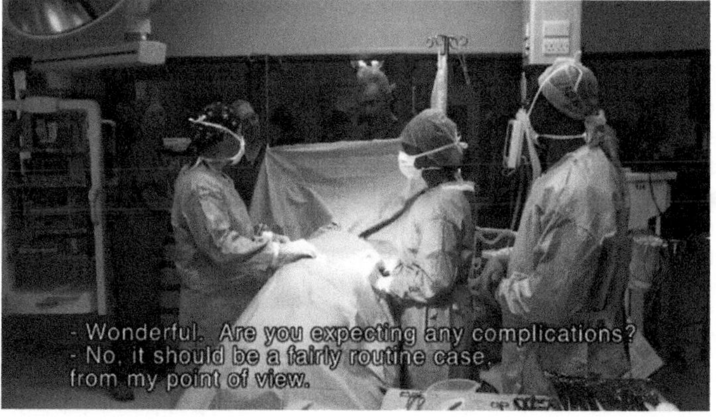


**Fig. 2.** Simulated video clip used in OTAS faculty workshop.

**Table 1**
**OTAS faculty development workshop: course content**

| | Content | Method of Delivery |
|---|---|---|
| Session 1: nontechnical skills and safe surgery | Definition of nontechnical skills<br>Relationship between nontechnical skills and adverse events/never events<br>Identification of key nontechnical skills in the OR | Lecture plus interactive forum |
| Session 2: recognition and assessment of nontechnical skills | Definition and components of assessment<br>Assessment process<br>Requirements of a good assessment<br>Biases and limitations of assessment<br>Common rating errors<br>Overcoming rating errors: rater error training | Lecture |
| Session 3: OTAS | Structure of OTAS<br>Teamwork behaviors and skills: definitions<br>OTAS rating scale<br>Exemplar behaviors<br>OTAS: tips for rating | Lecture plus video demonstration plus interactive forum |
| Session 4: OTAS training | Practical application of OTAS: hands-on practice observing and evaluating nontechnical and teamwork skills based on prerecorded simulated OR clips | Video observation and assessment plus interactive forum plus group discussion and feedback |
| Session 5: feedback and debriefing | Key elements of debriefing<br>Introduction to evidence-based debriefing guidelines<br>Integrating feedback/debriefing into practice | Lecture plus group discussion |

## INFORMATION-BASED SKILLS TRAINING

Several studies have been published in the literature describing information-based nontechnical skills training. These publications typically report the development, content, and delivery of classroom-based skills training sessions, in which theory, definition, and explanation are offered on what nontechnical skills are and how they apply to surgical practice. Some evaluation is offered, although typically skill application cannot be assessed within this context. One of the early training programs to be published using this approach was based on the NOTSS nontechnical skills taxonomy. The training was well received, with surgeons finding the content both interesting and relevant to surgical practice and patient safety.[18]

### *Critical Evaluation*

- Advantages: low cost compared with other training strategies; can be widely applied and delivered; well suited as an introductory approach to introduce the concept of nontechnical skills to surgeons; amenable to e-learning.

- Disadvantages: impact of such training confined to changes in attitudes and knowledge, because trainees do not have the opportunity to practice the taught skills.

## DEMONSTRATION-BASED SKILLS TRAINING

This is an extension to information-based training. The core idea here is that the skills are demonstrated to the trainees so that they can get a feel for what is required. These demonstrations can be live, for example via live role play within the training, or recorded, for example via simulated video clips that showcase appropriate or inappropriate team skills in the OR. An example of a demonstration-based approach was provided by Arora and colleagues,[19] who incorporated a half-day training session into regular general surgical residents' teaching rotations. Nontechnical skills were incorporated using the revised NOTECHS (Nontechnical Skills) framework into a training curriculum that covered basic safety skills, incident analysis, checklist usage, and briefings/debriefings in the OR. The demonstration element of the course was performed via video-clip demonstrations, analysis of surgical incidents in which nontechnical skills were found lacking in the OR, and via asking trainees to use the revised NOTECHS to self-reflect on cases they observed in their own ORs. This course too was well received and showed improvement in objective knowledge and attitudes.

### *Critical Evaluation*

- Advantages: low cost compared with practice-based training, although initial investment in producing demonstration materials is required; can be widely applied and delivered; well-suited as an introductory approach to introduce the concept of nontechnical skills to surgeons; amenable to e-learning; blends well with information-based training.
- Disadvantages: impact of such training confined to changes in attitudes and knowledge, because trainees still do not have the opportunity to practice the taught skills.

## PRACTICE-BASED SKILLS TRAINING

In surgery, practice-based training has more often than not been realized via simulation. Simulation has been suggested as an attractive and complementary training environment to clinical practice,[20] offering the advantage of allowing surgeons (and OR teams) to learn nontechnical and team skills in an structured and tailored learning environment, in which permission to fail is granted and mistakes, which can be frequent in the early phases of the learning curve, do not endanger patient safety. Simulators have radically evolved from simple bench-top models to fully immersive simulated ORs, thus affording an ideal arena to train nontechnical aspects of surgical performance (**Fig. 3**). Further, in situ simulation modules have been developed to bring the simulation into the clinical environment, which makes simulation more realistic (because it occurs within a team's usual work setting) and also addresses some of the barriers to bringing surgeons or entire teams into a simulation center.

Several early studies have shown the feasibility and value of this type of training to date.[21–23] The use of simulation-based training for nontechnical and teamwork skills was recently reviewed by Stefanidis and colleagues.[24] The findings are positive in that simulation-based training improved attitudes to teamwork, skills, and process-related metrics, like adherence to checklists.

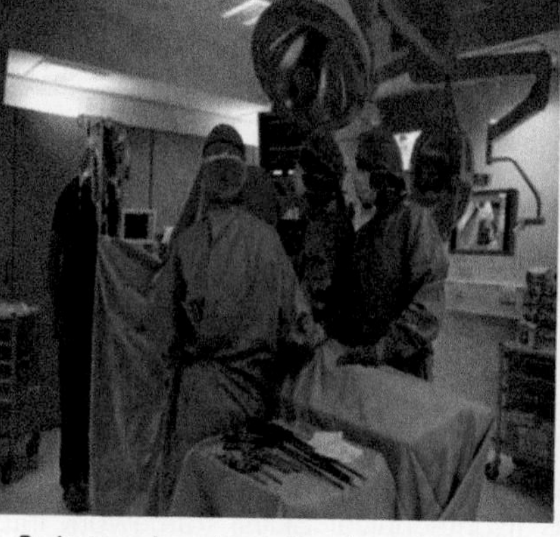
 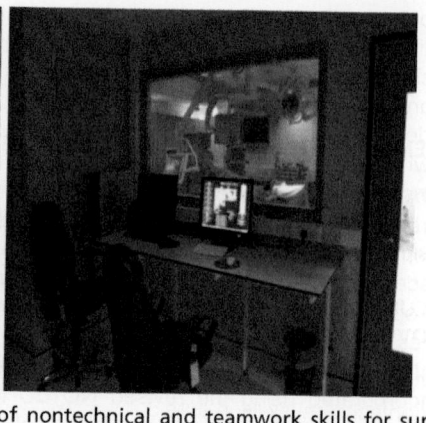

**Fig. 3.** Immersive simulation-based training of nontechnical and teamwork skills for surgeons and OR teams.

***Critical Evaluation***

- Advantages: ideally suited as hands-on approach to deliver basic and advanced nontechnical skills training; evidence-based; allows additional testing of hospital capabilities if delivered in situ; blends well with the other 2 approaches to training.
- Disadvantages: significant resource requirement, including financial and faculty; requires organizational commitment; requires experienced faculty to deliver and evaluate appropriately.

## INSTRUCTIONAL STRATEGIES: IS THERE A BEST APPROACH?

This article highlights a diverse range of instructional strategies to nontechnical skills training. There are numerous examples, including those referred to earlier, of diversity in how nontechnical skills are trained and, even if similar strategies are taken, there is still diversity in how different surgical programs or hospitals have implemented them.

Is there a best approach to use? If best is defined as the most effective and efficient instructional strategy to train nontechnical skills, then the answer remains unclear. Surgeons and surgical educators are currently faced with developing nontechnical skills training initiatives with uncertainty and a lack of consensus regarding how best to achieve effective and efficient training.

There are some practical considerations to take into account: a recent survey conducted among program directors (PDs) of accredited general surgery residency programs in the United States and Canada[25] found that PDs envisaged the ideal nontechnical and teamwork training to combine didactic training and opportunities for practice in simulation-based training methods (83%). Most PDs did not recommend training approaches that were exclusively simulation based (9%) or fully based on didactic methods (8%).

Blending different strategies seems a sensible route to take. Information-based and demonstration-based strategies can be used at early stages of the training to develop a basic understanding of the skills in question. Practice-based strategies can subsequently complement and consolidate the learning. Application of these approaches is likely to require ongoing review; the learning needs to go hand in hand with the clinical experience of the learners, so that the understanding of the relevance and application of specific nontechnical skills becomes fully embedded into the learners' clinical practice. Practically, and based on our own experience, this means, for example, that demonstrating the skills and team processes required to avoid wrong-side/wrong-site/wrong-patient procedures in the OR resonates much better with senior residents and attending surgeons than with second-year medical students because the residents and the attendings can directly link the skills to their own clinical experiences, whereas, to the students, operating on the wrong patient or organ is still inconceivable.

**Box 3** summarizes some basic practical principles on how best to train nontechnical skills.

## CURRENT PRACTICES IN NONTECHNICAL AND TEAMWORK SKILLS TRAINING: OVERVIEW AND CASE STUDIES

A recent systematic review[26] exploring the literature on current approaches to training nontechnical skills in surgical residency suggests that:

- Training in nontechnical skills typically centers on 5 aspects of nontechnical skill performance: patient-centered communication, teamwork, decision making, coping with stress, and patient safety and error management.
- Diversity of instructional strategies and methods used in training nontechnical skills in surgical residency, ranging from reading assignments and lectures to high-fidelity simulation.
- Training typically consists of a combination of several instructional strategies (eg, lecture plus simulation).

**Box 3**
**How best to train surgical nontechnical skills: a basic practical guide**

Use a blended approach to education and training

- Using a full simulation is expensive and unnecessary. Information and demonstration-based approaches are needed to explain what the skills to be taught are and their importance to safety, and to establish a minimum baseline for simulation-based training, which should come later. This approach keeps costs manageable and allows simulation to achieve its maximum impact.

Develop and follow a curriculum

- One-off or unstructured training sessions are unlikely to elicit lasting skills improvement. The training needs to have a logical structure, based on explicit learning objectives that are appropriate for the level of the trainees. This structure can be provided via a curriculum. A curriculum also allows faculty to be slotted in, so changes in faculty do not mean the training collapses or keeps changing based on faculty interests. The curriculum should ideally be long term and linked to clinical practice in the OR.

Implement an existing nontechnical skills framework (see **Box 1**)

- There are now multiple frameworks for the presentation and evaluation of nontechnical skills for surgeons, or even for entire surgical teams. One of these can be implemented as part of the training curriculum, because they offer an evidence-based structure for the relevant skills to be developed and also evaluated.

Invest in faculty development

- Skills training cannot be delivered without able faculty; including surgeons and/or educators, depending on the program/hospital. Faculty need to be able to deliver the curriculum, offer advice and support throughout, and also perform formative and summative evaluations and offer performance feedback and debriefing. Skills training is a skill in itself; unskilled faculty deliver low-quality training.

- Evidence exists that training in nontechnical skills improves surgical residents' attitudes, knowledge, and skills.

## CASE STUDY 1: THE ROYAL COLLEGE OF SURGEONS OF EDINBURGH TRAINING MODULES

The Royal College of Surgeons of Edinburgh (RCSEd) has created a range of resources to support and structure the education and training of NOTSS targeted at all levels of surgeons, from residents in the early stages of training to attending surgeons. These educational resources are briefly described later (more information is available on the RCSEd Web site: www.rcsed.ac.uk/education).

- Early stages of surgical training: NOTSS for Trainees

NOTSS for Trainees is an e-learning course for residents in the early stages of surgical training. The primary objective of this e-learning resource is to provide surgical trainees education in nontechnical aspects of safe surgical performance that currently are not taught in their undergraduate and postgraduate education. This resource, consisting of 6 modules, is free to complete for those with a registered account with the RCSEd.

- Senior residents and attending surgeons: NOTSS in a Box and NOTSS Masterclass

NOTSS in a Box is designed for senior residents and attending surgeons who are involved in training and assessing surgical trainees. This e-learning course contains an introduction to human factors and the NOTSS assessment instrument. The masterclass was described in more detail earlier.

## CASE STUDY 2: JUSTIFYING THE COST OF NONTECHNICAL SKILLS AND TEAMWORK TRAINING: THE VETERANS' HEALTH ADMINISTRATION'S MEDICAL TEAM TRAINING PROGRAM

To the best of our knowledge, the largest study to provide compelling evidence and a sound argument for training OR teams in nontechnical and teamwork skills is that of the Veterans' Health Administration (VHA), which recently reported the beneficial impact of a national OR team training program on patient outcomes.[27,28] Details of the costs and resources involved in developing and delivering the training, and also the effectiveness of the training, are provided later; this is the information required for justification of the resources required to deliver impactful nontechnical skills training programs and also to perform formal cost-effectiveness analyses in the future.

The costs and resources of the training:

- The Medical Team Training (MTT) program involved a 2-month preparation and planning period.
- Closure of ORs to allow surgical staff to attend, as a team, and a full-day training session.
- Training involved a mixture of lectures, group work, and video presentations to train surgical teams to work as a team, question one another when safety risks arise, perform checklist-guided preoperative briefings and postoperative debriefings, and implement other communication strategies (eg, recognizing red flags [risks], stepping back to reassess a situation).
- Implementation of the training was assessed and reinforced by 4 quarterly follow-up structured telephone interviews.

## THE BENEFITS OF THE TRAINING

- The intervention hospitals (n = 74) that completed the training experienced a significant reduction of 18% in mortalities ($P$ = .01) compared with a reduction of 7% ($P$ = .59) in the control hospitals that did not introduce the team training program.
- A reduction of 0.5 death per 1000 ($P$ = .001) occurred after each additional reinforcement session (thereby indicating a dose-response effect).
- A significant decrease of 17% in surgical morbidity rates ($P$ = .01) was observed in the intervention (trained) hospitals, compared with a decrease of 6% in morbidity in the control (nontrained) hospitals, which was not significant ($P$ = .11).
- After adjusting for surgical risk, a decrease of 15% in morbidity rates for intervention hospitals occurred, compared with a decrease of 10% for control hospitals (decline was 20% steeper in the trained group, which was significantly higher; $P$ = .001).

## LOOKING TO THE FUTURE: ADDRESSING THE CHALLENGES AND BARRIERS IN WIDESPREAD, SYSTEMATIC NONTECHNICAL SKILLS TRAINING

In spite of the increasing recognition of the importance of nontechnical and team skills, most surgeons and OR teams continue to lack formal, structured, and systematic training in these skills. It has been suggested that the low implementation of nontechnical skills and team training among general surgery residency programs implies a lack of clarity regarding the necessity of such training, and controversy regarding its effectiveness.[25] However, we argue that although this view may be held by a few individuals, in our experience of training and assessing OR teams, this issue is not necessarily the principal barrier. There are numerous barriers that prevent the systematic training and assessment of surgeons' nontechnical skills, despite the desire to do so, and reasonable evidence exists that doing so in a well-orchestrated manner would improve knowledge, skills, attitudes, and potentially also patient outcomes.

We thus argue that the evidence gap of the past decade has progressed to an implementation gap at present. A few years ago, there was a lack of evidence in terms of how nontechnical skills should be assessed or trained; some clinicians argued that such assessment can only be subjective and biased. Considerable progress has since been made: the knowledge base and training programs that are reviewed in this article offer proof of this fact. Arguably, the evidence gap is now closing rapidly; however, the gap has shifted to a lack of application of what is known to work within an OR and wider care pathway, and hence the gap is now one of implementation.

The American College of Surgeons/Association of Program Directors in Surgery (ACS/APDS) National Skills Curriculum is a case study of this implementation gap. The curriculum is designed as a standard guide for general surgery programs to structure their training. It consists of 3 phases: phases I and II cover basic and more advanced skills and tasks, respectively, and phase III covers nontechnical skills and teamwork competences.[29] A recent implementation analysis across US general surgery PDs showed that phase III was implemented in some way in only about 16% of them.[30] Barriers to implementation included lack of faculty, lack of protected time for clinical faculty, the limited working hours of residents, and financial constraints. This case study is important because it shows that even a curriculum explicitly designed with the ability to be implemented in mind can face severe problems when it comes to practically making it happen within a busy surgical service.

In light of the this, there follows an overview of challenges and barriers, as well as facilitators and opportunities, that are associated with the systematic integration of nontechnical skills training and assessment into surgical training:

***Barriers and Challenges***

- Lack of awareness of the importance of nontechnical and team-based skills and their relevance to surgical patient safety; also resistance from surgeons/OR teams
- Lack of resources to develop nontechnical skill training programs
- Cost and difficulty of releasing surgical residents to attend nontechnical skills training
- Resident work hour restrictions (48 hours per week European Working Time Directive; 80 hours per week in the United States)
- Cost of maintaining training (recurrent training, refresher courses, and reinforcement of training)
- Lack of faculty/surgical educators with necessary expertise to delivery training in nontechnical and teamwork skills
- Lack of guidance or understanding of how best to implement nontechnical skills training
- Lack of nontechnical skills benchmarks leading to difficulty in targeting training at the appropriate learner level

***Facilitators and Opportunities***

- Provision of education regarding importance of nontechnical skills to surgical safety leading to increased engagement
- Increased interest in nontechnical skills from surgeons, researchers, and patient safety campaigners and policy makers
- Clear evidence showing the effectiveness of nontechnical skills training (in improving skills and safety)
- Increasing emphasis on nontechnical and teamwork training from accreditation and certification bodies (eg, phase III of the ACS/APDS National Skills Curriculum, NOTSS adopted by the Royal Australasian College of Surgeons as part of their competence assessment and recommended by the Accreditation Council for General Medical Education for workplace assessment)
- Integrating nontechnical skills training into existing surgical training

This summary of barriers and facilitators makes it clear that there are different elements that require intervention; some are logistical, others are scientific, and others are financial. Further development of the evidence base on the value of nontechnical skills for safe surgery will provide further impetus for integration of these skills into existing curricula. With availability of metrics as reviewed in this article, we think that cost-effectiveness analyses will be required in the near future to make the business case for the integration of nontechnical training into the mainstay of surgical education and also service provision. In addition, formal implementation analyses need to be performed; these analyses often reveal local problems and cultural barriers and can inform a locally applicable implementation strategy. Senior surgical leaders will be needed to take on the role of championing nontechnical skills training.

## SUMMARY

Training and assessing surgeons' nontechnical and teamwork skills is not only a complex and challenging endeavor but also resource intensive. Over the past decade, significant progress in this area has taken place across the globe. However, despite the development and availability of comprehensive training programs and assessment instruments, diffusion has not been as widespread as was hoped. The successful implementation of structured nontechnical skills training and assessment into surgical training is an aspiration for the future that can only be accomplished if the barriers and challenges of implementing such training and assessment are understood and overcome. Achieving this will mark a culture change in modern surgical education and will reinforce the OR as a more open and safe clinical environment.

## REFERENCES


1. Yule S, Paterson-Brown S. Surgeons' non-technical skills. Surg Clin North Am 2012;92(1):37–50.
2. Vincent C, Moorthy K, Sarker SK, et al. Systems approaches to surgical quality and safety: from concept to measurement. Ann Surg 2004;239(4):475–82.
3. Calland JF, Guerlain S, Adams RB, et al. A systems approach to surgical safety. Surg Endosc 2002;16(6):1005–15.
4. Flin R, O'Connor P, Crichton M. Safety at the sharp end: a guide to non-technical skills. Aldershot (United Kingdom): Ashgate; 2008.
5. Sharma B, Mishra A, Aggarwal R, et al. Non-technical skills assessment in surgery. Surg Oncol 2011;20(3):169–77.
6. Undre S, Healey AN, Darzi A, et al. Observational assessment of surgical teamwork: a feasibility study. World J Surg 2006;30(10):1774–83.
7. Sevdalis N, Davis R, Koutantji M, et al. Reliability of a revised NOTECHS scale for use in surgical teams. Am J Surg 2008;196(2):184–90.
8. Yule S, Flin R, Paterson-Brown S, et al. Development of a rating system for surgeons' non-technical skills. Med Educ 2006;40(11):1098–104.
9. Mishra A, Catchpole K, McCulloch P. The Oxford NOTECHS System: reliability and validity of a tool for measuring teamwork behaviour in the operating theatre. Qual Saf Health Care 2009;18(2):104–8.
10. Robertson ER, Hadi M, Morgan LJ, et al. Oxford NOTECHS II: a modified theatre team non-technical skills scoring system. PLoS One 2014;9(3):e90320.
11. Steinemann S, Berg B, DiTullio A, et al. Assessing teamwork in the trauma bay: introduction of a modified "NOTECHS" scale for trauma. Am J Surg 2012;203(1):69–75.
12. Henrickson Parker S, Flin R, McKinley A, et al. The Surgeons' Leadership Inventory (SLI): a taxonomy and rating system for surgeons' intraoperative leadership skills. Am J Surg 2013;205(6):745–51.
13. Pucher PH, Aggarwal R, Singh P, et al. Ward simulation to improve surgical ward round performance: a randomized controlled trial of a simulation-based curriculum. Ann Surg 2014;260(2):236–43.
14. Hull L, Birnbach D, Arora S, et al. Improving surgical ward care: development and psychometric properties of a global assessment toolkit. Ann Surg 2014;259(5):904–9.
15. Russ S, Hull L, Rout S, et al. Observational teamwork assessment for surgery: feasibility of clinical and nonclinical assessor calibration with short-term training. Ann Surg 2012;255(4):804–9.
16. Baker D, Dismukes R. A gold standards approach to training instructors to evaluate crew performance. 2003. Available at: http://human-factors.arc.nasa.gov/flightcognition/Publications/GoldStandardsTM.PDF. Accessed May 11, 2015.

17. Hull L, Arora S, Symons NR, et al. Training faculty in nontechnical skill assessment: national guidelines on program requirements. Ann Surg 2013;258(2):370–5.
18. Flin R, Yule S, Paterson-Brown S, et al. Teaching surgeons about non-technical skills. Surgeon 2007;5(2):86–9.
19. Arora S, Sevdalis N, Ahmed M, et al. Safety skills training for surgeons: a half-day intervention improves knowledge, attitudes and awareness of patient safety. Surgery 2012;152(1):26–31.
20. Paige JT. Surgical team training: promoting high reliability with nontechnical skills. Surg Clin North Am 2010;90(3):569–81.
21. Paige JT, Kozmenko V, Yang T, et al. High-fidelity, simulation-based, interdisciplinary operating room team training at the point of care. Surgery 2009;145(2):138–46.
22. Undre S, Koutantji M, Sevdalis N, et al. Multidisciplinary crisis simulations: the way forward for training surgical teams. World J Surg 2007;31(9):1843–53.
23. Powers KA, Rehrig ST, Irias N, et al. Simulated laparoscopic operating room crisis: an approach to enhance the surgical team performance. Surg Endosc 2008;22(4):885–900.
24. Stefanidis D, Sevdalis N, Paige J, et al. Simulation in surgery: what's needed next? Ann Surg 2014;261(5):846–53.
25. Dedy NJ, Zevin B, Bonrath EM, et al. Current concepts of team training in surgical residency: a survey of North American program directors. J Surg Educ 2013;70(5):578–84.
26. Dedy NJ, Bonrath EM, Zevin B, et al. Teaching nontechnical skills in surgical residency: a systematic review of current approaches and outcomes. Surgery 2013;154(5):1000–8.
27. Young-Xu Y, Neily J, Mills PD, et al. Association between implementation of a medical team training program and surgical morbidity. Arch Surg 2011;146(12):1368–73.
28. Neily J, Mills PD, Young-Xu Y, et al. Association between implementation of a medical team training program and surgical mortality. JAMA 2010;304(15):1693–700.
29. Scott DJ, Dunnington GL. The new ACS/APDS Skills Curriculum: moving the learning curve out of the operating room. J Gastrointest Surg 2008;12(2):213–21.
30. Korndorffer JR Jr, Arora S, Sevdalis N, et al. The American College of Surgeons/Association of Program Directors in Surgery National Skills Curriculum: adoption rate, challenges and strategies for effective implementation into surgical residency programs. Surgery 2013;154(1):13–20.

# Using Simulation to Improve Systems

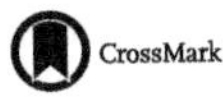

Peter W. Lundberg, MD, James R. Korndorffer Jr, MD, MHPE*

**KEYWORDS**

• Simulation • Systems • Surgery • Six Sigma • Team STEPPS

**KEY POINTS**

- Simulation technology provides an important opportunity to prospectively identify systemic problems with minimal risk to patient safety and quality.
- Health care systems are implementing simulation-based exercises on a more regular basis, especially in high-risk settings such as the emergency department and operating room.
- The adoption of simulation-based and other system-oriented improvement strategies by the health care industry, especially regarding quality and safety, was preceded by its development in the manufacturing and aviation sectors.

## INTRODUCTION

> *"Simulated disorder postulates perfect discipline; simulated fear postulates courage; simulated weakness postulates strength."*
>
> —*Sun Tzu, The Art of War*[1]

The notion that a simulated action, whether routine or rare, can improve the eventual real performance of that action has existed since the ancient Chinese strategist and philosopher, Sun Tzu,[1] applied it to warfare. What makes this idea transcendent for its time, and relevant to surgical safety, is its application beyond the idea that practice makes perfect and into the simulation of adverse circumstances (disorder, fear, weakness) wherein a person may confront adverse contingencies with no real consequence. Thus, when such adversities arise, they might be met with paradoxic discipline, courage, and strength, respectively, thanks to learning and experience empowered by simulation.

Department of General Surgery, Tulane University School of Medicine, 1430 Tulane Avenue, New Orleans, LA 70112, USA

* Corresponding author. Department of Surgery, Tulane University School of Medicine, SL-22, 1430 Tulane Avenue, New Orleans, LA 70112.

*E-mail addresses:* Korndorffer@tulane.edu; jkondo@tulane.edu

Surg Clin N Am 95 (2015) 885–892
http://dx.doi.org/10.1016/j.suc.2015.04.007
surgical.theclinics.com

Although Sun Tzu's[1] simulation was largely a mental one, the technological advances of the last several decades have enabled tangible implementation of this 2500-year-old idea. Its application to health care systems, particularly surgical systems, is best considered in light of simulation's sentinel adoption in other fields. Two decades after the introduction of Resusci-Anne for cardiopulmonary resuscitation in the 1960s, health care simulation entered the modern age with the development among anesthesiology departments of simulation-based systems training clinical management and teamwork.[2] Other early work addressed patient throughput following emergent and nonemergent admissions.[3] Correctly using simulation now requires it to be designed to answer particular questions about the system; common points of review are listed in **Box 1**.

When applied to improving system performance, simulations provide a venue for the combined practice of technical skills, decision making, communication, and leadership. In addition, team-based simulation affords instantaneous feedback and self-reflection among complementary individuals. Challenges to existing systems can thus be more quickly identified and improved, and the adoption of new systems can be streamlined.

This article reviews the evolution of simulation as a safety measure in the aviation industry, the process of team building and streamlining production that has gained popularity in industry and manufacturing, and the adoption of these measures into health care systems, particularly surgery.

## QUALITY IMPROVEMENT THROUGH SIMULATION

The last several decades have seen a profound reemphasis on the quality of care and safety within the health care industry, driven by changing market forces and government policy as much as internal forces. Health care is not unique in this regard, because other industries have used the practice of self-reflection for the sake of error reduction. A notable example is the development of the Six Sigma program by Motorola in which tolerance limits for defective products were set very high in order to limit defects to 3.4 events per million observable units (ie, a rate at 6 standard deviations from the mean). Motorola and others, notably General Electric, achieved considerable success simply by setting standards higher for quality. Some have advocated for the adoption of this policy within other industries,[4] including medicine. However, medical error rates are currently at levels that would represent a serious deterioration in the performance of other high-reliability industries. Applying this concept to medicine carries the dilemma of comparing apples with oranges. At a defect rate of 20%, for

**Box 1**
**Target issues in applying simulation to health care systems**

- Patient safety focus points
- Continuity of safety and quality throughout patient experience
- Simultaneous demands for patient safety and worker safety, efficiency, environmental sustainability, and disaster contingencies
- Adopting new medical devices, technology, and facility designs before their implementation?
- Checkout procedures to ensure clinician proficiency with new systems
- Diagnostic performance and patient throughput
- Stressful situations and decision making that mirror those of a clinical setting

instance (which roughly occurs in the use of antibiotics for colds), the credit card industry would make daily mistakes on more than 9 million transactions, and deaths from airplane crashes would increase 1000-fold.[5] Attempts continue to apply the same rigorous quality standards to health care throughout the world and with varying amounts of success.[6] However, the lack of blinding and randomization, as well as the nonequivalence of assembly lines and manufacturing infrastructure to the human body and interpersonal systems, currently limit the feasibility of Six Sigma as a realistic goal in modern medicine.[6]

Ways forward were initiated by the airline industry, which reacted to studies in the 1970s showing that more than 70% of crashes involved some measure of human error by developing standardized, simulation-based programs to improve communication and teamwork among aircraft crews.[7]

Nonetheless, medicine has moved away from a system that depended on idealized, subjective standards of performance requiring individual providers to perform tasks at levels of perfection that cannot be achieved by human beings. However, Lockheed Martin engineers identified a coincidence of criticality and complexity in the highest acuity units of a hospital (the emergency department, operating room, and intensive care unit) that makes traditional approaches to systems improvement very difficult in light of their simultaneous autonomy and interconnectedness: a system of systems.[8] As **Table 1** shows, identifying a problem and determining the utility of an improvement is difficult in a highly complex and/or critical setting, both of which conditions are present in modern health care. Boosman and Szczerba[8] also point out that traditional simulation-based technologies, wherein environments can be modeled and experiments run within them, are inadequate in fully recreating complex clinical systems without constant validation of simulations to their real-world equivalents thereby changing the simulation while it is being conducted.

Aviation is perhaps the best example of an industry that combined real-world behaviors of multiple human actors within a simulation-based methodology that offered sufficient technical realism while obviating the potential for harm to arise. After the introduction of basic flight simulators to accelerate training for new recruits in World War II, successes in machinery and industry standards led to increasing emphases on competency assessment and contingency planning.[9] Ruffell-Smith's[10] seminal 1979 study showed that the predominant role was the human element (both in individual and group decision making) that contributed to crashes and near misses in aviation. Within the following decade, Crew Resource Management (CRM) simulation-based training had evolved to test flight teams in the management of nonroutine and emergency situations[11] with coincident emphasis on open channels of communication between all those involved, regardless of rank.

**Table 1**
**Complexity and criticality in the clinical environment**

| | Complexity | Criticality |
|---|---|---|
| Source or nature of the issue | Use of ad hoc, incremental, accretive, proprietary, noninteroperable systems | Failure in care, especially high-acuity care, can lead to injury, disability, or death |
| Effect on engineering and integration | Traditional systems processes are incomplete at best, inaccurate at worst | Traditional experimentation processes are difficult at best, impossible at worst |

*From* Boosman F, Szczerba RJ. Simulated clinical environments and virtual system-of-systems engineering for health care. I/ITSEC. Orlando, Nov 29-Dec 2, 2010; (paper #10230). p. 4; with permission.

## THE USE OF SIMULATION IN HEALTH CARE SYSTEMS

Just as flight simulation led to documented benefits in pilot training as well as saving countless resources and lives,[12] the increased implementation of simulations in health care systems grew with improved technology. By the mid-1990s, operative models and screen-based simulations were being added to the cadre of cadavers, mannequins, and standardized patients in medical school curricula.[9]

Anesthesiology was at the forefront of simulation-based training and education, with the adoption of computer-based mannequins that could accurately reflect human physiology and its response to various interventions.[13,14] Given the limitation of these mannequin-only simulation models in reflecting the myriad variables of the operating room, a paradigm shift occurred wherein naturalistic decision making was applied to this particular complex dynamic world (**Table 2**).[15] Simulation-based training using a fully realized operating room quickly arose that involved providers at all levels and roles, emphasized team communication and avoidance of blame, and mandated prompt review and frequent repetition.[16] With similar extensions into the intensive care unit, emergency department, delivery room, and other hospital departments, it became possible to simulate increasingly complex systems.

Aside from the obvious benefit of rehearsing a new or updated clinical practice before implementation (ie, a safety net), increasingly complex scenarios with multiple variables can be integrated into increasingly sophisticated models that can emulate complex systems that often cannot be effectively analyzed using other methods. Whether this means using a computer model to accurately predict the effects of staffing, room availability, wait time, examination time, and patient presentation and illness severity on care in emergency departments,[5] or building a mock operating room complete with actual surgical and anesthesia instruments, trained staff, and the myriad nonverbal cues present within a surgical scenario, simulation-based training can produce far more reliable data than the mentally driven thought experiments of an individual or committee. Benneyan[5] published in 1997 such a study driven by computer-based simulation, using 10 independent variables to determine 25 output measures in studying patient care in a pediatric emergency room that were remarkably congruent with their real-world observations. **Fig. 1** highlights the steps in designing such a project, emphasizing regular data review and adjustment of objectives, creating a feedback loop of experimental redesigns and data to accommodate evolving scenarios.

Computer-modeled simulation of medical systems remains common, and is particularly well suited to the emergency department where so-called discrete event simulation models can accurately describe outcomes in linear, queue-based systems given varying input variables.[17] A characteristic example published in 2007 used data recorded from the throughput of more than 500 emergency department patients as well as staffing and supply data to establish a digital model of the entire department.[18] Several a priori scenarios were then applied to the model, each representing a

**Table 2**
**Criteria of a complex dynamic system**

| | |
|---|---|
| Problems are ill-structured | The environment is dynamic |
| The environment is full of uncertainty | The are multiple players |
| Goals are ill-defined, shift, and compete with each other | Personnel operate under strong organizational and cultural norms |
| Action/feedback loops are tightly coupled | The stakes are high |

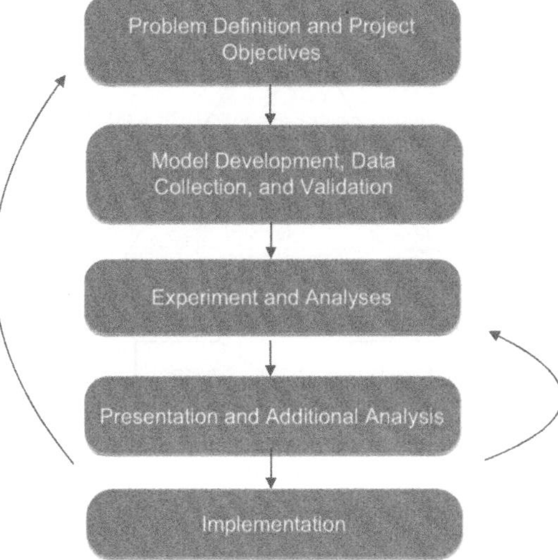


**Fig. 1.** Steps in a simulation study.

significant investment of financial or personnel resources that, absent a simulation, would have had only anecdotal evidence in favor of one or another. This design can also apply to nondigital simulations. For instance, a 2008 study described real-time simulations wherein nurses and technicians working in the operating room or the central sterilization department systematically reenacted and refined the process by which instruments were sterilized while adjusting the amount and distribution of staff and supplies to maximize cost-effectiveness.[19] Admittedly, this example has the disadvantage of needing to organize dozens of individuals to perform a simulation rather than needing only 1 person to enter data parameters and digitally simulate the same scenario. However, its greatest benefit is that the live simulation is conducted by those who will directly benefit from the changes being tested. This learning and team building within a simulation rather than post hoc is a feature owed largely to the aforementioned CRM model.

By the mid-2000s, CRM-style training was being progressively applied to multiple health care specialties, including the Military Health Service (MHS). To improve on the discord of nonstandardized protocols between several branches of the military, the US Department of Defense developed TeamSTEPPS (Team Strategies and Tools to Enhance Performance and Patient Safety). In addition to training MHS personnel in all branches using the same program, TeamSTEPPS focused on implementing evidence-based data related to enhancing team-based performance and interaction, engaging trainees with interactive learning, sustaining team behaviors on the job, and conducting regular evaluation of desired goals.[20] Although initially developed to reduce hospital errors and improve patient safety, TeamSTEPPS has been applied to venues throughout and beyond health care by training individuals more on the means to improving systems (ie, supportive interpersonal behaviors and organization [**Fig. 2**]) than on the end goals of patient safety (although it remains regularly used to this end). Simulation-based methodology is an important, albeit nonfoundational, aspect of this team training that relies on multiday workshops to organize a system's leadership, identify areas of need and training resources (including simulation of potential interventions), and develop means of integrating and maintaining change.[20,21]

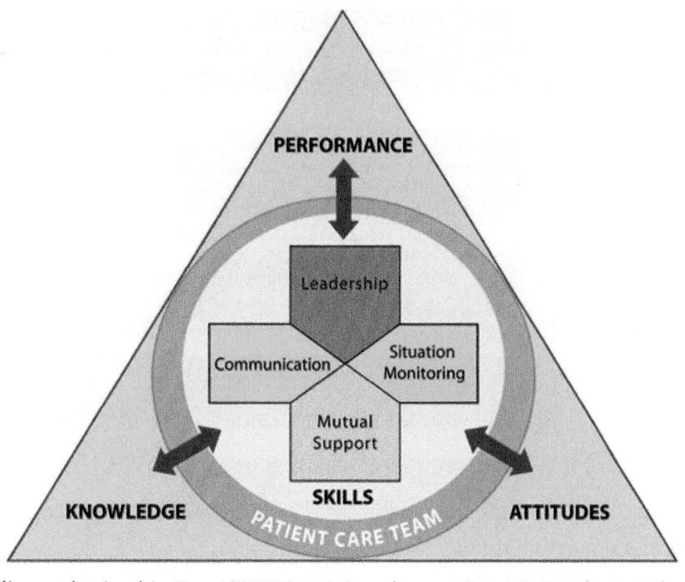


**Fig. 2.** Skills emphasized in TeamSTEPPS training. (*From* King HB, Battles J, Baker DP, et al. TeamSTEPPS: team strategies and tools to enhance performance and patient safety. In: Henriksen K, Battles JB, Keyes MA, et al, editors. Advances in patient safety: new directions and alternative approaches (vol. 3: performance and tools). Rockville (MD): Agency for Healthcare Research and Quality (US); 2008. p. 11; with permission.)

For surgical providers, the operating room team dynamic is increasingly being applied to TeamSTEPPS and training simulations. Particular to trainees, patient hand-offs and technical competency, when supervised with appropriate leadership and reinforced over time, show promise for low-stakes, high-value systematic improvement.[22]

The use of simulated scenarios and the TeamSTEPPS philosophy has also been successfully applied to root cause analysis (RCA) of adverse events within the operating room.[23,24] Before simulation, RCA at this institution was done retrospectively and with a bias toward identifying errors made by individuals rather than systemic error, correction of which holds far greater promise for improving quality, safety, and cost. By recreating as many variables as possible within a dedicated simulation facility and by involving and empowering all involved parties (surgeon, anesthesiologist, nurses, technicians, and residents), this experiment in recreating an RCA event identified several options for improvement in patient flow and staff distribution; corrections to systems-based errors rather than individual errors. Simulation-based analyses such as described in this study have the potential advantage of scrutinizing an entire system a priori, enabling the identification of causes rather than symptoms of systemic error.

## CLOSING THOUGHTS

The last few decades' increasing interest in simulation within health care is of little wonder. Technological advances, willingness to incorporate the successes of other industries, a premium on resident work hours, national focus on patient safety, emphases on performance-based and competency-based training, and the omnipresent concern to reduce associated costs are constants of developing and maintaining a health care system. Such motivations have already borne notable advances.

Simulation centers are ubiquitous in medical and nursing schools. The Accreditation Council for Graduate Medical Education, the governing body for postgraduate medical education in the United States, has advocated for using simulation to help satisfy the 6 core competencies: patient care, medical knowledge, practice-based learning and improvement, interpersonal and communication skills, professionalism, and system-based practice. Starting in the early 2000s, the United States Agency for Healthcare Research and Quality has offered substantial grants dedicated to projects that use simulation to improve technical skills, team performance, system performance, accreditation, and issues of an educational or methodological nature.[2] The Society for Simulation in Healthcare was founded in 2004, publishes its own journal, holds yearly conferences, and is a driving force for the expansion and refinement of simulation techniques in health care on an international level.[25]

As the technical abilities of simulation have evolved with increasingly complex procedures, a paradox has arisen within health care delivery that today's patients can be harmed in the training of tomorrow's practitioners. To confront this dilemma, the idea of "see one, do one, teach one" has been changed to "see one, do many with simulation, teach one" by proponents of simulation-based techniques. The emergence of new techniques and delivery systems, particularly those dedicated to minimally invasive surgery, further highlights the potential benefit of simulation-based training and education to extend not only to younger practitioners in their early training but also to experienced health care professionals learning new ideas. Furthermore, with simulation being more and more customizable and detailed to better reflect the realities of a practitioner's experience level and the circumstances of a workplace, providers with a wide range of abilities and backgrounds can achieve improvement in the quality of their care of patients through an entirely personalized simulated exercise.

## REFERENCES


1. Tzu S. The Art of War. Oxford: Oxford University Press; 1963.
2. The Agency for Healthcare Research and Quality. Improving patient safety through simulation research: funded projects. Available at: http://grants.nih.gov/grants/guide/pa-files/PA-14-004.html. Accessed January, 2015.
3. Roberts SD, England WL. Survey of the application of simulation to healthcare. Simulation 1981;10(1):1–15.
4. Harry MJ. Six Sigma: a breakthrough strategy for profitability. Qual Progr 1998;31(5):60–4.
5. Benneyan JC. An introduction to using computer simulation in healthcare: patient wait case study. J Soc Health Syst 1997;5(3):1–15.
6. Mason SE, Nicolay CR, Darzi A. The use of Lean and Six Sigma methodologies in surgery: a systematic review. Surgeon 2015;13(2):91–100.
7. Helmreich RL. Managing human error in aviation. Sci Am 1997;276:62–7.
8. Boosman F, Szczerba RJ. Simulated clinical environments and virtual system-of-systems engineering for health care. I/ITSEC. Orlando, Nov 29-Dec 2, 2010; (paper #10230). p. 1–9.
9. Ziv A, Small SD, Wolpe PR. Patient safety and simulation-based medical education. Med Teach 2000;22(5):489–94.
10. Ruffell-Smith HP. A simulator study of the interaction of pilot workload with errors, vigilance, and decisions. NASA-Ames Research Center, NASA Technical Memorandum #78482, public document. 1979.
11. Weiner EL, Kanki BJ, Helmrech RL. Cockpit resource management. San Diego (CA): Academic Press; 1993.

12. Leedom DK, Simon R. Improving team coordination: a case for behavior-based training. Mil Psychol 1995;7:109–22.
13. Gaba D. The human work environment and anesthesia simulators. In: Miller R, editor. Anesthesia. 5th edition. New York: Churchill Livingstone; 1999. p. 2613–69.
14. Smith B, Gaba D. Simulators. In: Lake C, Hines RL, Blitt CD, editors. Clinical monitoring: practical application for anesthesia and critical care. Philadelphia: WB Saunders; 2001. p. 26–44.
15. Orasanu J, Connolly T. The reinvention of decision making. In: Klein G, Orasanu J, Calderwood R, editors. Decision making in action: models and methods. Norwood (NJ): Ablex; 1993. p. 3–20.
16. Gaba DM, Howard SK, Fish KJ, et al. Simulation-based training in anesthesia crisis resource management (ACRM): a decade of experience. Simulat Gaming 2001;32:175–93.
17. Eitel DR, Rudkin SE, Malvehy MA, et al. Improving service quality by understanding emergency department flow: a white paper and position statement prepared for the American Academy of Emergency Medicine. J Emerg Med 2010;38(1):70–9.
18. Hung GR, Whitehouse SR, O'Neill C, et al. Computer modeling of patient flow in a pediatric emergency department using discrete event simulation. Pediatr Emerg Care 2007;23(1):5–10.
19. Lin F, Lawley M, Spry C, et al. Using simulation to design a central sterilization department. AORN J 2008;88(4):555–67.
20. Alonso A, Baker DP, Holtzman A, et al. Reducing medical error in the Military Health System: how can team training help? Hum Resource Manag Rev 2006;16:396–415.
21. King HB, Battles J, Baker DP, et al. TeamSTEPPS™: team strategies and tools to enhance performance and patient safety. In: Henriksen K, Battles JB, Keyes MA, et al, editors. Advances in patient safety: new directions and alternative approaches. Performance and tools, vol. 3. Rockville (MD): Agency for Healthcare Research and Quality (US); 2008. p. 5–20.
22. Sanfey H, McDowell C, Meier AH, et al. Team training for surgical trainees. Surgeon 2011;9:S32–4.
23. Simms ER, Slakey DP, Garstka ME, et al. Can simulation improve the traditional method of root cause analysis: a preliminary investigation. Surgery 2012;152(3):489–97.
24. Slakey DP, Simms ER, Rennie KV, et al. Using simulation to improve root cause analysis of adverse surgical outcomes. Int J Qual Health Care 2014;26(2):144–50.
25. The Society for Simulation in Healthcare. About SSH. Available at: http://www.ssih.org/About-SSH. Accessed January, 2015.

# Simulation for Maintenance of Certification

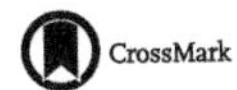

Brian K. Ross, PhD, MD*, Julia Metzner, MD

**KEYWORDS**

• Maintenance of certification • Simulation • High-stakes assessment

**KEY POINTS**

- Maintenance of certification is a process by which health care practitioners can remain current, expand their knowledge and technical expertise, and improve their quality of care and patient safety.
- Simulation takes many forms: part-task trainers, virtual computer worlds, complex procedure-based simulators, full-scale computer-based human patient simulators, standardized patients and family members, or hybrids of any of the simulator types.
- The use of simulation technologies is slowly making inroads into the high-stakes assessment world of maintenance of certification.

## INTRODUCTION

The privilege to practice medicine places on practitioners the onus to show and maintain competence in their areas of expertise, not on just 1 occasion but throughout a career. This continuous process is particularly important in current medical practice because the necessary body of knowledge combined with the technical expertise needed to function effectively is increasing exponentially. Because of these constantly escalating requirements, public scrutiny of the status of practitioners' skills throughout their careers is growing. Over the past several decades, public trust has been further eroded by the increased awareness of the complexity of the health care system and the concomitant adverse events associated with it as well as well-publicized stories regarding fraudulent practitioners who abuse the system.

Studies suggest that board-certified physicians provide improved quality of patient care and better clinical outcomes than those physicians without board certification.[1] For example, patients treated by board-certified physicians after heart attacks show

Department of Anesthesiology and Pain Medicine, University of Washington, Box 356540, Seattle, WA 98195, USA
* Corresponding author.
*E-mail address:* bkross@uw.edu

Surg Clin N Am 95 (2015) 893–905
http://dx.doi.org/10.1016/j.suc.2015.04.010 surgical.theclinics.com
0039-6109/15/$ – see front matter 

a 15% reduction in their mortality.[2] However, a recent meta-analysis showed a decline in physician performance associated with the time elapsed since the physician's initial training.[3] Such findings show that physicians need to participate in continuing medical education (CME) programs in order to keep current with medicine's expanding knowledge base and technical advances, and to apply this knowledge to quality improvement in their medical practice. Thus, state and national accreditation and regulatory bodies have developed stronger and more complex licensing requirements, statutes, and review boards. These bodies have developed tools that are thought to define, assess, and ensure more clearly maintenance of physician competence.

The maintenance of certification (MOC) concept, which grew out of the CME program, originated with The American Board of Medical Specialties (ABMS) in 1999 as a professional response to the need for public accountability and transparency of practice improvement initiatives by physicians. MOC allows practitioners to show to the public that they are continually improving their practice by documenting the steps that they are taking to do so. MOC may also help meet payer, regulatory, and consumer demands for quality in the future. Besides medical knowledge, MOC recognizes that several essential elements involved in delivering quality care exist that physicians must develop, maintain, and be regularly assessed on throughout their careers. These elements often include basic technical skills, skills around new and evolving technologies, and such softer skills as professionalism, team work, and team communication.

In terms of the civic interest, most current MOC programs have similar basic structures that have been developed to assure the public that practitioners are up to date with knowledge related to their specialties; that they hold unrestricted medical licenses, are respected in their practices by peers and patients, show professionalism as physicians, and are willing to evaluate and continually improve their practices. In terms of practitioners, participation in a MOC program should provide some assurance that it will lead to better care for patients, may help the practitioner meet regulatory and consumer demands for quality, shows their commitment to providing quality care to their patients, and acknowledges their keeping up to date with the latest advances in care in their specialties.

For postgraduate practitioners, MOC uses 4 unique program elements to assess the 6 core competencies required for satisfactory completion of residency training as identified through the Accreditation Council for Graduate Medical Education (ACGME) Outcome Project (http://www.acgme.org/Outcome/). These competencies are patient care and procedural skills, medical knowledge, practice-based learning and improvement, interpersonal and communication skills, professionalism, and system-based practice. Unlike the MOC process, the ACGME has provided residency programs with a toolbox of methods, techniques, and devices that are used to teach and assess these competencies (**Box 1**).

Although MOC represents a standard 4-part process known as the ABMS MOC process (**Box 2**), each board is left to determine the specific components of MOC that ensure specialist competency. By 2005, all 24 boards overseen by the ABMS became time limited and required physicians to participate in MOC activities to satisfy recertification every 6 to 10 years. Before this period, most specialty board certifications were permanent.

Having defined competence in terms of the 6 core ACGME competencies, including those often called softer skills, such as communication and professionalism, identifying a variety of tools to teach and assess competence or maintenance of competence became essential, because performance on a test of knowledge was no longer adequate to satisfy MOC. As a result, both the ACGME and the ABMS began

**Box 1**
**ACGME toolbox assessment tools**

- 360° evaluation instrument
- Chart stimulated recall oral examination
- Checklist evaluation of live or recorded performance
- Global rating of live or recorded performance
- Objective structured clinical examination
- Procedure, operative, or case logs
- Patient surveys
- Portfolios
- Record review
- Simulations and models
- Standardized oral examination
- Standardized patient examination
- Written examination (multiple-choice questions)

*Data from* Accreditation Council for Graduate Medical Education (ACGME) Outcome Project. Available at: http://www.acgme.org.

seriously considering that the use of simulation, in all its forms, might be an effective way to teach and assess all of the competencies, both soft (eg, professionalism) and hard (eg, medical knowledge).

## SIMULATION AND HEALTH CARE EDUCATION

Simulation-based health care education to train physicians had its beginnings in the early 1920s with intensivists and anesthesiologists attempting to improve patient safety in the operating room. Their efforts can be traced to the anatomy laboratory of John Lundy, MD, head of anesthesiology at Mayo Clinic. Dr Lundy developed a method to educate surgical fellows about anatomic structures to improve their performance of regional anesthesia as part of an effort to interest them and other physicians

**Box 2**
**General MOC program elements**

1. Professional standing: validation of unrestricted licensure to practice medicine and confirmation of good standing in their local practice community.
2. Lifelong learning and self-assessment: use of examinations and other assessment methods developed by the ABMS member boards' medical societies to allow physicians to assess their clinical and practical knowledge; usually require documentation of such activities.
3. Cognitive expertise: required to pass a proctored examination in a specialty.
4. Practice performance assessment and improvement: tools to self-assess performance in medical practice with emphasis on patient care and quality improvement.

*Data from* American Board of Medical Specialties. Available at: http://www.abms.org/board-certification/steps-toward-initial-certification-and-moc/.

in its use. Initially surgical residents used this clinic, but it ultimately became a multidisciplinary laboratory.[4,5] The laboratory allowed the surgical fellows to practice procedures, learn anatomy, and receive feedback about their performance, which before this was difficult or impossible because all of the training occurred in the operating room.[6] Since that time, anesthesia has led other health care specialties in both patient safety and the use of simulation-based technologies for training and, now, assessment. In the past 2 decades, interest in technologies around simulation have expanded exponentially. More and more medical schools, nursing schools, allied health care programs, and hospitals have been building simulation programs.

Several events in the history of simulation are worthy of mention, because they have played key roles in the process of simulation gaining its place in the toolbox of the health care educator. As early as the 1950s, interest in patient safety and efforts to improve outcomes after cardiac arrest motivated Peter Safar, MD, an intensivist, to lead the development of a new resuscitation method that revolutionized the world of post–cardiac arrest resuscitation (ie, mouth-to-mouth resuscitation). This new technique made it possible to oxygenate and ventilate arrest victims.[7,8] Dr Safar worked with Bjorn Lind, MD, an anesthesiologist, and with Asmund S. Laerdal, a toy manufacturer, to create the simulator known as Resusci Anne.[9] Evidence of the importance of closed chest massage prompted Dr Safar to advise Laerdal to add an internal spring mechanism to permit training in proper cardiac compression.[10] This simulator is still in use as a platform for training and certifying trainees in life support skills.

In the 1960s, Stephen Abrahamson, a medical educator and engineer, in conjunction with Judson Samuel Dens, MD, an anesthesiologist, constructed the Sim One anesthesiology simulator. This device was the earliest computer-controlled mannequin simulator representing the entire patient. The simulator had an anatomically shaped chest that moved with respiration, eyes that were able to blink, pupils that dilated and constricted, and a jaw that opened and closed. Sim One was used for airway training and for educating residents in critical anesthesia-related events. It showed for the first time that trainees who learned skills on Sim One achieved performance criteria in real patients in less time and with fewer attempts than those who did not use the simulator.[11,12] The mannequin required a separate room for the computer, was about 2 decades ahead of its time, and was never produced commercially.[12,13]

Over the next several decades, major advances in simulation had to wait for the ideal conditions of evolution of medical technology and the birth of acute care specialties; increased understanding of the structure and function of the human body (ie, disease, aging); and the extraordinary growth of computer hardware/software that could provide improved mathematical models of human physiology, drug pharmacology, and human tissues. Also playing a central role in the advancement of simulation was a revolution in synthetic materials, allowing construction of not only modern computers but also the part-task trainers and realistic full-scale human patient mannequins. The final impetus to move medical simulation forward was the recognition by non–health care industry of the importance of incorporating simulation into their training as a way of improving industrial safety (eg, aviation, nuclear power, military defense). Accelerating the recent more widespread incorporation of simulation into medical education has been the birth of worldwide communication (Internet) and the design of virtual worlds. Regulatory agencies pushing the evolution in health science education and evaluation toward a student-centered, competency-based method, and eventually the public demand have facilitated this transition.

The goal of simulation in training is to replicate patient care scenarios in an immersive, realistic environment to facilitate feedback and assessment.[14] Public expectations, a push for improved patient safety, a reduction of house-staff duty hours, and the ethical implications of practicing on real patients have all contributed to fewer patient encounters and have continued to shrink the clinical opportunities in which nursing students, medical students, residents, and fellows can be trained. The National Council of State Boards of Nursing has continually supported the usefulness of a variety of forms of simulation for prelicensure nursing students. Until recently, the nursing regulatory bodies explicitly stated that simulation cannot take the place of actual patients. However, this opinion may be changing with the publication of a comprehensive multicentered nursing study. The study showed that, when up to 50% of traditional clinical experience in the undergraduate nursing program was replaced by simulation, no significant differences in end-of-program nursing knowledge; clinical competency; overall readiness for practice; NCLEX (National Council Licensure Examination) pass rates; and new graduate managers' assessments in thinking, clinical competency, and overall readiness for practice were noted.[15] A survey of the Association of American Medical Colleges (AAMC) shows that most (52%) medical schools and 39% of teaching hospitals use simulation-based methodologies through the 4-year medical school curriculum (standardized patients, full-scale mannequins, part-task trainers, and screen-based virtual reality simulators). Simulation-augmented training is most frequently seen in internal medicine, pediatric emergency medicine, and anesthesiology clerkships. In recent years, several resident review committees (anesthesiology, internal medicine, surgery, and surgical critical care) have followed the lead of the AAMC and have added a simulation-based component to their program requirements to assess core competencies (**Table 1**). Emergency medicine counts simulated patient-centered scenarios as being identical to patient care encounters for their experience quotas.

Theoretically, simulation should translate into improved learner performance, but this finding has been shown only in isolated settings. Training associated with specific procedures has tended to be more readily transferable; this transfer to practice has been most apparent in studies in which the rates of complications from central line placement were significantly decreased after residents were trained using simulation-based techniques.[16] In a second study, simulation-trained anesthesiology residents weaned patients from cardiopulmonary bypass better than residents taught through didactic methods.[17] In addition, high-fidelity simulations have also been

**Table 1**
**ACGME simulation requirements for graduate education**

| | |
|---|---|
| Anesthesiology | Residents must participate in at least 1 simulated clinical experience each year (effective July 2011) |
| Emergency medicine | Encounter guideline numbers include both patient care and laboratory simulations |
| Family medicine | Type of experience not specified |
| Internal medicine | Must provide residents with access to training using simulation (effective July 2009) |
| Neurology | Type of experience not specified |
| Obstetrics and gynecology | Type of experience not specified |
| Pediatrics | Type of experience not specified |
| Surgery | Program must include simulation and skills laboratories addressing acquisition and maintenance of skills with a competency-based method of evaluation |

shown to improve care during the management of shoulder dystocia and the management of cardiac arrests.[18,19] A recently published meta-analysis showed large effects on knowledge, skills, and behaviors and moderate effects on patient-related outcomes when simulation-based training was compared with no intervention.[20]

## WHAT IS SIMULATION?

It is important to clarify what is meant by simulation. Simulation, in its broadest sense, is an instructional process, not a particular technology. The intent is to either substitute for or amplify real-life experiences through thoughtfully constructed curricula and mentored experiences, in an attempt to evoke real-life interactive responses from the trainee. When constructed around particular single tasks or complicated patient care scenarios, in settings that contextually duplicate real clinical environments, simulation can be a very effective educational experience. It moves learning out of the classroom and away from lectures and the excessive use of PowerPoint into a realm that is conducive to adult learning. Leading this new process in health care education are expensive, computer-driven devices that can mimic, at the basic level, the salient portions of simple to very complex tasks[21–23] or, at the other extreme, an entire patient and clinical event.[24–26] Low-technology simulation might involve using a partial-task trainer to practice a clinical examination or procedure, such as endotracheal intubation, interosseous line placement, vaginal ultrasonography, or central venous catheter placement. In contrast, high-technology simulation often involves expensive, highly realistic, computer-driven mannequins that can mimic the physiology of a real patient. The fidelity of experiences is depends primarily on the curriculum in which the simulator serves as 1 small part.

Simulation-based experiences may involve a single learner or may include a full team of health care providers experiencing an interprofessional activity. Matching the equipment and the environment to both the learners and the educational goals and objectives is critical. Expensive equipment and elaborate programs are not always the correct solution.[26] The advantages of simulation-based experiences are that the educators can choose the appropriate simulators and educational techniques to create a realistic, predictable, standardized, safe, and reproducible clinical environment. Students are able to make mistakes, recognize when they are about to make a mistake, and learn from their successes and errors without putting patients at risk.[27] Simulation-based technologies encompass a wide array of devices from very simple part-task simulators to very complicated, high-fidelity, computer-driven, full-scale human mannequins (**Box 3**).

Because simulation-based experiences are being designed and developed for either primary training or, even more importantly, MOC, several important factors must be considered. First, a thoughtful needs assessment must be done around the task to be taught or the goals and objectives for the training or assessment to be conducted. The correct piece of simulation-based technology must be matched carefully with the assessment need, be it a part-task trainer, a computer-based virtual trainer, or a full-scale mannequin-based simulator. Second, consideration must be given to whether the training/assessment will be sufficiently robust if a part-task trainer versus a full-scale immersive experience is used. The fidelity of simulation required escalates as the level training of the trainee/participant advances. Fully trained health care providers frequently require equivalently higher levels of fidelity in their simulation-based technologies. In addition, as providers advance in their training and clinical practice, they become very contextual in their requirement of the environment in which the simulation is being conducted. In situ simulation, which is simulation-based training

**Box 3**
**General categories of simulators**

Part-task trainers: mannequin-based trainers that represent anatomic body parts for teaching and/or evaluating skills (synthetic airways for intubation, arms for intravenous or intra-arterial line placement, necks for central line placement, necks and thorax for chest tube placement or emergent cricothyroidotomy placement).

Full-scale mannequin-based simulators: computer-driven mathematical model–driven, realistic human mannequins; have palpable pulses, breaths sounds, reactive pupils, dynamic airway anatomy; capable of recognizing both intravenous and inhaled medications; interact with a variety of medical devices; output vital signs via physiologic monitors.

Standardized patients: simulated patients played by trained actors, used alone or in conjunction with part-task or full-scale mannequin-based simulators.

Immersive environments: often involve a combination of standardized patients, computer-driven mannequins, and high-fidelity and low-fidelity part-task trainers to create an immersive environment of multimodality simulation in which entire teams of health care providers can train to perform tasks, manage potentially deadly scenarios, and improve teamwork skills, including leadership, communication, delegation, and prioritization.

Hybrid simulation: combining any 2 of the general categories described earlier, most frequently a part-task simulator or full-scale mannequin with a standardized patient or family member.

physically integrated into the clinical environment, has gained in popularity and importance as simulation-based methodologies have been used to train and assess board-certified/eligible experienced practitioners. Context becomes increasingly important with this group of providers.

## SIMULATION AND MAINTENANCE OF CERTIFICATION

What role does simulation play in Maintenance of Certification in Anesthesiology (MOCA)? Has the world of simulation matured enough that it can play a major role in the MOC process, in which the assessment tools are difficult to define and validate, and the consequences of failure are potentially catastrophic for the practitioner? This question must be balanced against the potential benefit that both the practitioner and patient may gain from a process based in simulation, in which a greater degree of granularity might be provided in the training, and more in-depth information might be gained around the assessment and competency of the practitioner being evaluated.

High-stakes simulation-based assessment for licensure and specialty board certification is already more common than most people realize (ie, advanced cardiovascular life support or hospital required training modules that provide continual remediation until passed). These examples involve high-stakes examinations that, if failed, could greatly impact a practitioner's ability to practice a specialty. The confusion around the role that simulation plays in these arenas may result from the misconception that simulation must include the use of a full-scale, immersive, high-fidelity simulated environment, with expensive mannequins. This belief is not the case. Even though some form of task-based or mannequin-based simulation technology is often used in these settings, they are often viewed as being neither high stakes nor simulation.

The United States Medical Licensing Examination involves successful completion of all its steps as a requirement for graduation and moving on to residency training. Several simulation-based technologies are used during these examinations, such as computer-based simulations (Clinical Knowledge) as well as interactions with standardized patients (Clinical Skills). The computer-based examinations include multiple-choice question (MCQ) examinations combined with a set of computer-based simulated patients requiring care. In step 3, more complex MCQs as well as computer-based case simulations are used. During the simulations, the examinees encounter interactive time-based scenarios with repercussions associated with poor or dangerous physical examination and/or intervention decisions.

Even though simulation-based education and evaluation seem to be gaining traction in the worlds of medical student and residency education, the situation with postlicensure specialty boards is different. To date, only 2 specialty boards require simulation for primary certification: Anesthesiology remains the only specialty having a simulation-based requirement for recertification (MOC). In the area of anesthesia, simulation has been shown as an effective tool for pre–board certification training and assessment of softer skills, such as communication, teamwork, and professionalism, as well as evaluating several of the ACGME competency domains, such as systems-based practice, and practice-based learning.[28–30]

## SURGERY

Surgical education, assessment of competency, and physician certification and MOC is slowly undergoing a paradigm shift. The apprenticeship model of see one, do one, teach one, used for more than 100 years, is being replaced by objectives-based training assessment methods founded on competency achievement that incorporates basic tenets of modern learning theory. Very simple to highly sophisticated part-task trainers, realistic computer-based skills trainers, and high-fidelity full-scale human patient simulators are increasingly being incorporated into resident and fellow training in several surgical fields.

The use of high-fidelity simulation seems to be particularly well matched with minimally invasive surgery. The digital image nature of laparoscopic surgery makes it possible to teach and evaluate objectively essential technical skills by recording and breaking down key components of the skill.

The American Board of Surgery (ABS) voted a formal simulation requirement for primary certification into place in 2008. As part of this requirement, surgical residents are required to successfully complete 2 curricula involving simulation-based exercises: the Fundamentals of Laparoscopic Surgery (FLS; Society of Gastrointestinal and Endoscopic Surgeons and American College of Surgeons) and Advanced Trauma Life Support (ATLS).[31] The FLS assessment consists of a 2-part proctored examination of both cognitive and technical skills, using a computer-based MCQ examination and the FLS Laparoscopic Trainer Box respectively. FLS and ATLS use a variety of simple task trainers and standardized patients. To add a team communication component, many organizations are using sophisticated human patient simulators to assess physician performance.

Specialty-specific simulation-based technologies are used in many surgical specialties for training. In contrast, the surgical specialty leadership has yet to incorporate simulation-based evaluations into their initial certification or MOC process. A recent review of the posted requirements for board certification and recertification from the American Board of Obstetrics and Gynecology, American Board of Orthopedic Surgery, American Board of Urology, and the American Board of Thoracic Surgery showed that they continue to base their certification on the traditional MCQ examination followed by an oral examination. Nonetheless, the ABS does require completion of FLS in order to sit for the qualifying examination.

## ANESTHESIOLOGY

In general, anesthesiology has led health care in both patient safety and the use of simulation-based technologies for training and assessment. Since July of 2011, anesthesiology residents have been required to participate at least once yearly in a simulated intraoperative clinical experience.[32] Those anesthesia practitioners who received their board certification after 2000 are no longer certified for life by the American Board of Anesthesiology (ABA); instead, recertification is required every 10 years. Between 2000 and 2014, diplomates have been able to elect, but are not required, to satisfy part 4 of the MOC with an immersive simulation-based experience. As of 2014, simulation-based education is now a mandatory prerequisite for all newly trained anesthesiologists as well as those seeking recertification. These requirements reflect the current ABMS standards. The specific requirements of anesthesiology MOCA simulation courses are outlined in **Box 4**.[33]

As a result of the success of this MOCA program using simulation-based training, the ABA is now considering requiring 2 subspecialty boards (ie, pain medicine and critical care) to incorporate simulation-based immersive experiences into their recertification programs.

A critical assessment of the ABA high-stakes MOCA process reveals that the use of high-fidelity computer-based mannequin simulators helps to provide a realistic immersive environment in which the trainees are allowed to function in teams to manage patients experiencing critical life-threatening problems common to the practice of anesthesia. The performance during these simulations is assessed only in a self-reflective, formative way during the postscenario debriefing. However, results from the first 2 years of experience with this simulation-based MOC suggest that physician participants found the experiences educationally valuable and clinically

**Box 4**
**Anesthesiology MOCA part 4 simulation requirements**

- Course length: minimum of 6 hours
- Management of patient scenarios
- Significant hypoxemia from any cause
- Difficult airway
- Hemodynamic instability

*Active participation in patient scenarios*

- Must be the primary anesthesiologist in 1 scenario
- Emphasis on teamwork and team communication during scenarios
- Participation in postscenario debrief
- Participation in a postcourse survey
- Participation in an online practice improvement plan (PIP) (personal, departmental, institutional)

Within 3 months of attending the course, diplomates must provide an online narrative description on the successful implementation of the PIP or outline barriers they experienced that prevented or hindered the successful implementation of the plan.

*Data from* American Society of Anesthesiologists. Available at: http://education.asahq.org/PPAI.

relevant, transferring knowledge and skills from their simulated experiences that led to changes in their real-world practice.[34]

To date, formal assessment tools are not used during the ABA simulation-based MOCA courses to pass or fail the participants. Thus, the well-choreographed simulation-based experiences do not qualify as a high-stakes assessment component of the MOCA; the simulation-base training is a technique, an immersive experience, that leads to a self-reflective practice improvement process. Why is this the case? The literature is devoid of well-designed research studies that validate the use of high-fidelity simulation as a high-stakes assessment tool in situations like the MOC process.

Many of the same factors that pushed the development of simulation-based methodologies in the aviation and nuclear industries are present in health care. Commercial pilots take their first flight only after a rigorous simulation-based training program, and operators of nuclear power plants train on simulators for several critical emergencies before taking their seat as the lead operator. For the most part, the extent of simulation used in both these industries has not been driven by evidence, but by intuition and common sense. As mentioned earlier, a small body of literature has shown that adding a simulation-based component to training improves health care education, the practice of medicine, and ultimately patient safety. Dr Dave Gaba,[34] a founding father of health care simulation, has opined that "… no industry in which human lives depend on skilled performance has waited for unequivocal proof of the benefits of simulation before embracing it."

## INTERNAL MEDICINE

One of the largest regulatory boards in the United States is the American Board of Internal Medicine (ABIM), which provides board certification in internal medicine and approximately 20 other medical subspecialties. Although the initial internal medicine and subspecialty certification does not include a simulation-based component, the ABIM introduced simulation into the interventional-cardiology assessment in 2008 as an option for the diplomates to satisfy partial completion of the self-evaluation of medical knowledge requirement of MOC.[35] The simulations use very high-fidelity simulation-based platforms, which require the participants to go to Medical Simulation Corporation's SimSuite centers during, preconference or postconference training sessions associated with national ABIM meetings. SimSuite provides an opportunity to manage 5 specifically developed cases in a replica of a catheterization operation, which is the ultimate in high fidelity. Under the umbrella of ABIM, other subspecialties will imbed some level of simulation into their MOCA process. Other ABIM specialty areas that seem particularly well matched for incorporation of simulation-based components are those specialties with significant technical components, like gastroenterology and pulmonary medicine. High-fidelity simulators currently exist that could easily support a simulation-based component for gastroenterology.

## FAMILY MEDICINE

The American Board of Family Medicine (ABFM) requires completion of 2 self-assessment modules (SAMs) from a list of 13 medical topics as part of its MOC. These modules incorporate a knowledge assessment on a chosen topic (eg, diabetes, hypertension, asthma, coronary artery disease) and are followed by screen-based clinical simulation-based scenarios. The condition of simulated patients unfolds over time as a result of the participant's management skills and therapeutic interventions. As of April 2005, more than 7000 ABFM diplomates had completed SAMs in the topic of hypertension and diabetes mellitus. The evaluations of these simulation-based patient scenarios provided by users were generally favorable, and 55% of the participants stated that the experience would lead to changes in their future practice.[36]

## WHERE IS SIMULATION GOING FOR MAINTENANCE OF CERTIFICATION IN ANESTHESIOLOGY?

Licensing, certification, and credentialing bodies are quickly adopting simulation-based techniques for health care practitioner assessment. This trend is occurring despite a paucity of evidence for improved medical outcomes from such use[37] because the public is demanding a different model for qualifying health care professionals. In addition, federal agencies, national accreditation, licensing organizations, state licensing bodies, educational accrediting bodies, specialty medical boards, medical schools, and local credentialing committees are signaling the obvious advantage of simulation as an assessment technology.[38,39] Even though the current national certification model allows older providers to have permanent, lifelong licensure and certification, these same providers may soon be asked to show their commitment to lifelong learning and sustained competence in a simulated environment. Simulation is currently being used extensively in the early education, training, and assessment of new health care providers. The future for training and assessment clearly involves the use of multimodal immersive simulation for the assessment of health care providers throughout the educational continuum.

Patients allow health care providers into their lives at their most fragile moments, entrust them with their well-being, and enter into a relationship in which they believe their providers to be not just competent but expertly trained in their areas of specialty. A reasonable extension of this thought might be that using simulation for training and assessment before a real patient encounter not only for basic, routine procedures but also before the use of new technologies reduces a patient's exposure to professionals who are not trained in a similar fashion. Thus, patients receive a higher quality of care than they would otherwise get from those health care providers who had received their training in the age-old apprentice-based see one, do one, teach one system and were assessed on paper-based or oral examinations. The conventional assessment system may overestimate the experience and skill of the provider. This conclusion is supported by observations in other high-risk fields such as aviation and the nuclear power industry, in which simulation is a central component of training and assessment; their safety records are clearly superior to those found in modern health care systems.

## REFERENCES

1. Chen J, Rathore SS, Wang Y, et al. Physician board certification and the care and outcomes of elderly patients with acute myocardial infarction. J Gen Intern Med 2006;21(3):238–44.
2. Norcini J, Lipner R, Kimball H. Certification status of generalist physicians and the mortality of their patients after acute myocardial infarction. Acad Med 2001;76(10 Suppl):S21–3.
3. Choudhry NK, Fletcher RH, Soumerai SB. Systematic review: the relationship between clinical experience and quality of health care. Ann Intern Med 2005; 142:260–73.
4. Lundy JS. Anatomy service report, February 14, 1929. In the collected papers of John S. Lundy. Rochester (MN): Mayo Foundation Archive; 1929.
5. Ellis TA 2nd, Bacon DR. The anatomy laboratory: a concept ahead of its time. Mayo Clin Proc 2003;78:250–1.

6. Lundy JS. Twenty-one months' experience in operating a dissecting room under the Mayo Foundation. In the collected papers of John S. Lundy. Rochester (MN): Mayo Foundation Archive; 1927.
7. Safer P, Escarrage LA, Elam JO. A comparison of the mouth-to-mouth and mouth-to-airway methods of artificial respiration with the chest-pressure armlift methods. N Engl J Med 1958;258:671–7.
8. Tjomsland N. From Stavanger with care: Laerdals' first 50 years. Stavanger (Norway): Laerdal; 1990.
9. Tjomsland N. Saving more lives together. Stavanger (Norway): Laerdal; 2005.
10. Safer P, Brown TC, Holtey WJ, et al. Ventilation and circulation with closed-chest cardiac massage in man. JAMA 1961;176:574–6.
11. Abrahamson S. Human simulation for training in anesthesiology. In: Ray CE, editor. Medical engineering. Chicago: Yearbook; 1974.
12. Denson J, Abrahamson S. A computer-controlled patient simulator. JAMA 1969; 208:504–8.
13. Abrahamson S, Denson J, Wolf R. Effectiveness of a simulator in training anesthesiology residents. J Med Educ 1969;44:515–9.
14. Okuda Y, Bryson EO, DeMria S, et al. The utility of simulation in medical education: what is the evidence? Mt Sinai J Med 2009;76(4):330–43.
15. Hayden JK, Smiley RA, Alexander M, et al. The NCSBN National Simulation Study: a longitudinal, randomized, controlled study replacing clinical hours with simulation in pre-licensure nursing education. J Nurs Reg 2014;5(2 Suppl): S1–64.
16. Barsuk JH, McGaghie WC, Cohen ER, et al. Simulation-based master learning reduces complications during central venous catheter insertions in a medical intensive care unit. Crit Care Med 2009;37:2697–701.
17. Bruppacher HR, Alam SK, LeBlanc VR, et al. Simulation-based training improves physicians' performance in patient care in high-stakes clinical setting of cardiac surgery. Anesthesiology 2010;112:985–92.
18. Draycott TJ, Crofts JF, Ash JP, et al. Improving neonatal outcome through practical shoulder dystocia training. Obstet Gynecol 2008;112:14–20.
19. Wayne DB, Didwania A, Feinglass J, et al. Simulation-based training improves quality of care during cardiac arrest team responses at an academic teaching hospital: a case-controlled study. Chest 2008;133:56–61.
20. Cook DA, Hatala R, Brydges R, et al. Technology-enhanced simulation for health professions education: a systematic review and meta-analysis. JAMA 2011; 7(306):978–88.
21. Seymour N, Gallagher A, Roman S, et al. Virtual reality training improves operating room performance. Ann Surg 2002;236:458–64.
22. Dawson SL, Cotin S, Meglan D, et al. Designing a computer-based simulator for interventional cardiology training. Catheter Cardiovasc Interv 2005;51:522–7.
23. Goldman K, Steinfeldt T. Acquisition of basic fiberoptic intubation skills with virtual reality airway simulator. J Clin Anesth 2006;18:173–8.
24. Gaba DM, DeAnda A. A comprehensive anesthesia simulation environment: recreating the operating room for research and training. Anesthesiology 1988;69: 387–94.
25. Cooper JB, Taqueti VR. A brief history of the development of mannequin simulators for clinical education and training. Qual Saf Health Care 2004;13(Suppl 1): i11–8.
26. Sinz EH. Anesthesiology national CME program and ASA activities in simulation. Anesthesiol Clin 2007;25:209–23.

27. Scerbo MW, Dawson S. High fidelity, high performance? Simul Healthc 2007;2: 224–30.
28. Devitt H, Kurrek MM, Cohen MM, et al. Testing the instrument: internal consistency during evaluation of performance in an anesthesia simulator. Can J Anaesth 1997;44:924–8.
29. Schwid HA, Rooke GA, Carline J, et al, Anesthesia Simulator Research Consortium. Evaluation of anesthesia residents using mannequin-based simulation: a multi-institutional study. Anesthesiology 2002;97:1434–44.
30. Buyske J. The role of simulation in certification. Surg Clin North Am 2010;90: 619–21.
31. Fundamentals of laparoscopic surgery. Available at: http://www.flsprogram.org. Accessed December 20, 2010.
32. Levine A, Flynn B. Simulation-based Maintenance of Certification in Anesthesiology (MOCA) course optimization: use of multi-modality educational activities. J Clin Anesth 2012;24:68–74.
33. McIvor W, Burden A, Weinger M, et al. Simulation for maintenance of certification in anesthesiology: the first two years. J Contin Educ Health Prof 2012;32:236–42.
34. Gaba DM. Improving anesthesiogists' performance by simulating reality. Anesthesiology 1992;76:491–4.
35. American Board of Internal Medicine. Available at: http://www.abim.org. Accessed December 20, 2010.
36. Hagen MD, Ivins DI, Puffer JC, et al. Maintenance of certification for family physicians (MC-FP) self assessment modules (SAMs): the first year. J Am Board Fam Med 2006;19:398–403.
37. Kassebaum DG, Eaglen RH. Shortcomings in the evaluation of students' clinical skills and behaviors in medical school. Acad Med 1999;74:842–9.
38. Langsley DG. Medical competence and performance assessment: a new era. JAMA 1991;266:977–80.
39. Hatala R, Kassen BO, Nichikawa J, et al. Incorporating simulation technology in a Canadian internal medicine specialty examination: a descriptive report. Acad Med 2005;80:554–6.

# Index

*Note:* Page numbers of article titles are in **boldface** type.




Surg Clin N Am 95 (2015) 907–918
http://dx.doi.org/10.1016/S0039-6109(15)00101-2
0039-6109/15/$ – see front matter


surgical.theclinics.com

## D



## E

**F**

## G



## H



## I

**K**



**L**



**M**

## O



## P

## Q



## R



## S

**T**

## U



## V



## W



## Z

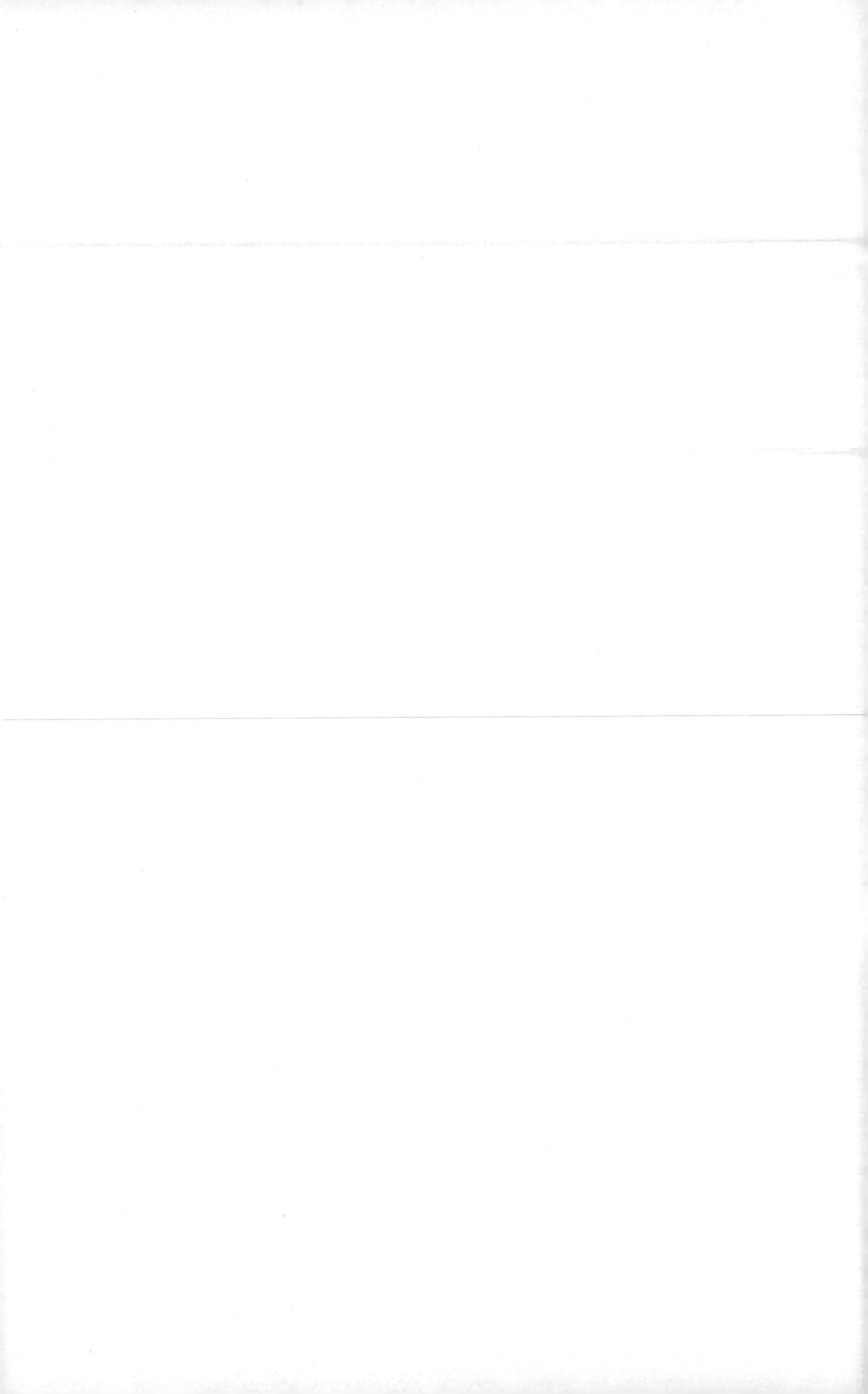